SURGICAL MANUAL
of
SKULL BASE SURGERY

Dr. Produl Hazarika MS, DLO, FACS, FRCS, FAIO

Professor & Head of ENT & Head & Neck Surgery - UNIT I
Kasturba Medical College, Manipal, India
Senior Consultant ENT Surgeon, **New Medical Centre**, Abu Dhabi
E-mail : produl_ent@rediffmail.com

Co-Authors
Dr. Kailesh Pujary MS, DNB
Associate Professor
Dept. of ENT, Kasturba Medical College

Dr. Rohit Singh MS, DNB
Asst. Professor
Dept. of ENT, Kasturba Medical College

Dr. Sunil Ramnani MS
Asst. Professor
Dept. of ENT, Pdt. JN Medical College
Raipur

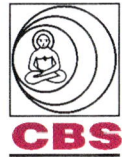

CBS

CBS PUBLISHERS & DISTRIBUTORS PVT. LTD.
NEW DELHI • BANGALORE • PUNE • COCHIN • CHENNAI (INDIA)

ISBN : 978-81-239-1612-5

First Edition : 2008
Reprint : 2012

Published by Satish Kumar Jain and produced by V.K. Jain for
CBS Publishers & Distributors Pvt. Ltd.,
CBS Plaza, 4819/XI Prahlad Street, 24 Ansari Road, Daryaganj,
New Delhi - 110002, India.   • Website: www.cbspd.com
e-mail: delhi@cbspd.com, cbspubs@airtelmail.in
Ph.: 23289259, 23266861, 23266867   • Fax: 011-23243014

Branches:
• *Bengaluru:* Seema House, 2975, 17th Cross, K.R. Road,
  Bansankari 2nd Stage, Bengaluru - 560070
  • Ph.: +91-80-26771678/79 • Fax: +91-80-26771680
  • E-mail: cbsbng@gmail.com, bangalore@cbspd.com
• *Pune:* Bhuruk Prestige, Sr. No. 52/12/2+1+3/2,
  Narhe, Haveli (Near Katraj-Dehu Road By-pass), Pune - 411041
  • Ph.: +91-20-64704058/59, 32342277   • E-mail: pune@cbspd.com
• *Kochi:* 36/14, Kalluvilakam, Lissie Hospital Road,
  Kochi - 682018, Kerala • Ph.: +91-484-4059061-65
  • Fax: +91-484-4059065   • E-mail: cochin@cbspd.com
• *Chennai:* 20, West Park Road, Shenoy Nagar, Chennai - 600030
  Ph.: +91-44-26260666, 26208620   • Fax: +91-44-42032115
  • E-mail: chennai@cbspd.com

Printed at :
Swastik Packagings, Delhi

Senior Author dedicated this book
to his wife
Mrs. Madhurima Hazarika,
Son Mr. Mrinmoy Hazarika
Daughter Dr. Manali Hazarika
and Son in law Dr. Rohit Singh

Foreword

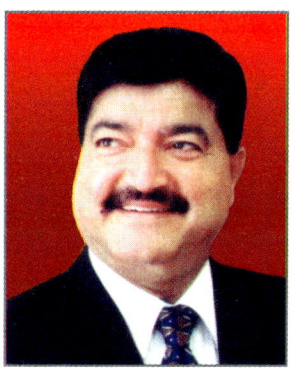

It is said ëknowledge percolates knowledgeí and to this end documenting the abstract and concepts in the form of a book is a noblest thing one can do. Capturing the wisdom and years of research has translated into a fine work of ìSurgical Manual of Skull Base Surgeryî by Prof. Produl Hazarika is highly commendable.

Prof. Hazarika is ably supported by Dr. Kailesh Pujary, Dr. Rohit Singh and Dr. Sunil Ramnani. These stalwarts have immortalized the fundamentals and concepts involved in the field of Skull Base Surgery, wnich I am sure will serve as a reference book and collection issue.

The lucid illustrations and clear narration of the various details involved go a long way in conveying un-equivocally total comprehension of the professional expertise, the author has gained over a period of time under various complex situations.

I take this opportunity to acknowledge that Prof. Hazarika will be joining our institution shortly as Consultant ENT Surgeon to further enhance our Super Specialty Hospital in UAE. †

With best regards,†

Dr. B.R. Shetty
Managing Director & CEO
NEW MEDICAL CENTRE
P O Box 6222, Abu Dhabi

June 8, 2007

Foreword

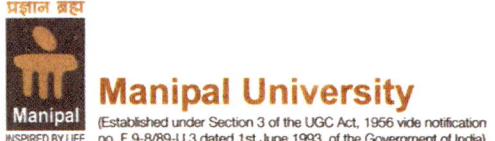

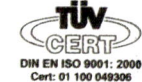

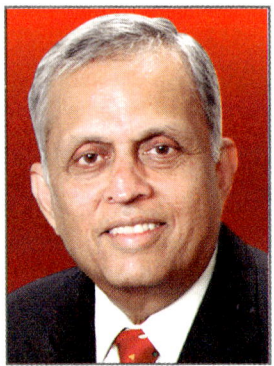

Dr Hazarika and his team is to be complimented on producing this very well written book with clear and simple description of many complicated procedures and diagnostic dilemmas. Dr Hazarika has been a leader in the super specialty of Skull-base surgery and has developed a great reputation for himself and the team at Manipal. This book reflects their knowledge, surgical skills and dedication to teach the unique knowledge and skills they posses. This well written book with vast information & simple diagrams could be of great value to all postgraduates, practicing surgeons and maxillofacial surgeons. The administration, faculty and students of Manipal University wish to congratulate Dr Hazarika and his team in their endeavor to publish this book.

With best regards,†

Dr Raj Warrier
Vice Chancellor
Manipal University

Preface

The manual of skull base surgery is a unique book highlighting the anatomical and surgical methodology in dealing with the skull base tumors. The skull base tumors always require a multidisciplinary approach. So in order to establish a good skull base unit requires a great deal of cooperation and understanding among the various consultants of the specialized departments. Not many Indian authors have written a comprehensive and systematic text book on skull base surgery.

The present author has made an effort along with the contributing authors from different specialities to bring out this book. The systematic organization of the chapters is necessary to retain a sensible balance. While our knowledge has expanded in some areas more than others it would be rewarding for the authors if the book becomes a resource of information for the readers and helps in generating interest to pursue this field of speciality

The knowledge acquired from this book will definitely help the management of skull base tumors. This is critical to avoid diagnostic and surgical pitfall while providing safe and effective care.

Acknowledgement

It is now only after completion of our work that we realize the immense necessity of writing this page, in an effort to acknowledge those who in all their possible ways have helped us in carrying out and completing this book. Of course, this small return in a few words is only a fraction of what we were given by them.

We take the privilege to express our profound sense of gratitude to late Prof. B.R. Das, MBBS, DLO, FRCS (Edin), FRCS (Glas), Assam Medical College who had a towering and divine influence in initiating this project of ours. We have the pleasure to place on record the concise and concrete suggestions as well as the goodwill offered to us by Dr. B. R. Shetty, Managing Director of New Medical Center Group of Hospitals from U.A.E. in response to a few of our queries in connection with this book. We owe a deep sense of gratitude to this great personality and pioneer of our time.

We are grateful to our founder Dr. T.M.A. Pai, our beloved president of MAHE, Dr. Ramdas M. Pai, Dr. Raj Warrier, Vice Chancellor of MAHE, Dr. R.S.P. Rao, Dean of KMC, Manipal who kindly permitted us to carry out this book in this institution lacking which we scare, it would not have been possible to bring this work to light.

We do always have an indebted honour for Dr. Peddhibottala Kumararaja, Assistant Professor, Dept. of ENT, Medical College, Karimnagar for his many fold help throughout this work.

Senior author shall be failing in his duties if he does not offer his hearfelt gratitude to his parents late Mr. and Mrs. L.C. Hazarika.

Our secretary Mrs. Thulasi also deserves our thanks for her help in association with non-teaching staff of the department Mr. Seetharam, Mrs. Mangala, Mr. Bhaskar, Mr. Sudhakar and sister Mrs. Shanthi, Mrs. Malathi, Mrs. Mohini, Mrs. Usha, Mrs. Baby, Mrs. Vasanthi and Mrs. Bhavani.

We shall be failing in our duties unless we offer our gratefulness to our patients who so optimistically offer themselves to our surgical mutilation.

Contributing Authors

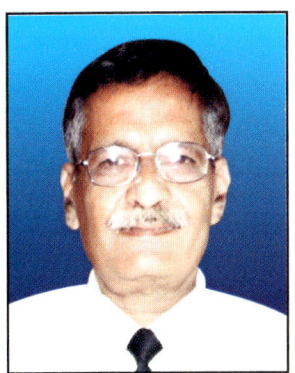

Prof A Raja MS (Neurosurgery)
Prof & Head
Department of Neurosurgery
KMC, Manipal

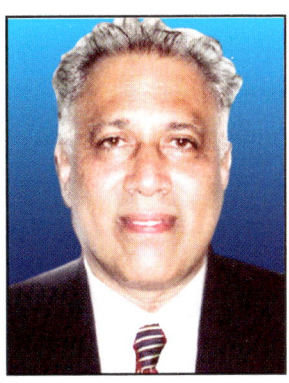

Dr K.M Cariappa MDS, MOMS,
RCPS (Glasgow)
Prof & Head, Department of
Oromaxillofacial Surgery
KMC, Manipal

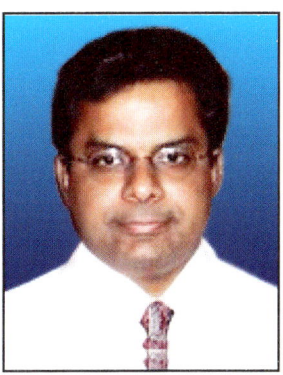

Dr C Rayappa FRCS,DLO
Senior Consultant
ENT, H&N, Skull Base Surgeon
Apollo Hospital, Chennai

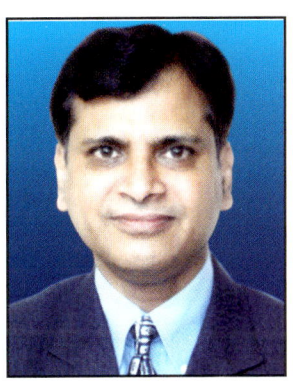

Prof D.R. Nayak MS,FICS,FIAO
Prof & Head
Department of Otolaryngology &
Head & Neck Surgery
KMC, Manipal

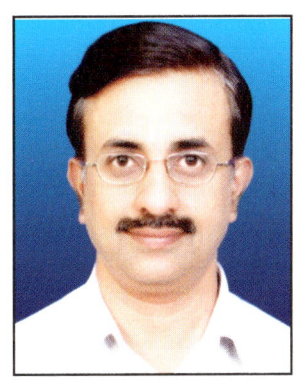

Prof Balakrishna R MS, DNB
Department of Otolaryngology &
Head & Neck Surgery
KMC, Manipal

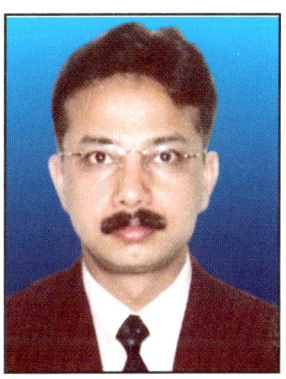

Dr Roopjyothi Hazarika
MS, MCH (Neurosurgery)
KMC, Manipal

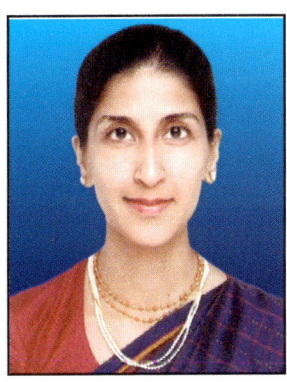

Dr Parul Pujary MS
Associate Professor
KMC ,Manipal

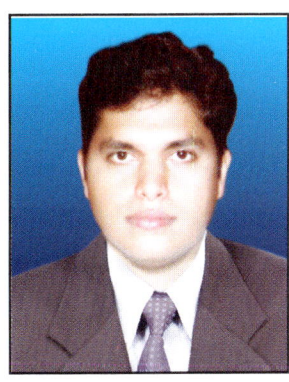

Dr Mahesh SG MS ,DNB
Assistant Professor
KMC, Manipal

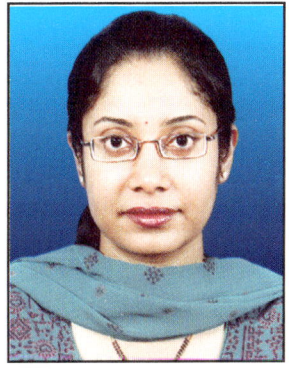

Dr Pallavi Pavithran MS, DNB
Assistant Professor
KMC, Manipal

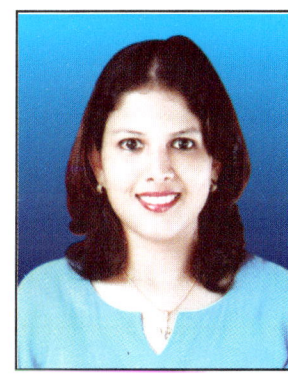

Dr Manali Hazarika MBBS
Resident in Opthalmology
KMC, Manipal

Contents

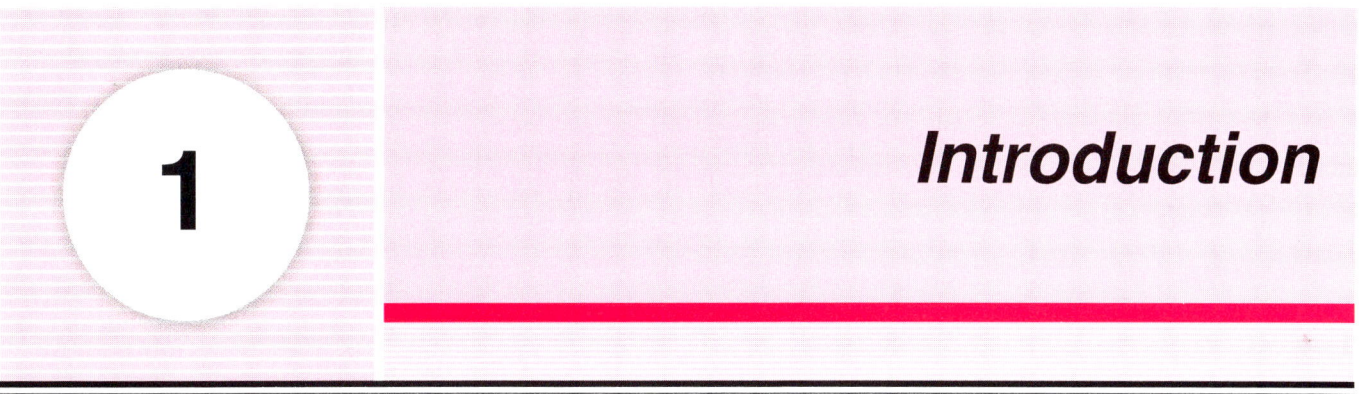

Tumor involvement of the skull base is not an uncommon clinical entity in otolaryngological practice. The skull base may be involved in the primary tumor. However, secondary tumor involvement extending from the ENT and head and neck area is very common. Clinicians face various diagnostic and therapeutic problems, due to the lack of clinical and surgical experience and also because of the rarity of these tumors in this complex anatomical region.

Skull base was a no mans land a decade ago. Nowadays, fortunately, this area is being explored by various surgical specialities thereby making this area ideal for a multidisciplinary approach. This surgical group dealing with this area is known as skull base surgeons; consisting of specialists like:

- Otolaryngologist
- Neurosurgeon
- Oromaxillofacial surgeon
- Ophthalmologist
- Plastic surgeon
- Neuro-anaesthesiologist
- Radiation oncologist
- Medical oncologist
- Interventional radiologist

Earlier surgical attempts for removal of the skull base tumor was associated with very poor prognosis, and a high mortality and morbidity. Now with the application of a multi-disciplinary approach, better knowledge of micro anatomy of this area, tremendous improvement in anesthesia, technical improvement in reconstructive procedures and various innovative surgical approaches have made the skull base procedures more safe. The quality of surgical removal of the tumor has improved with good prognosis, reduced morbidity and very little mortality. Surgical results of maxilloethmoidal complex malignancy has gone up by 10 to 12% after introduction of anterior skull base approach for resection of these tumors. Craniofacial resection has become the GOLD STANDARD for lesions that involve the roof of the ethmoid sinus or the superior nasal vault (cribriform plate) as visualization from above (cranial) and below (facial) became possible. Knowledge of the surgical anatomy of the skull base is very important to select the proper surgical approach or approaches for tumor exposure and its complete or piece meal removal. Too many surgical approaches have been described. A good understanding and hands on experience of all the approaches will definitely help in making a versatile skull base surgeon. Any approach which gives an adequate exposure of the skull base, allowing identification and preservation of vital neurovascular structures, safe and complete removal of the tumor with preservation of function and aesthetics, followed by restoration of appropriate barriers between the neurocranium and the nasosinus regions is considered to be an excellent approach.

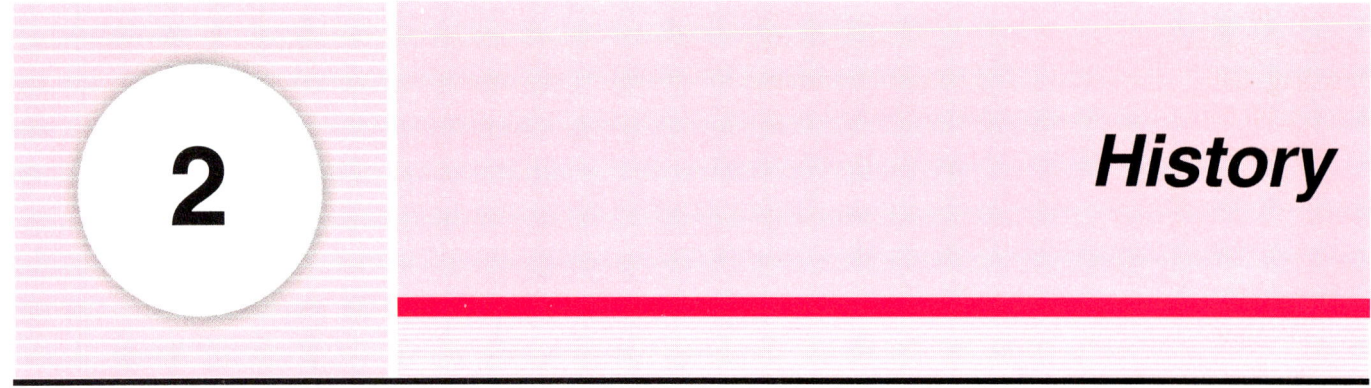

Skull base surgery first started with pioneers in the field of head and neck surgery and neurosurgery who, with no blood transfusion or antibiotics, intrepidly attempted to resect selected lesion in this formidable area.

The evolution of surgical techniques have been paralleled by developments in diagnostic radiology. History and evolution of anterior, lateral and posterior skull base have been described separately.

History of anterior fossa and pituitary surgery

Surgical adventure to explore the anterior skull base started with pituitary surgery. Caton and Paul first attempted operating on the pituitary by performing a temporal lobe decompression. Victor Horsley performed the first transfrontal operation for pituitary in 1899. Anterior transfrontal subdural techniques were demonstrated experimentally by Krause I and Killiani in the first decade of the 20th century in 1912. Frazier used this approach in one of his patients. An extracranial attempt on the pituitary was first described by the Italian surgeon Giordano.

In 1909, Cushing II described his first attempt via the transnasal approach to the pituitary. In 1914, he described the sublabial approach that has many features which is similar to the present day transseptal transsphenoidal operation. At the same time that Cushing described the transnasal route to the pituitary, a similar approach was being used by the Viennese otolaryngologist, Oskar Hirsch. Initially, the procedure was done entirely transnasally in three stages. Eventually, in 1911, he combined the stages through a midline sub labial approach.

The first recorded anterior craniofacial resection for a tumor was by Dandy in 1941. While removing an orbital tumor through an anterior cranial fossa approach, he entered the ethmoid bloc in an attempt to improve exposure and achieve complete resection. However, the landmark article in anterior cranial base surgery that involved a coordinated transfacial and transcranial approach to tumor removal was published in 1954 by Klopp, a head and neck oncosurgeon who teamed up with Smith and Williams to do a planned procedure to remove what was described as a cancer of the frontal sinus.

Ketcham et al launched skull base surgery for malignant lessions by using Anterior craniotomy and Weber Ferguson approach in 1966. In 1976, *Sisson et al* reported their experience with craniofacial resection for paranasal sinus malignancies. In 1986, *Cheesman et al* reported their 10 year experience on craniofacial resection of ethmoid carcinomas with intracranial spread using a small 'window' craniotomy.

Attempts were made to improve the exposure of the anterior fossa, especially at its most posterior extent. This often was difficult to achieve without aggressive retraction of the frontal lobes using the standard craniotomy. Based on this experience of removal of fronto-orbital tumors Bandeau and Tressier extended the indication of craniofacial surgery for correction of congenital craniomaxillary anomalies *Derome et al[1]* described the low frontoorbital technique for spheno-ethmoid tumors. The extended anterior subcranial approach was developed by Raveh in 1978 to manage intracranial trauma and then adapted it to tumor resection and is excellent for midline lesions. **Mid Facial Degloving** was originally proposed by Rouge in 1974 Casson rediscovered this approach which was popularized by Price in 1986. In 1859 Von Langenberg initially reported the **Le–forte technique**. The level of high maxillary and midfacial osteotomies has been named according to the fracture classification proposed by LeFort in 1901. In 1867 Cheever made early attempts for excision of nasopharyngeal polyp by this approach. The Facial translocation approach was discovered by *Janecka P et al* in 1990.

In India initial work in anterior skull base surgery was done in KMC Manipal by a group of surgeons headed by P Hazarika in 1980s and 90s. He published in 1985, a case of Primary Malignant Fibrous Histiocytoma of Ethmoid Sinus in Indian Journal of Cancer. In 1990, Hazarika and Murty published Combined craniofacial approach for Fronto-Maxillo-ethmoidal Lesions in Indian Journal of Otolaryngology. D. R Nayak, Hazarika and Raja published similar paper entitled Malignant tumours of the skull base and CFR and Olfactory Neuroblastoma - our experience in proceedings of Asia-pacific congress, International federation of Head and Neck Oncologic Societies, sponsored by Indian Society of Head and Neck Oncology, Mumbai, 1997 Balakrishnan R., Hazarika P., Nayak D.R. & Raja A. published a case of Anterior Skull Base Surgery – our experience in The Indian Journal of Otolaryngology and Head & Neck Surgery. Olfactory Neuroblastoma - our experience published in The Indian Journal of Otolaryngology and Head & Neck Surgery, Vol. 51, No.1, Jan-March 1999, P. 68 – 73 by S. Sharma, J. Sahota, P. Hazarika.

History of posterior fossa-acoustic tumors

Another major area of skull base surgery was surgical development for excision of lesions of the posterior cranial fossa. In the early 20th century, the removal of acoustic neuromas was first done in a systematic manner by Harvey Cushing. In London in 1894, Ballance and Beevor reported the removal of an acoustic tumor with a favorable result. Prior attempts by Starr and McBurney for a posterior fossa exploration for such a tumor was unsuccessful. In the years before Cushing successfully resected these lesions, a common practice was to insert a dissecting finger between the tumor and the pons in an attempt to enucleate it. In his own report, Cushing found that with increasing experience, his mortality rate diminished from the death of his first patient to 20%.

Dandy's 1942 description of acoustic tumor removal by a modified Retrosigmoid approach remained the standard approach until the introduction of the operating microscope in 1961.

The operating microscope was first used in clinical surgery by Nylen in 1921 to drain an acute suppurative otitis media by myringotomy. This was a uni-ocular microscope that lacked the three-dimensional visualization what surgeons enjoy today. Holmgren, who had been doing labyrinthine procedures for otosclerosis, developed the binocular microscope for middle ear surgery in 1922. In 1953, the Zeiss Company produced a prototype of the operating microscope that is universally used today.

In 1904, Panse developed an approach through the temporal bone, with a radical mastoidectomy. It was followed by removal of the labyrinth, cochlea, and facial nerve with a gouge. Profuse bleeding and cerebrospinal fluid leak predictably accompanied these procedures.

William House an otologist and B. B. Doyle, a neurosurgeon were the first to successfully resect an acoustic neuroma using the microscope. Because it was unprecedented for an otolaryngologist to do this type of surgery, the neurosurgery community presented resistance to House's desire to remove this tumor. After considerable debate an otoneurosurgical skull base team headed by William House did the operation through the middle fossa approach. At that time the middle fossa appeared to be a good route for facial nerve exposure, but inadequate for tumor removal. After eight attempts through the middle fossa route, sometimes accompanied with the suboccipital approach, house decided to redesign the operation and modified the original approach of Panse using the microscope, drill and suction irrigation. He was able to preserve the facial nerve, the posterior canal wall, and the tympanic membrane. William Hitselberger then joined with House to form the solid, long-lasting relationship that was the nucleus of the first true skull base surgical team.

The transotic approach destroys hearing as the removal of the bony and membranous labyrinth eliminates all vestiges of hearing on that side. However, by the time the diagnosis was made most patients had little or no useful hearing in the affected ear. The loss of remaining hearing acuity was of little consequence (a position voiced by numerous otologists even today). As clinicians became more aware of this diagnosis, the computed tomography and magnetic resonance imaging improved their ability to detect small tumors in patients whose hearing was intact or minimally affected hence hearing preservation now became more important. The translabyrinthine approach developed by House preserved facial nerve function in most cases Sterkers began hearing preservation surgery in 1969 and reported only a 10% favorable hearing result when he and his team used either the middle fossa or retrosigmoid approach. Cochlear and brain stem implants are the other alternatives to improve the hearing acquity in patients whose hearing has been sacrificed during this procedure.

History of lateral skull Base

A history of modern skull base surgery would be very much amiss without mention of one of the premier skull base surgeons, Ugo Fisch. With his background as head and neck oncologic surgeon, he extended the limits of otologic surgery into the area of the infra-temporal fossa. He and his neurosurgical colleague, Gazi Yasargil, combined their skills to develop an approach through the infratemporal fossa to lesions that approached or invaded middle fossa dura. The uniqueness of this approach lays in that; the lesion could be adequately exposed and resected with minimal temporal lobe retraction. Fisch is particularly known for his pioneering work in the resection of juvenile nasopharyngeal angiofibroma with massive infratemporal fossa and middle fossa extension. He then turned his attention to resection of jugular foramen tumors, producing a workable classification of glomus jugular tumors and a systematic solution to their extirpation.

A number of modifications of Fisch's approach have been made. The most notable one is by Victor Schramm and Laligam Sekhar in 1987. Refinements of Fisch's technique enabled wider exposure and more definitive resection of invasive meningiomas of the anterior and middle cranial fossae with extracranial extension and carcinomas arising in the upper aerodigestive tract invading the intracranial cavity by using subtemporal preauricular infratemporal approach.

Schramm and Myers 1978 described the lateral rhinotomy approach. Biller described the transmandibular approach to skull base in 1981. Janecka introduced facial translocation procedure and the midfacial split approach in 1991. Holliday in 1986 described lateral transtemporal sphenoid approach. Panje and Pitcock in 1991 described the extended Rhytidectomy approach. Sewall in 1926 devised transantral approach to the pterygopalatine fossa for sphenopalatine ganglionectomy. Seiffert in 1928 ligated internal maxillary artery by transantral approach. Golding – Wood contributed to transantral approach to pterygopalatine fossa with his work on vidian neurectomy in vasomotor rhinitis. Fairbanks-Barbosa (1916) were the first to report an infratemporal fossa (ITF) approach, indicated for advanced tumors of the maxillary sinus. In 1992, P. Hazarika & A. Kumar removed Schwannoma of Jugular Foramen by Infra Temporal Fossa approach – published in Indian Journal of Otolaryngology and Head and Neck. In 1993 Surgical Treatment of Lateral Skull Base Tumours - our Experience has been published in Indian Journal of Otolaryngology and Head and Neck Surgery, Vol. 2, No.1, 19-22. In 1995 Congenital Internal Carotid Artery Aneurysm was removed by infratemporal fossa approach and published in International Journal of Paediatric Otorhinolaryngology (USA). Osteogenic Sarcoma of Sphenoid Bone - An extended lateral skull base approach was published in The Journal of Laryngology and Otology, Vol. 109, 1101-1104 by P. Hazarika, D.R.Nayak. Osteolipoma of the skull base: a case report was published in The Journal of Laryngology and Otology, U.K. Vol. 115, PP.136-139, Feb. 2001 by P. Hazarika, Kailesh Pujary, which was approached by Billers transcervical transmandibular approach.

Surgery-related anatomy

The 5 bones that make up the skull base are the ethmoid, sphenoid, occipital, paired frontal and paired temporo-parietal bones.

Classification

To have a comprehensive knowledge regarding the surgical approaches, a clear cut classification of this area is mandatory (Fig. 3.1 & 3.2).

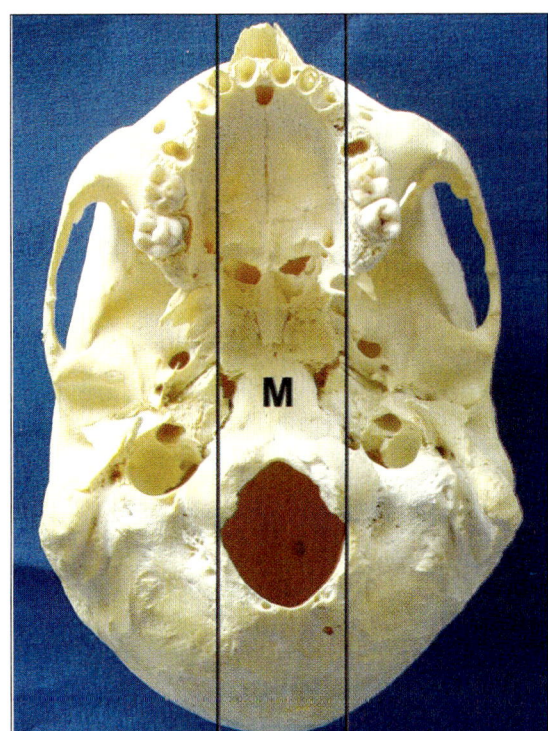

Fig. 3.1 Cranial base is divided classically into anterior, middle and posterior segments

The cranial base is classically divided into

- Anterior
- Middle and
- Posterior segments

The importance of classifying these regions is:

- To have a comprehensive knowledge regarding the surgical approaches, and
- For successful skull base surgery without undue complications.

From the diagnostic and therapeutic point of view, the Anterior and the Middle Cranial Base are considered together because

- They contribute commonly to the 'craniofacial junction' which is an important area in which the neurocranium and viscerocranium meet.
- Both share anatomical relations with the orbit, the nasal airway, and the paranasal sinuses and are therefore affected by several similar pathological processes.

The anterior and middle cranial base regions are commonly approached using craniofacial disassembly techniques.

Glasscock et al and Som *et al* defined the skull base, as the part of cranium, formed by the greater wing of sphenoid, temporal bone and occipital bone to the midline thereby highlighting only the middle and posterior cranial fossae. This may be because anterior cranial fossa cannot be visualized as clearly as the corresponding surface of middle and posterior cranial fossa from an extracranial approach.

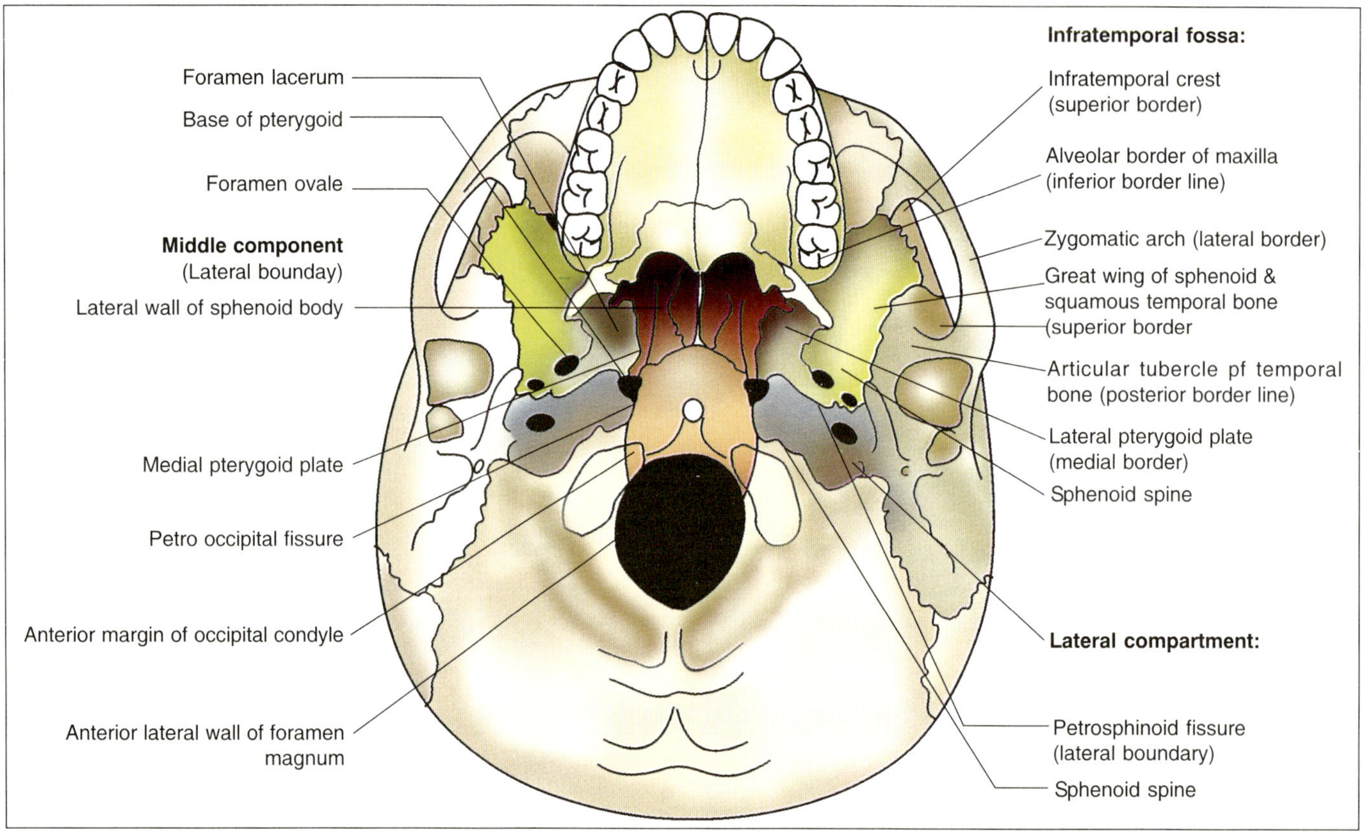

Foramen lacerum

Base of pterygoid

Foramen ovale

Middle component
(Lateral bounday)

Lateral wall of sphenoid body

Medial pterygoid plate

Petro occipital fissure

Anterior margin of occipital condyle

Anterior lateral wall of foramen magnum

Infratemporal fossa:

Infratemporal crest
(superior border)

Alveolar border of maxilla
(inferior border line)

Zygomatic arch (lateral border)

Great wing of sphenoid &
squamous temporal bone
(superior border

Articular tubercle pf temporal
bone (posterior border line)

Lateral pterygoid plate
(medial border)

Sphenoid spine

Lateral compartment:

Petrosphinoid fissure
(lateral boundary)

Sphenoid spine

Fig. 3.2 The basal view of the skull divided into various compartments and showing the foramens and the contents of the foramen

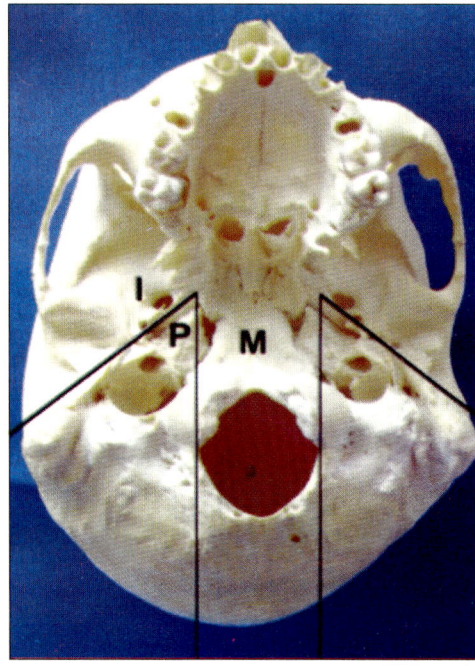

Fig. 3.3 Cranial base divided into Central and Lateral compartment, Lateral compartment further divided into infratemporal compartment and petrotemporal compartment

The floor of the anterior cranial fossa is formed by the extra cranial surface of the orbital roof laterally and the roof of ethmoid labyrinth medially and posterior wall of frontal sinus anteriorly.

Kumar & Vulvasori1 (1986) have described a different classification which can be followed to select the proper surgical approach. Viewing the skull base from inferiorly, this irregular and anatomical complex extra cranial skull base surface was subdivided by them by using two para sagittal lines.

First line: Two imaginary para sagittal straight lines are drawn, one on each side through the medial pterygoid plate anteriorly and the occipital condyle posteriorly, thereby dividing the skull base into a central and two lateral compartments (anteriorly the two lines correspond with the medial wall of each orbit). The central compartment contains the nasion, roof of nose, ethmoid labyrinth, sphenoid sinus, basisphenoid and basiocciput.

The **second line** is drawn from each medial pterygoid plate to the glenoid fossa thereby dividing the lateral compartment into two subdivisions:

1. Anterolateral to the line - infratemporal compartment.

2. Posteromedial to the line - petrotemporal compartment.

   Therefore the middle cranial base may be further subdivided into a single central, two lateral compartments.

ANTERIOR CRANIAL BASE ANATOMY

The anterior cranial base can be defined as that portion of the skull base adjacent to the anterior cranial fossa.

The extracranial surface

The Anterior cranial fossa cannot be visualized as clearly as the corresponding surface of the middle and posterior cranial fossa from an extracranial approach.

Topographically it is related to the nasal cavities, ethmoid sinuses, sphenoid sinus and the orbits.

- The floor of the anterior cranial fossa is quite uneven with downward slopping of the orbits. This places the ethmoid roof lower and the cribriform area at a still lower level in the floor of anterior cranial fossa. This non planer arrangement is important during transethmoid extracranial approaches to the cribriform plate. An axial plane of dissection along the roof of the ethmoid may risk injury to the dura and frontal lobes if extended medially to encompass the region of the cribriform plate.

- The anterior and posterior ethmoid foramina mark the level of the *frontoethmoid suture line and serve as a landmark for the level of the ethmoid roof and anterior fossa floor.* They also encompass anterior and posterior ethmoidal arteries.

- The superior orbital fissure transmits the cranial nerve III, IV, V-1, VI, and the ophthalmic vein. It directly communicates with the middle cranial fossa.

- The inferior orbital fissure contains the maxillary nerve (V-2) and communicates with the pterygopalatine fossa. *The lateral end of this fissure is an important landmark for the placement of lateral orbital osteotomies.*

- The optic canal transmits the optic nerve and the ophthalmic artery. In most of the cases the optic canal is 4-7 mm posterior to the posterior ethmoidal foramina. *The optic foramen lies at the posterior limit of the anterior cranial base.*

- The roof of the orbit is formed by the orbital process of the frontal bone. The greater and lesser wings of the sphenoid form the apex and lateral wall of the orbits. The zygomatic bone marks its lateral wall. The lacrimal, ethmoid, palatine and sphenoid bones comprise the medial wall of the orbit.

THE INTRACRANIAL SURFACE OF ANTERIOR CRANIAL BASE

Boundaries

Anteriorly: by the frontal bone, which contains the Frontal sinus and Supraorbital foramina.

Superiorly

- Frontal lobe

Posteriorly

- Anterior clinoid process
- Lesser sphenoid wings
- Optic canal

The floor

The floor of the anterior cranial fossa is formed by the crista galli, cribriform plates, orbital roof and planum sphenoidal (Fig. 3.4).

Frontal sinus is located in the frontal bone and is extremely variable in size and must be dealt with in most of the anterior cranial base surgeries.

Supraorbital foramen transmits the supraorbital nerves and vessels. These vessels contribute a major portion of blood supply to the galea and the pericranium of the frontal region. They must be preserved in order to be used in the reconstruction of anterior cranial base defects.

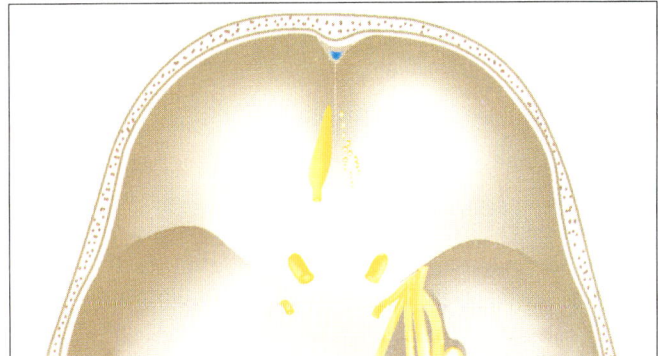

Fig. 3.4 Showing important structures of intracranial surface of anterior skull base

The foramen caecum is in the midline behind the frontal bone. Its posterior and lateral boundaries are formed by the ethmoid bone. This is the site of communication between the veins of the nasal cavity and the origin of the superior saggital sinus.

The crista galli is an osseous ridge arising from the midline of the ethmoid bone. It provides attachment to the falx cerebri. It is the only intracranial air cell.

The cribriform plate which is on either side of the crista, contains the olfactory foramina through which olfactory nerves travel. The dura mater over the cribriform plates is thin.

The planum sphenoidale is the smooth surfaced area behind olfactory foramina. It forms the roof of sphenoid sinus.

The anterior clinoid process and lesser wings of sphenoid delineate the posterior limit of the anterior cranial base.

Blood supply

The blood supply to the anterior cranial fossa is from the anterior and posterior ethmoidal arteries, middle meningeal artery and ICA via the ophthalmic artery.

MIDDLE SKULL BASE ANATOMY

The middle cranial base may be further subdivided into a

- Single central
- Two lateral compartments.

Single central compartment

Boundaries of middle skull base form the floor of the middle cranial fossa. From an intracranial perspective the middle cranial base begins anteriorly at the posterior edge of the lesser wing of sphenoid and posteriorly it ends at the posterior superior edge of the petrous part of the temporal bone. The intracranial surface is formed by the greater wing and the body of sphenoid bone as well as the petrous and squamous portions of the temporal bone. This forms the roof of the infratemporal fossa, middle ear, mastoid, and condylar fossa. The floor of the middle cranial fossa has several important foramina. The lateral wall is formed by the greater wing of the sphenoid anteriorly and the squamous portion of the temporal bone posteriorly. The body of the sphenoid makes up the central portion of the middle fossa.

LATERAL COMPARTMENT

1. Infratemporal (anterolateral) compartment

- Infratemporal fossa
- Pterygopalatine fossa
- Posterior wall of maxilla
- Floor of middle cranial fossa

2. Petrotemporal (posteromedial) compartment

As many lateral skull base approaches involve the infratemporal fossa, this anatomical region deserves special mention.

The ITF is a potential space bounded:

- Superiorly by the temporal bone and the greater wing of the sphenoid bone;
- Medially by the superior constrictor muscle, the pharyngobasilar fascia, and the pterygoid plates;
- Laterally by the zygoma, mandible, parotid gland and masseter muscle;
- Anteriorly, by the pterygoid muscles; and
- Posteriorly by the articular tubercle of the temporal bone, glenoid fossa, and styloid process.

By this definition, the ITF comprises the contents of both the parapharyngeal space (i.e., internal carotid artery [ICA], internal jugular vein [IJV], cranial nerves [CN] IV to XII) and the masticator space (i.e., V3, internal maxillary artery [IMA], pterygoid venous plexus, pterygoid muscles).

The ITF communicates with the middle cranial fossa via the neurovascular foramina (i.e., carotid canal, jugular foramen, foramen spinosum, foramen ovale and foramen lacerum). Medially, the ITF communicates with the pterygopalatine fossa via the pterygomaxillary fissure, which is contiguous with the inferior orbital fissure and, thus, the orbit.

Surgical implications for exposure of the infratemporal fossa

In the lateral approach for surgical exposure of the infratemporal fossa, structures are encountered in the following anatomical order:

1. Skin
2. Parotid gland and duct, transverse facial artery and branches of CN VII
3. Masseter muscle

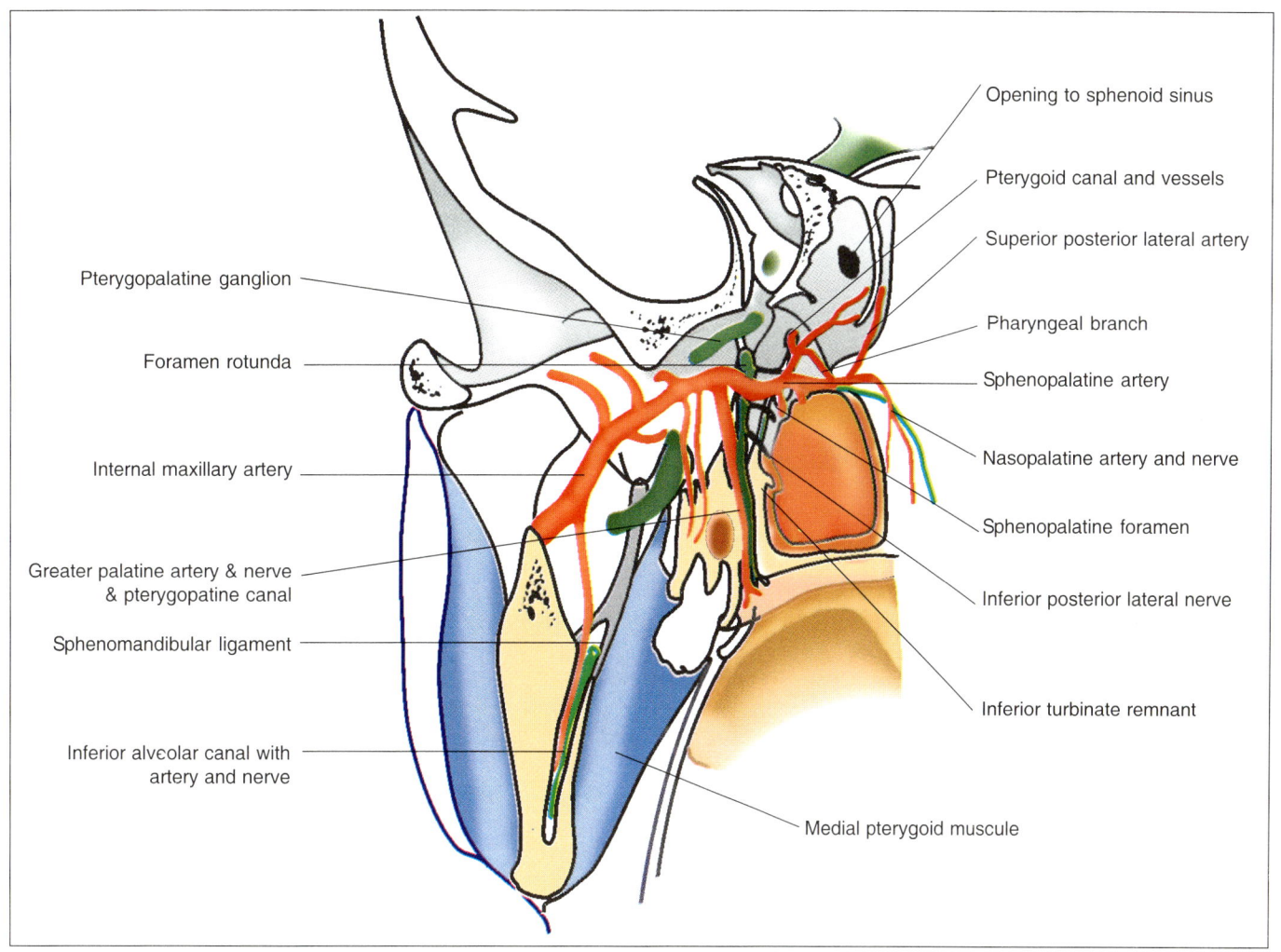

Fig. 3.5 Showing the coronal cut of the infratemporal fossa

4. Ramus of the mandible and temporalis muscle.

5. Internal maxillary artery and branches.

6. Lateral (external) pterygoid muscle.

7. Mandibular division of CN V and its branches.

8. Medial (internal) pterygoid muscle inferiorly and lamina of the pterygoid superiorly.

9. Pharynx (medial boundary of the infratemporal fossa).

Pterygopalatine fossa

It is a space in lateral skull base just medial to infratemporal fossa, distributing nerves and vessels to the middle third of face.

The boundaries are

Anteriorly - Posterior wall of maxilla (superomedial part).

Posteriorly - Root of pterygoid process.

- Anterior part of greater wing of sphenoid.

Medially - Perpendicular plate of palatine bone.

Laterally - Pterygomaxillary fissure connecting it to infratemporal fossa.

Superiorly - Body of sphenoid.

Inferiorly - Junction of anterior and posterior walls leading to greater palatine canal (Fig. 3.5).

Sphenopalatine foramen lies between perpendicular plate of palatine bone, body of sphenoid (superiorly) orbital process (anteriorly) and sphenoidal process (posteriorly). The foramen opens into the nasopharynx.

The fossa contains terminal branches of maxillary artery, (infraorbital, descending palatine, sphenopalatine branches), maxillary branch of trigeminal nerve, pterygopalatine ganglion.

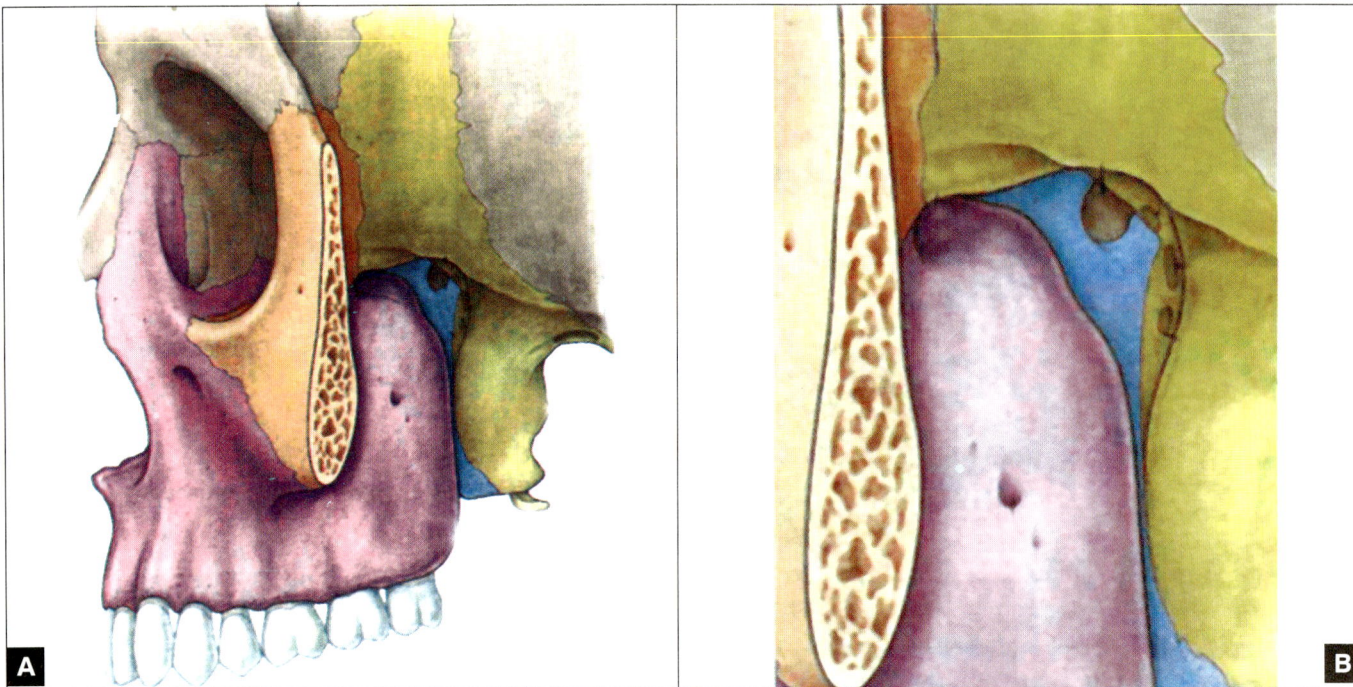

Fig. 3.6 A. Showing pterygopalatine fossa in lateral view of skull. **B.** Closeup view

2. PETROTEMPORAL (POSTEROMEDIAL) COMPARTMENT

1. Petrous part of temporal bone
2. Mastoid
3. Infralabynthine part of petrous
4. Foramen lacerum
5. Jugalar foramen

The temporal bone is surrounded by many important structures. It articulates with five other cranial bones: the frontal, parietal, sphenoid, occipital and zygomatic (Fig. 3.6).

It can be divided into four parts and four surfaces:

Parts: Squamous, Mastoid, Petrous and Tympanic.

Surfaces: Superior, anterior, posterior cerebellar and inferior.

a. *Squamous portion:* The lateral surface defines the boundary of the middle cranial fossa. It extends medially to join the superior surface of the petrous bone in the region of the tegmen.

b. *Mastoid portion:* Pneumatization within the mastoid process is variable. The squama of the temporal bone forms the lateral wall of the central air containing space, the antrum, which communicates with middle ear by the aditus. The suprameatal spine and cribriform area provide important landmarks for surgical access

wall of the middle ear cavity contains the basal turn of the cochlea.

d. *Tympanic portion:* The tympanic part of the temporal bone forms the anterior and inferior walls and part of the posterior wall of the external auditory meatus. It is separated anteriorly from the squamous bone by the tympanosquamous suture more medially from the petrous bone by the petrotympanic fissure and posteriorly from the mastoid portion of the petrous bone by the tympanomastoid fissure. The inner part of the tympanic ring is grooved and is called the tympanic sulcus, which accomodates the tympanic membrane annulus. The inferior aspect of the tympanic bone is elongated into a vaginal process immediately anterior to the styloid process (Fig. 3.7).

SURFACES

Superior and anterior surface

This forms part of the middle cranial fossa. The foramen lacerum is found between the apex of the petrous bone and sphenoid bone and contains, but does not transmit the ICA. Near the apex is a small depression which lodges the trigeminal ganglion. The arcuate eminence of the petrous bone overlies the superior semi-circular canal. The tegmen

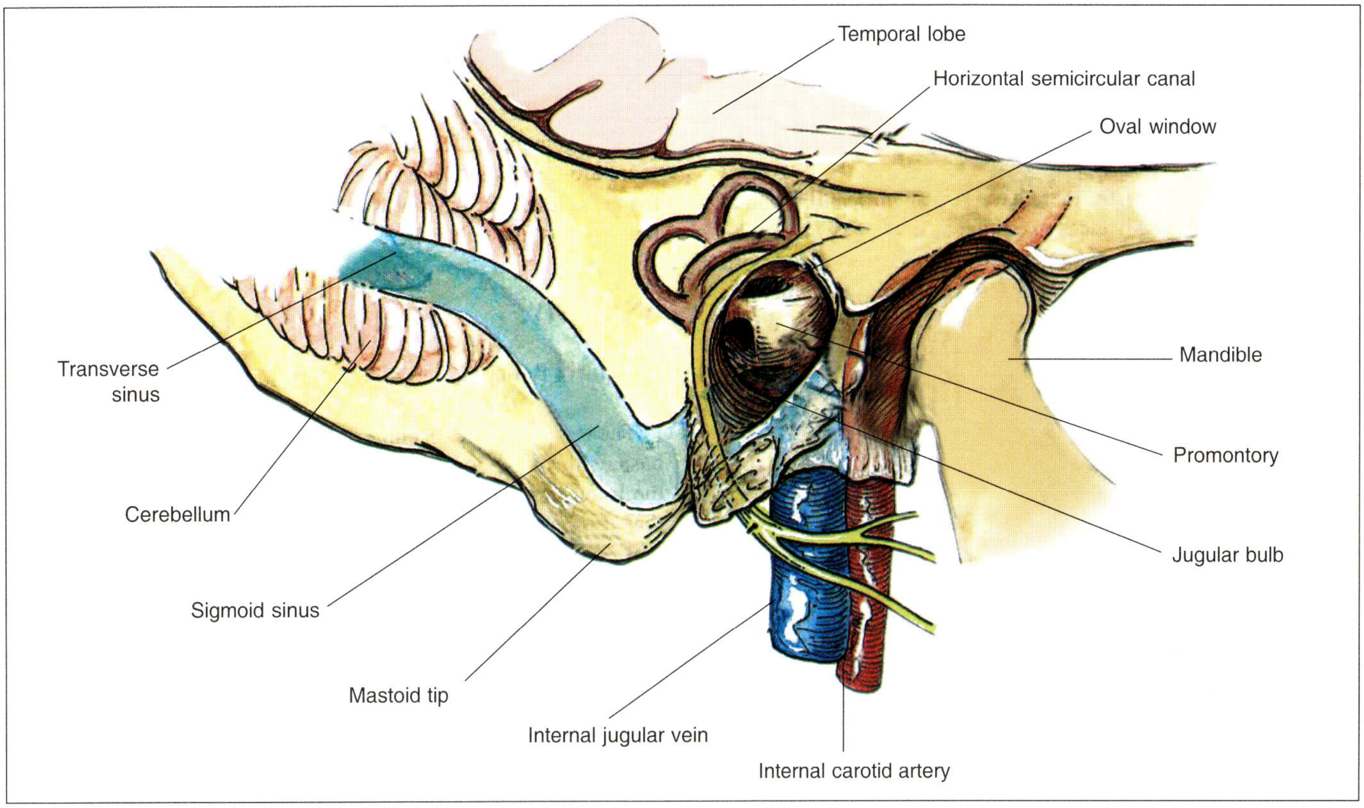

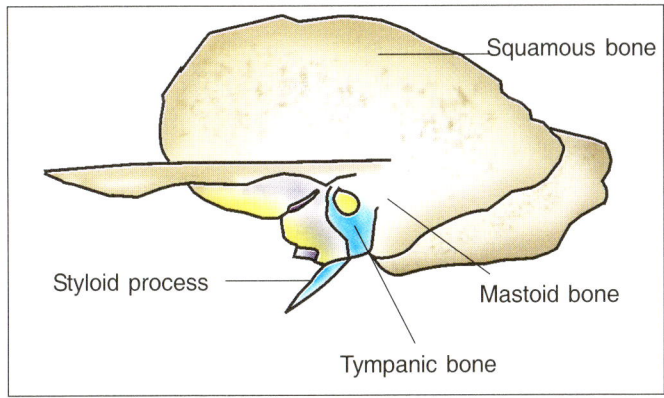

Fig. 3.7 Temporal bone showing relationships of major vessels, brain, mandible and middle ear.

[Fig. 3.7 labels: Temporal lobe, Horizontal semicircular canal, Oval window, Mandible, Promontory, Jugular bulb, Internal carotid artery, Internal jugular vein, Mastoid tip, Sigmoid sinus, Cerebellum, Transverse sinus]

Fig. 3.8 Osseous components of temporal Bone

[Fig. 3.8 labels: Squamous bone, Mastoid bone, Tympanic bone, Styloid process]

petrosal sinus defines its superior border. Posteriorly it articulates with the occipital bone. Approximately midway between the apex and the anterior border of sigmoid sulcus is the IAM. It is a short canal which begins medially at the internal acoustic pore. A bony plate which is also part of tympani is lateral to this eminence. The opening of the hiatus of the facial canal is anterior and medial to the arcuate eminence; this transmits the superficial petrosal branch of the middle meningeal artery and the greater petrosal nerve.

Posterior cerebellar surface

Posterior surface of the petrous bone forms the anterolateral surface of the posterior fossa. A sulcus for the superior

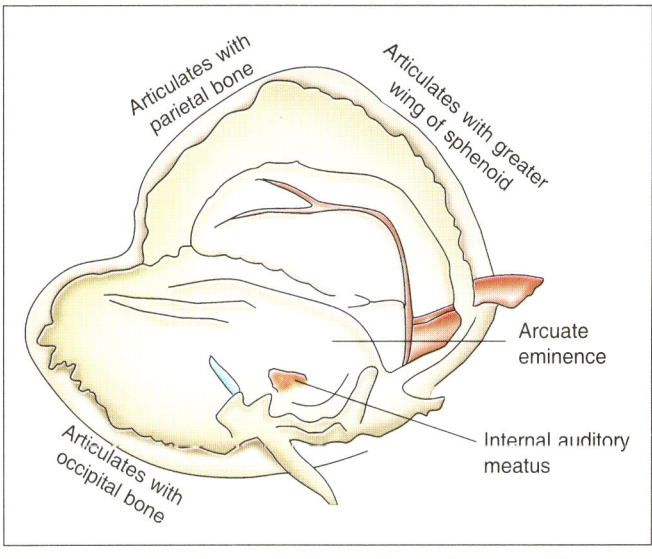

Fig. 3.9 Posterior cerebellar surface of temporal bone

[Fig. 3.9 labels: Articulates with parietal bone, Articulates with greater wing of sphenoid, Arcuate eminence, Internal auditory meatus, Articulates with occipital bone]

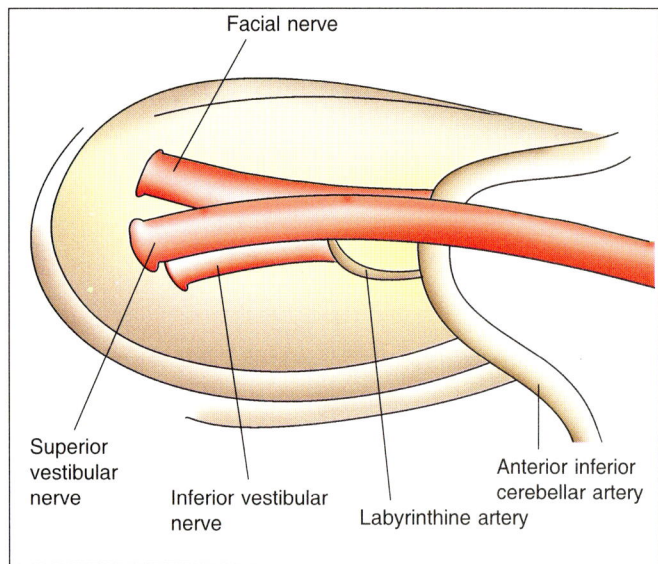

Fig. 3.10 Internal auditory meatus

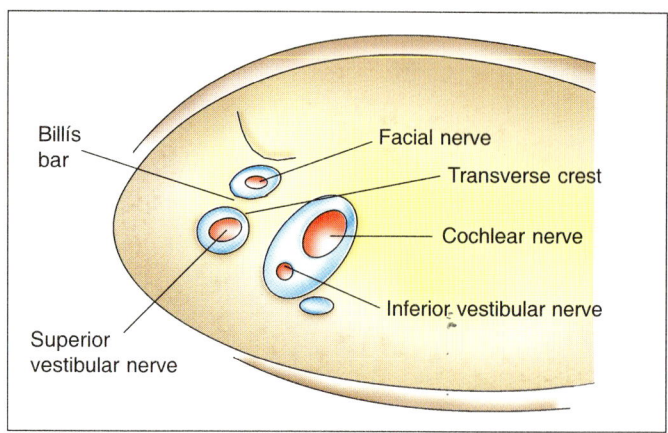

Fig. 3.11 Fundus of internal auditory meatus

the medial wall of the cochlea and vestibule closes the lateral end. A horizontal ridge of bone, the transverse crest, divides the pore into upper and lower areas. The anterior portion of the superior division contains the facial nerve which is separated from the superior vestibular nerve by a small, vertical crest of bone, known as 'Bill's bar'. It serves as an important landmark during the translabyrinthine approach. The cochlear nerve lies in the anterior portion and the inferior vestibular nerve in the posterior portion of the lower division. Midway between the meatus and sigmoid sulcus, is the vestibular aqueduct which transmits the endolymphatic sac and duct.

Inferior surface

It is the most irregular area of the petrous bone's surfaces. The opening of the carotid canal is about midway between the apex and base; this is the entrance for the ICA and its plexus of veins and sympathetic nerves. The canal courses in a cephaloid direction along the anterior wall of the tympanic cavity to the bony eustachian tube and then bends horizontally, ending at the apex of the petrous bone and the occipital bone. Carotid ridge is a sharp bone separating the carotid and jugular foramen. The lateral part of the foramen contains the sigmoid portion of the transverse sinus; the medial part contains the inferior petrosal sinus and the glossophayrngeal, vagus and accessory nerve. Anterior to the lateral compartment is the broad fossa for the jugular bulb. Posterior and lateral to it is the styloid process. Lateral to its base is the stylomastoid foramen transmitting the facial nerve.

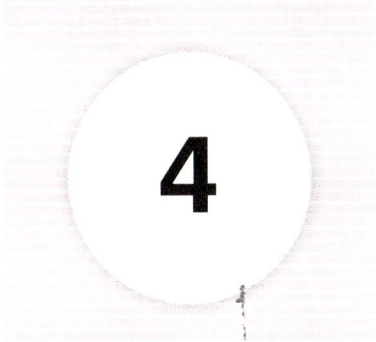

4

Common Skull Base Lesions and Clinical Features

COMMON ANTERIOR SKULL BASE TUMORS

A diverse type of tumors can involve the anterior cranial fossa: Primary benign tumors with rare malignant potential include meningioma and pituitary adenoma. Primary malignant tumors include chordoma, chondrosarcoma, osteogenic sarcoma and invasive pituitary tumor. Malignant tumors with secondary involvement include carcinoma of the paranasal sinuses. Others include lymphoma arising from the nasopharynx, minor salivary gland neoplasms, paragangliomas, olfactory neuroblastoma, mucoepidermoid carcinoma, and osteosarcoma. Histologically benign tumors include angiofibroma and inverted papilloma. Metastasis from renal, breast, and lung carcinoma can also involve the anterior cranial fossa. Teratocarcinoma is rare in this region. Lastly, paranasal sinus infections can extend into the anterior skull base.

Benign tumors

- Olfactory meningioma
- Recurrent invasive inverted papilloma (extending into cribriform plate)
- Fibro-osseous tumors
- Angiofibromas
- Giant frontoethmoidal mucocele
- Benign mixed tumor of minor salivary gland
- Aspergilloma of PNS
- Chromophobe adenoma (pituitary)

Malignant tumors

- Squamous cell carcinoma

- Malignant tumors of minor salivary glands e.g. adenoid cystic, oncocytoma
- High mucoepidermoid carcinoma, arising from mucosa of PNS nasal cavity or lacrimal apparatus.
- Esthesioneuroblastoma.
- Chondrosarcoma
- Haemangiopericytoma
- Invasive basal cell carcinoma of skin involving facial bones of skull.
- Nasopharyngeal carcinoma
- Rhabdomyosarcoma

Benign tumors of anterior skull base

Encephalocoeles of the anterior cranial fossa

Encephalocoeles are extensions of intracranial structures outside the normal confines of the skull. Their incidence is approximately 0.2 per 1000 live births and fetal deaths. These lesions can be classified into sincipital and basal encephaloceles. Sincipital encephaloceles can be further subdivided into frontonasal, ethmoidal and orbital subtypes. Basal encephaloceles may be sphenoorbital, maxillary, ethmoidal, or transethmoidal.

Surgery-related strategies for repair of anterior cranial fossa encephaloceles usually require a bicoronal scalp incision, frontal craniotomy, and bilateral orbitotomy. The dural defect is defined at the anterior skull base, and the dura is then opened. Normal-appearing herniated brain tissue can sometimes be restored to the intracranial compartment: However, frequently this tissue is dysplastic and irretrievable. The dura is closed in a watertight fashion, and the craniofacial skeleton is reconstructed in conjunction with the craniofacial surgeons along with cosmetic repair of the facial skin defect. In cases in which marked hypertelorism has resulted, an orbital translocation procedure may be required. In contrast to occipital encephaloceles, which are frequently associated with hydrocephalus, marked herniation of brain tissue, and microcephaly, management of encephaloceles of the anterior cranial base usually does not require CSF diversionary procedures for hydrocephalus.

Olfactory meningioma

About 8%-18% of all intracranial meningiomas are olfactory meningiomas. Their growth is usually slow. Due to their location they often reach a very large size (>4 cm) before the diagnosis is made. Although anosmia is thought to be an early symptom, surprisingly few patients complain of olfactory dysfunction.

This may be due to the fact that (1) the decline in olfactory function is gradual, similar to what is seen in elderly patients, and (2) in most of the patients only one side of the nose is affected such that the olfactory function is maintained by the contralateral side. Thus, lateralized anosmia is extremely difficult to detect during routine clinical examination in patients in whom it is the only neurological symptom before the tumour becomes large enough to affect the other structures. The diagnosis is made by coincidence on the basis of MRI which is performed and not as a consequence of olfactory evaluation. To detect an olfactory meningioma, lateralized testing of olfactory function seems to be necessary.

Benign mixed tumor of the salivary gland

It is also known as pleomorphic adenoma. These tumors arise from minor salivary gland nests located within the nasal cavity, paranasal sinuses, nasopharynx, and paranasopharyngeal space. Histologically, they contain multiple neoplastic tissue types, including both epithelial (glandular) and mesenchymal (collagenous) components. Although pleomorphic adenomas are the most common tumors of the major salivary glands, they are less common than malignant salivary neoplasms within other sites of the aerodigestive tract. Pleomorphic adenomas do not metastasize but demonstrate variable rates of local growth.

Nasal papillomas (Inverted papillomas)

Papillomas of the sinonasal tract arise from squamous or schneiderian epithelium. They can be grouped into inverting,

fungiform, and cylindrical subtypes (based on histologic architecture). Inverting papillomas, also known as schneiderian papilloma, originate in the lateral nasal wall, antrum, and ethmoid sinus. They involve the skull base more commonly than other types of nasal papilloma, demonstrating a progressive local growth with a significant risk of malignant transformation 15%. Treatment is complete surgical en bloc resection because piecemeal removal is associated with an unacceptable recurrence rate (50%). Radiation therapy is believed to stimulate malignant changes.

Pituitary adenoma

These adenomas are benign neoplasms of the anterior hypophysis. They can be functional, in which case the hormone related to the cell of origin is hypersecreted or nonfunctional (null cell adenoma). Progressive growth, bone destruction, and compression of parasellar structures can occur. Surgical treatment is recommended with either an attempt at complete removal or debulking, depending on the lesion.

Fibro-osseous tumors

This group of lesions encompass fibrous dysplasia and ossifying fibroma. Giant cell lesions (*e.g.*, reparative giant cell granuloma, giant cell tumor of bone) can also be considered fibro-osseous lesions. Fibrous dysplasia is a hamartomatous process characterized by proliferation of immature woven bone. Monostotic and polyostotic forms can be found, depending on single or multiple site involvement. Growth typically progresses through puberty and then slows or stops at the time of skeletal maturity. Lesions can reach considerable size with associated disfigurement, and symptoms are related to gradual encroachment on vital structures (*e.g.*, orbit, optic nerve, frontonasal duct). Ossifying fibroma is a true neoplasm and can be difficult to distinguish histologically from fibrous dysplasia.

These fibromas tend to behave more aggressively than fibrous dysplasia, can exhibit very rapid growth, and continue growing if left untreated. Juvenile ossifying fibroma is a form that occurs early in life (early childhood) and demonstrates rapid local enlargement. Treatment of ossifying fibroma requires an attempt at complete removal to reduce the chances of recurrence.

Juvenile angiofibroma

Angiofibromas are composed of dual neoplastic elements, consisting of a dense fibrous mass interlaced with variable amounts of thinly walled endothelial-lined vascular spaces, more popularly known as embryonic vessels. These lesions are exclusively found in adolescent boys and originate in the mucosa around the sphenopalatine foramen, from where they enlarge to present as nasopharyngeal mass with extension into the paranasal sinuses, orbit, pterygomaxillary space, and cavernous sinus. Patients with angiofibroma usually present with sinonasal symptoms, commonly with epistaxis. Although their growth eventually ceases with adolescence, they can quickly reach very large proportions and compress adjacent structures.

Mucocele and mucopyocele

Obstruction of mucociliary drainage from the paranasal sinuses can lead to expansile mucoceles capable of progressive growth and bony distortion. Maxillofacial trauma is the most common predisposing factor. Lesions of the frontal and ethmoid sinuses involve the skull base.

MALIGNANT TUMORS OF THE ANTERIOR SKULL BASE

Nasopharyngeal carcinoma

Nasopharyngeal carcinoma arises from the surface epithelium of the nasopharynx and commonly metastasizes to the lymph nodes. As many as 82% of the tumors arise in the lateral wall of the nasopharynx in the fossa of Rosen Muller (pharyngeal recess), 12% in the midline, and 6% in normal-appearing mucosa.

Nasopharyngeal carcinoma has a bimodal age distribution with peaks in the second and sixth decades of life. It occurs predominantly in males. Patients with nasopharyngeal carcinoma may present with variable nonspecific symptoms, the most common of which is painless upper deep cervical adenopathy. Lateral pharyngeal node involvement may result in pain with ipsilateral neck rotation or ear pain. Unilateral conductive hearing loss resulting from serous effusions due to poor eustachian tube function commonly occurs. Nasal obstruction occurs late in the course of the disease profuse epistaxis is rare. Dysphonia, difficulty in swallowing and diplopia may also occur. Physical examination may reveal maxillary nerve dysfunction. Extension of the tumor into the lateral pharyngeal wall results in ninth and 10th cranial nerve palsies. Proptosis and trismus are rarely associated with these malignancies.

Nasopharyngeal carcinoma is associated with bone destruction which can be demonstrated on CT scan. Intense homogeneous enhancement of the lesion is seen following contrast administration. The lesion can invade the middle fossa either by erosion through the greater wing of the sphenoid or extension through the foramen ovale. In advanced cases, the cancer can reach the clivus and violate areas of the posterior fossa. Adenoid cystic carcinomas are also associated with bone destruction. Postcontrast MR imaging may reveal perineural spread of the malignancy particularly along the V2 and V3 distribution.

Esthesioneuroblastoma of the anterior cranial fossa

Esthesioneuroblastomas or olfactory neuroblastomas are tumors of neuroectodermal origin believed to arise from the mitotically active basal layer of the olfactory epithelium normally located within the superior one third of the nasal septum, cribriform plate, and superior turbinates. Resection alone or in combination with radio- and/or chemotherapy is the treatment of choice performed in their management. The Kadish system for staging depends on the extent of disease. In Kadish Stage A, the tumor is limited to the nasal cavity; Stage B, the tumor is localized to the nasal cavity and paranasal sinuses; and Stage C, tumor extends beyond the nasal cavity and paranasal sinuses. Five-year survival rates in patients with Stage A, B, and C diseases have been reported to be 75, 60, and 41%, respectively.

Their clinical manifestations and treatment results were reviewed to identify possible prognostic factors. Whereas the overall 5-year survival rate in all patients was 69%, with low-and high-grade tumors was 80 and 40%, respectively. Surgery alone was advocated in cases of low-grade tumors if tumor-free margins could be obtained. Radiotherapy was recommended in cases of low-grade tumors when margins are close, in those of residual or recurrent disease, and in those of all high-grade cancers. The addition of chemotherapy was suggested in the management of patients with high-grade tumors.

Chemotherapeutic agents have been used to treat patients with recurrent, metastatic, or inoperable disease.

Paranasal sinus and nasal cavity cancers

Nasal/paranasal sinus cancers are rare tumors, comprising of approximately 3% of all head and neck cancers. They affect patients primarily between the age of 60 and 70 years of age. There is a slight male preponderance that may reflect occupational risks and exposure. Most common sites include the maxillary sinus (60%), the nasal cavity (20%), and the ethmoid sinuses (16%). Predisposing factors include occupational exposure to nickel, wood dust, and asbestos. In addition, smoking and using snuff has been known to increase the incidence of paranasal sinus cancers and have been implicated in the pathogenesis of head and neck cancers in general. These tumors present commonly with nasal obstruction, epistaxis, and/or nasal discharge. In addition, they can present with facial pain, proptosis, diplopia, and anosmia. Because of the similarity in presentation with sinusitis, it is imperative that these symptoms in patients over 50 years of age who present with these symptoms for over 6 weeks duration be investigated by an otolaryngologist.

Histologically, the majority of nasal/paranasal sinus cancers are squamous cell carcinomas (50%), which tend to arise primarily in the maxillary antrum. Adenocarcinomas occur in approximately 35% and primarily arise in the ethmoid sinuses or in the upper nasal cavity. Approximately 11% of tumors in this region are adenoid cystic carcinomas arising from minor salivary glands. They are known for their diffuse infiltration and their propensity for perineural extension. Less than 1% of paranasal sinus cancers arise in the sphenoid or frontal sinus.

Sinonasal undifferentiated carcinoma

It is a rare and aggressive malignancy. Sinonasal undifferentiated carcinomas are usually diagnosed late and commonly involve the orbit, multiple sinuses, and anterior cranial fossa. Resection followed by radiotherapy is the preferred treatment despite poor prognosis. Some surgeons will not consider resection because of the poor prognosis. Unresectable tumors are treated with concurrent chemoradiation.

Adenoid cystic carcinoma

Arising in sinonasal minor salivary gland tissue, adenoid cystic carcinomas tend to be slow but steady-growing lesions that are destructive and have a high propensity for perineural spread. Trigeminal nerve involvement is most common in nasal/paranasal sinus tumors. Regional lymphatic spread is rare, while distant metastasis is more common, averaging 40%. Bone and/or lungs are frequently involved. Systemic metastasis is most often secondary to failure of local control. Recurrence can occur as late as 10 to 20 years following treatment. Primary treatment is surgical, usually followed by radiation treatment in advanced stage lesions.

Rhabdomyosarcoma

Rhabdomyosarcomas of the head and neck were first reported in 1854 by Weber and not histologically classified until 1947. These tumors occur predominantly in the pediatric population. Children younger than age 5 years harbor the aggressive embryonal variant and older patients the pleomorphic variant. Approximately 40% of patients have head and neck involvement, which can be orbital, nonparameningeal / nonorbital, and parameningeal.

Magnetic resonance imaging reveals a soft-tissue mass in the sinonasal region, infratemporal fossa, or nasopharynx with significant contrast enhancement. Computerized tomography scanning commonly demonstrates bone destruction. Five-year survival rates is 94% in cases of orbital tumors and 50% in cases involving other head and neck regions as reported in 1983.

In recent years, improved outcomes have been associated with early provision of chemoradiation therapy and resection. Recurrences when resection is not performed are common. Rhabdomyosarcomas have a propensity to metastasize prior to operative intervention. Pulmonary metastases are associated with the worst prognosis.

Hemangiopericytoma

Hemangiopericytoma is an uncommon vascular tumor formed by the proliferation of vascular pericytes of Zimmerman. They should be considered malignant, not in terms of a 5-year survival rate, but over the patient's lifetime. Vascular pericytes are of mesenchymal origin that spiral around capillaries and postcapillary venules. They are believed to be capable of differentiating into smooth muscle cells. They possess contractile properties that are able to change the lumen of blood vessels and regulate blood flow.

Hemangiopericytoma is a mysterious tumor. Histopathologic studies have yet to generate reliable and reproducible criteria to distinguish the malignant from the benign types. The tumor behavior is inconsistent with respect to its pathologic and ultrastructural characteristics. Lesions with a benign appearance have been found to recur and metastasize. The recurrence rate is 25-50%, and the metastasis rate is 11-65%. Hence, the benign or malignant nature of a hemangiopericytoma is determined not histologically, but clinically, with lifelong follow-up observation. At initial workup, hemangiopericytoma should be regarded as potentially malignant.

The malignant behavior of the tumor is speculated to be closely related to tumor location and anatomic dimension, rather than the histologic feature. In the paranasal sinuses and nasal cavity, hemangiopericytoma tends to be indolent; conversely, those that arise around the cribriform plate are more likely to metastasize. Lesions smaller than 6.5 cm in greatest dimension have a low potential to metastasize.

The tumor can appear in persons of any age, with 80-95% of patients older than 20 years. Approximately 15-30% of hemangiopericytomas develop in the head and neck region; sinonasal presentation is rare. Approximately 10% of hemangiopericytomas are found in children. Their prognosis is more favorable than the prognosis in adults.

Optimal treatment is wide excision with negative margins. Tumor cells may be left behind with enucleation. For unresectable or incompletely excised tumors, radiotherapy has an important role.

Hemangiopericytomas metastasize via lymphatics and blood streams to the lung, bone, liver, and local lymph nodes. Regional lymph node involvement at presentation is unusual. Lung and bone are the most frequent sites for distant metastases.

Mucosal melanoma

Mucosal melanomas of the head and neck are, in general, rapidly lethal neoplasms. Most nasal mucosal melanomas arise from the mucosa of the septum and the lateral nasal wall rather than from the sinuses. The overall incidence is low; mucosal melanomas account for less than 1% of all malignant melanomas. In addition to symptoms typical of a nasal mass, gross pigmentation is present with 50% of sinonasal melanomas. The cause of melanoma in solar-hidden mucosa is unclear, although smoking may have a role in the activation of preexisting melanocytes, leading to melanogenic metaplasia.

Nasal and paranasal sinus melanomas are usually advanced when they are discovered. The possibility of regional or distant metastases must be considered, and metastases are frequently found at initial presentation. Involvement of regional lymph nodes strongly suggests distant spread, which is often not preceded by lymphatic spread. For both cutaneous and mucosal melanomas, the single most powerful predictor of survival is the status of regional lymph nodes. Once spread to regional lymph node has occurred, prognostic information derived from the primary melanoma, such as depth of invasion, helps little in comparison with the number of, not the size of, the involved lymph nodes. Mucosal melanoma tends to follow a more rapidly lethal course than its cutaneous counterpart. This rapid course is due in part to the advanced stage at discovery in terms of regional and distant metastases and deeper invasion at the primary site. Other factors include failure of early detection and possible unknown intrinsic tumor biology of mucosal melanoma.

Surgical resection offers the best treatment, although its effectiveness is questionable. The incidence of local recurrence is high, even with fresh frozen section to ensure complete excision. More radical excision, which includes the removal of the eye, palate, or external portion of the nose, may not significantly decrease the incidence of local recurrence. Local recurrence and even metastasis do not necessarily imply death within the near future; some patients with both have survived for several years. If possible, vigorous secondary local excision may be worthwhile. Radiotherapy is often used as adjuvant therapy, although the tumor is relatively radio insensitive. Adjuvant therapies, which include interferons and tumor-specific melanoma vaccine, are under investigation.

COMMON LATERAL SKULL LESIONS

Benign

- Schwannoma
- Paraganglioma
  - Carotid body tumor
  - Glomus jugulare
  - Vagale
  - Sympathetic ganglia
- Meningioma
- Neurofibroma
- Benign lesions of deep lobe of parotid
- Primary cholesteatoma
- Petrositis

Malignant

- Sarcoma
- Neurogenous sarcoma
- Neuroepithelioma
- Malignant granular cell tumor
- Malignant lesions of deep lobe of parotid

Primary cholesteatoma (epidermoid cyst)

Primary cholesteatomas arise from epithelial rests within the temporal bone or cerebellopontine angle. They are slow-growing masses filled with keratin debris and usually manifest with cranial nerve (CN) palsy or auditory system involvement due to compression of adjacent CNS and temporal bone structures.

Cholesterol granulomas

A cholesterol granuloma, the most common primary lesion of the petrous apex, results from chronic obstruction of pneumatized air cells. The pathway for ventilation of petrous apex cells is circuitous, eventually reaching the middle ear space to communicate with the nasopharynx via the eustachian tube. When edema occurs, negative pressure develops within the lumen of apex cells leading to fluid transudation and hemorrhage. It is believed that the red blood cells break down releasing cholesterol from their cell membranes which form crystals and incites a sterile inflammatory reaction. Granulation tissue forms secondary to repeated hemorrhage, thus creating an expansile / expanding lesion. Mass effect typically produces hearing loss, tinnitus, vertigo, or facial twitching.

On HRCT, these lesions appear as smoothly delineated expansile masses located in the anteromedial portion of the apex. The density is similar to that of surrounding brain. There is no enhancement of these lesions with contrast. HRCT provides essential information in determining the most favorable route for drainage of these lesions either via an infralabyrinthine, infracochlear, or transsphenoid routes.

MRI provides the diagnosis is virtually all cases. These lesions are markedly hyper intense on both T1- and T2-weighted images, likely secondary to the sub acute and chronic hemorrhages with associated breakdown products. They do not enhance further after the administration of gadolinium. MRI also plays a key role in assessing for recurrent lesions. Serous fluid, mucous, or scar tissue that fills a drained cholesterol granuloma will not produce the expansile mass effect and will have a much lower T1-weighted signal on MRI. Recurrence of a cholesterol granuloma should be suspected when cyst fluid contents demonstrate renewed hyper intensity on T1-weighted scans.

Aneurysms

Aneurysms of the petrous portion of the carotid artery are extremely rare. They are, however, an entity that must be differentiated from other lesions affecting the petrous apex. Their etiology is likely a congenital weakness of the artery wall but may also occur as a sequelae to trauma or infections. On HRCT, aneurysms have the appearance of a smoothly marginated bone-eroding lesion. With contrast, the lesion may be homogeneous and dense, or heterogeneous, depending on the amount of flowing blood and thrombus.

On MRI, intrapetrous aneurysms can be complex with flow voids. Relative intensity on T1- and T2-weighted images depends on the amount of thrombus present and the age of the aneurysm. Angiography may be required to confirm the diagnosis and MRA may be a useful adjunct.

Paraganglioma

Paraganglia are derived from neural crest cells of the dorsal root ganglia and are distributed widely throughout the head and neck with the highest concentration being found in near the carotid sheath. Head and neck paraganglia closely resemble carotid bodies and are comprised of two cell types: granule-storing chief cells and Schwann like satellite cells. Tumors of the internal jugular vein paraganglia (glomus jugulare) and the vagus nerve (glomus vagale) are the most common lesions involving the skull base, although glomus tumors may rarely arise in paraganglia of the orbit and nasopharynx.

Schwannomas

Schwannomas of the temporal bone and the skull base are benign neoplasms that arise from the sheaths of cranial nerves. Schwannomas in this location can be categorized as facial, trigeminal, or jugular foramen tumors, depending on the primary nerve involved. Vestibular schwannomas are by far the most common comprising 7% of all intracranial tumors and 80% of CPA tumors. These tumors usually expand centrally from the internal auditory canal into the CPA and may compress the pontine brainstem and cerebellum. Thus, the most common symptoms are unilateral hearing loss, tinnitus, and dysequilibrium. Large tumors extending anteriorly may compress the trigeminal nerve producing facial hypesthesias or may compress the brainstem producing hydrocephalus.

Facial nerve schwannomas can arise anywhere along the course of the facial nerve, however these most commonly arise in the perigeniculate, tympanic, or mastoid segments. Facial weakness or paralysis that progresses is the most common presentation.

Trigeminal schwannomas usually originate from the gasserian ganglion and may expand into the middle cranial or posterior fossa. Patients usually present with facial neuralgias, paresthesias, or hypesthesias in one or more divisions of the trigeminal nerve.

Jugular foramen schwannomas arise from the jugular fossa from the nerve sheaths of cranial nerves IX, X, and XI. The vagus nerve seems the most common however it is difficult to ascertain the nerve from which the tumor is derived. Patients typically present with dysphagia, hoarseness, and shoulder weakness.

Physical examination can reveal functional deficits, however diagnosis is most often made with radiographic studies. HRCT may show expansion of fallopian canal, or jugular fossa depending on the etiology of the disease. They can reveal inhomogeneous enhancement with contrast. MRI with the use of gadolinium permits definitive diagnosis in the vast majority of cases. MRI shows a low signal intensity on T1-weighted images that enhances markedly with intravenous gadolinium administration.

Facial nerve schwanomma

Schwannomas of the facial nerve can occur along any segment, but they frequently involve the geniculate ganglion and extend proximally or distally from there. Presentation of facial schwannomas is variable and depends on the segment of the facial nerve from which the tumor arises. Symptoms can range from facial palsy to progressive hearing loss resulting from ossicular interference and sensorineural hearing loss due to effects on cochlear nerve in the internal auditory canal which is less common (Fig. 4.1a & b).

External auditory canal malignancy

Cancer of the EAC has been found to be more common in women than men. The median age of onset is 55 years. There is generally believed to be a higher incidence in patients with preexisting ear inflammation such as otitis externa, chronic otitis media, or cholesteatoma. The most common histologic types of EAC cancer are squamous cell (90%), basal cell, and glandular tumors including adenoid cystic, mucoepidermoid and adeno carcinoma. Other rare lesions include sarcomas, melanoma, sebaceous cell carcinoma and metastatic lesions.

COMMON POSTERIOR SKULL BASE LESIONS

Benign: (Described earlier)

- Acoustic tumor
- Epidermoids
- Dermoids
- Chordomas
- Chondromas

Malignant

- Chondrosarcoma

Acoustic neuromas (Vestibular schwannoma)

Acoustic neuromas are intracranial extra-axial tumors that arise from the Schwann cell sheath investing either the vestibular or cochlear nerve. As acoustic neuromas increase in size, they eventually occupy a large portion of the cerebellopontine angle. Acoustic neuromas account for approximately 80% of tumors found within the cerebellopontine angle. The remaining 20% are principally meningiomas.

The vast majority of acoustic neuromas develop from the Schwann cell investment of the vestibular portion of the vestibulocochlear nerve. Less than 5% arise from the cochlear nerve. The superior and inferior vestibular nerves appear to be the nerves of origin with more frequency in superior vestibular nerve. Overall, 3 separate growth patterns can be distinguished within acoustic tumors, as follows: (1) no growth or very slow growth, (2) slow growth (i.e., 0.2 cm/y on imaging studies), and (3) fast

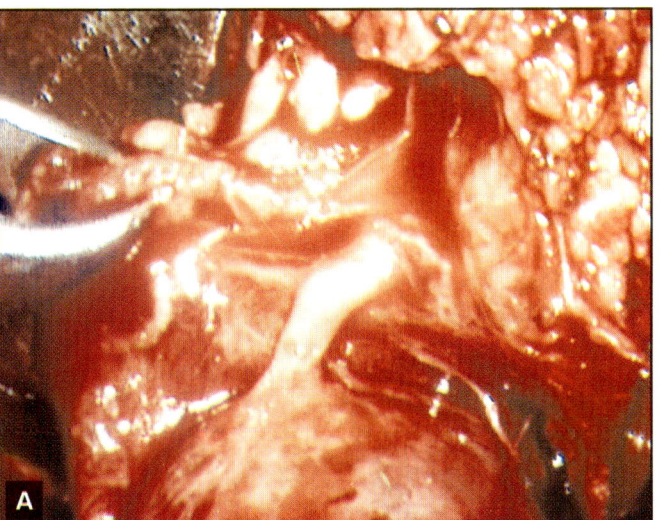
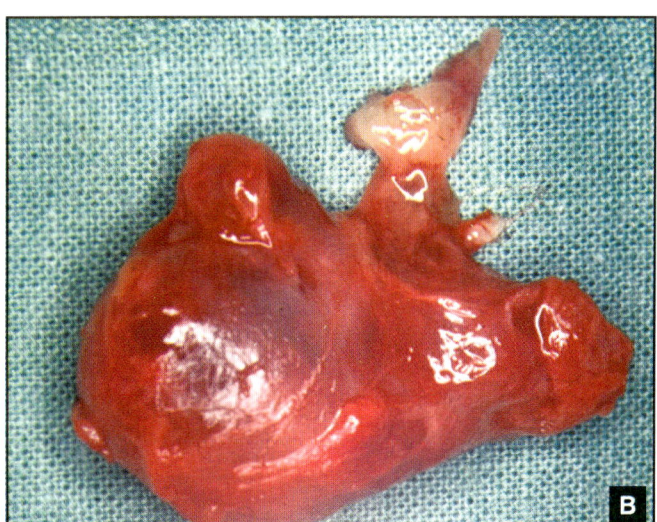

Fig. 4.1 Showing the intraoperative picture of facial nerve schwanomma

growth (i.e., >1.0 cm/y on imaging studies). While most acoustic neuromas grow slowly, some grow quite quickly and can double in volume within 6 months to a year.

While some tumors adhere to one or another of these growth patterns, others appear to alternate between periods of no or slow growth and rapid growth. Tumors that have undergone cystic degeneration (presumably because they have outrun their blood supply) are sometimes capable of relatively rapid expansion because of enlargement of their cystic component. Because acoustic tumors arise from the investing Schwann cell, tumor growth generally compresses vestibular fibers to the surface. Destruction of vestibular fibers is slow; consequently, many patients experience little or no dysequilibrium or imbalance. Once the tumor has grown sufficiently large to fill the internal auditory canal, it may continue growth either by eroding bone or by spilling out into the cerebellopontine angle. Growth within the cerebellopontine angle is generally spherical. Acoustic tumors, like other space-occupying lesions, produce symptoms by any of the four recognizable mechanisms: (1) compression or distortion of the spinal fluid spaces, (2) displacement of the brain stem, (3) compression of vessels producing venous or arterial infarction, or (4) compression and/or attenuation of nerves.

Because the cerebellopontine angle is relatively empty, tumors can continue to grow until they reach 3-4 cm in size before they come in contact with important structures. Growth is often sufficiently slow that the facial nerve can accommodate to the stretching imposed by tumor growth without clinically apparent deterioration of function. Tumors that arise within the internal auditory canal may produce relatively early symptomatology in the form of hearing loss or vestibular disturbance by compressing the cochlear nerve, vestibular nerve, or labyrinthine artery against the bony walls of the internal auditory canal. As the tumor approaches 2.0 cm in diameter, it generally comes to abut against the lateral surface of the brain stem. Further growth can occur only by compressing or displacing the brain stem toward the contralateral side. A 4.0-cm tumor often extends sufficiently far anteriorly to compress the trigeminal nerve and produce facial hypesthesia. Growth over 4.0 cm generally results in progressive effacement of the vestibular aqueduct and fourth ventricle with eventual development of hydrocephalus.

Chondrosarcomas

Chondrosarcoma of the skull base is thought to arise from embryonic rests of cartilage that occur near the foramen lacerum and petrous apex. Patients usually present with headaches or symptoms suggestive of multiple cranial nerve compromise. Although benign chondromas may also occur, chondrosarcoma appears to be much more prevalent.

On HRCT, benign chondroma has been described as a non-enhancing, relatively regular, lytic lesion. In the more common chondrosarcoma, irregular bone destruction is seen with areas of contrast enhancement. Multiple calcifications may occur which gives a "popcorn" appearance.

On MRI, chondrosarcoma enhances markedly with gadolinium. Differentiating chondrosarcomas with chordomas may be difficult. However, chondrosarcomas tend to arise more laterally (within the petrous apex) as compared to chordomas.

Chordomas

Skull base chordomas are low to intermediate grade malignancies that result from defective embryonic remnants of the notocord. While the notocord is typically a midline structure, lateral projections of notocordal tissue may reside in the medial aspect of the petrous apex. Thus, while most chordomas arise in the clivus and spread into the petrous apex, they may also develop entirely within the petrous apex. Headache, diplopia from abducens palsy, and visual deficits are the typical complaints of patients. Diagnosis can be made from radiographic imaging and from cytological or histological evaluation in which the typical "soap bubble" or physaliphorus cells are seen. HRCT images show a destructive lobulated soft tissue mass often containing foci of calcification. There is typical erosion of the clivus and basiocciput that may extend laterally to the petrous apex. Enhancement is typical with intravenous contrast.

On MRI, chordomas are hypointense on T1-weighted images and markedly hyperintense on T2-weighted images. They usually enhance with administration of gadolinium. Given their location and propensity for bony erosion, and imaging characteristics, chordomas may be difficult to differentiate from the chondrosarcomas discussed earlier.

CLINICAL FEATURES OF SKULL BASE TUMORS

The clinical features involving the skull base will have varied symptoms, which can be described as follows:

- Anterior skull base lesions predominantly presents with orbitorhinoneurological symptoms.

- Lateral skull base lesions predominantly presents with otoneurogical symptoms.

- Posterior skull base lesions presents predominantly with neurological symptoms.

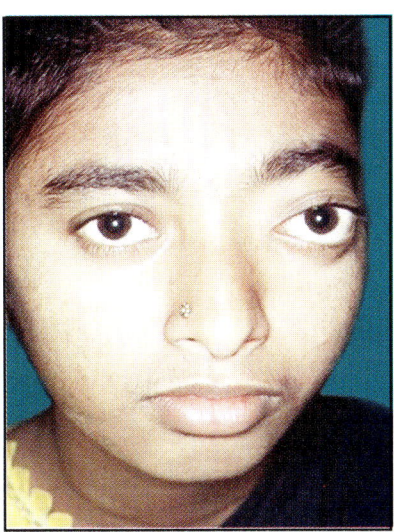

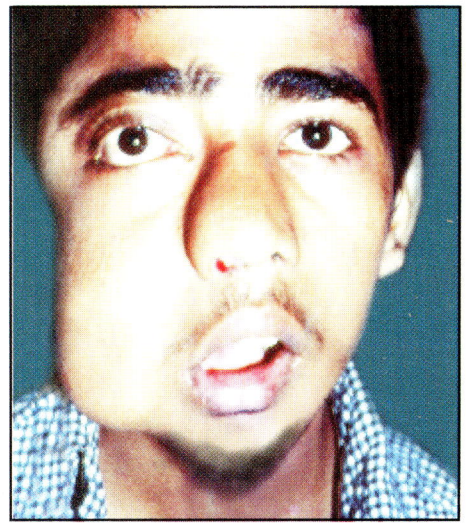

Fig. 4.2 A. Ethmoidal tumor presented with proptosis of the left eye   **B.** Angiofibroma presented with Cheek swelling

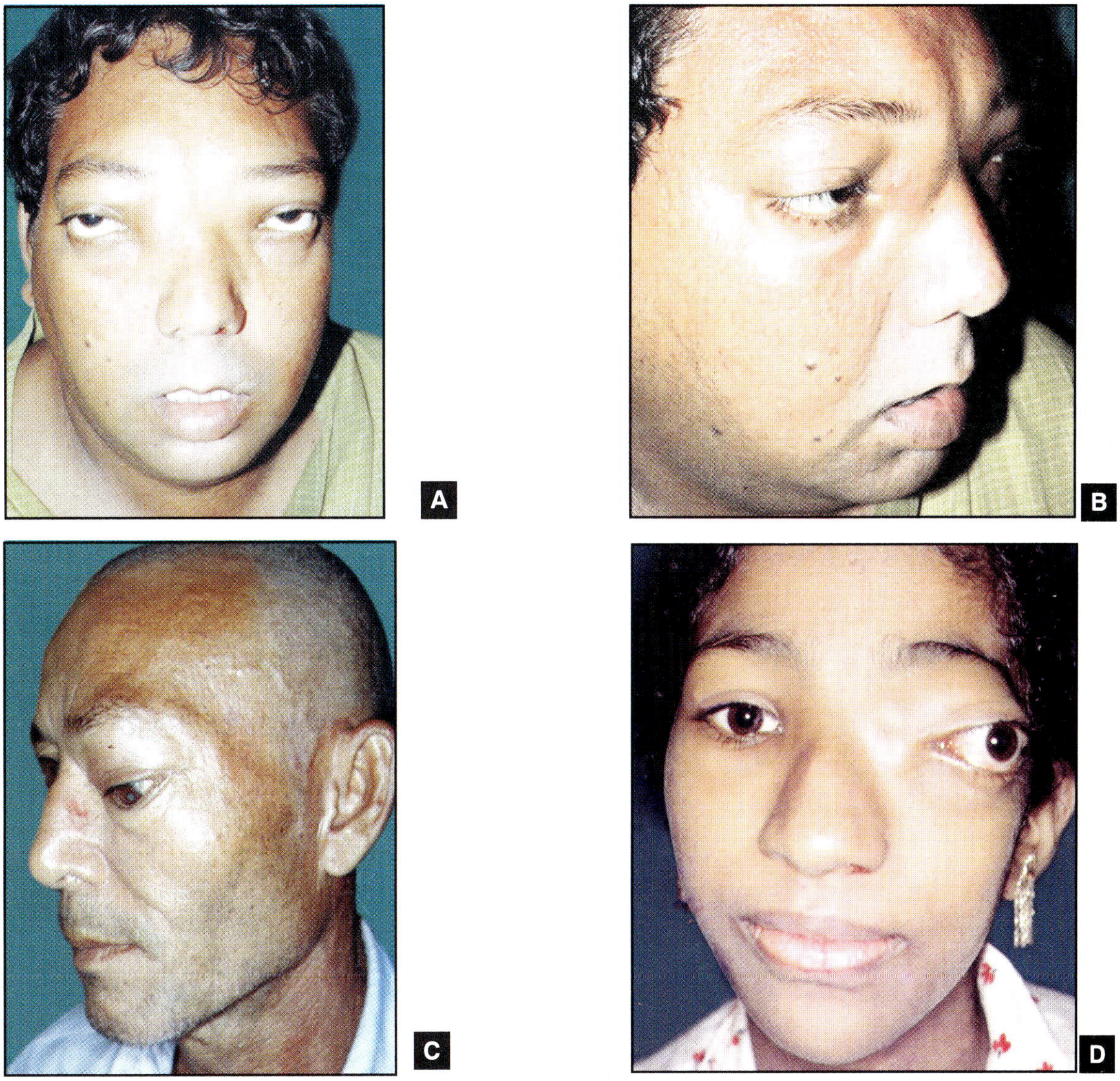

Fig. 4.3A, B, C, D Many of these tumors can be demonstrated on nasopharyngeal examination

Presenting features of anterior skull base

Anterior fossa tumors can manifest with a number of different symptoms, including nasal obstruction and congestion, epistaxis, rhinorrhea, hyposmia or anosmia, headache, seizure, and psychological changes. Paraesthesia in the distribution of the V1 or V2 divisions of the trigeminal nerve may occur. Invasion into the sella turcica can cause loss of endocrine function, or invasive pituitary tumors can be responsible for over production of corticosteroids, growth hormone, or prolactin. Visual loss can be unilateral or bilateral.

Associated ocular symptoms include diplopia, orbital pain, exophthalmos, and retroorbital headaches (Fig. 3.11a & b)

Presenting Features of Middle Skull Base Lesions

Clinical presentation of lateral skull base

Symptoms of glomus tumor are insidious in onset. Because of the location and the vascular nature of these tumors, it is not surprising that the most common complaint of symptomatic patients is pulsatile tinnitus. Its believed that the tinnitus is secondary to mechanical impingement on the umbo is most cases. Other common symptoms are aural fullness, and (conductive) hearing loss.

On physical examination, the hallmark of a jugulotympanic glomus tumor is a red or reddish-blue mass seen behind the tympanic membrane. The diagnosis of glomus tympanicum can only be entertained if the examiner can see a full 360 degrees around the perimeter of the lesion, otherwise the presumptive diagnosis must be a glomus jugulare. The finding of a middle ear mass is fairly reliable, with 94 - 100% of untreated cases demonstrating this in reviews of large series of patients. Brown's sign (blanching of the mass with positive pressure pneumotoscopy) is often mentioned, but the frequency of this finding is not clear. Rarely, a friable or bleeding mass in the EAC may be the presenting sign with larger tumors. HTN, tachycardia, tremor, or complaints of vascular headaches should alert for the possibility of a functional tumor.

Cranial nerve deficits are seen primarily with larger tumors. Reports cite compression or invasion of CN's IX, and X most commonly, with CN's VII, VIII, XI, and XII affected less often. The presence of lower cranial nerve deficits rules out an isolated middle ear glomus tympanicum. Isolated deficits of CN's VII and VIII are more likely to be secondary to a tympanicum.

Patients with cancer of the temporal bone most often present above the age of 60 years although any age group, including children, can be affected. Common presenting symptoms include chronic otalgia, otorrhea, bleeding, and hearing loss. Physical findings include otorrhea, mass lesion, facial swelling, facial paresis, and other cranial nerve (CN) deficits. Patients often present after many years of symptoms.

Symptoms and signs of temporal bone lesions are summarized as follows:

- Otalgia (80-85%)
- Otorrhea (40-75%)
- Facial paralysis (25%)
- Hearing loss (45-80%)
- Tinnitus (8-10%)
- Vertigo
- Auricular lesion
- External canal mass (10%)
- Parotid mass (19%)
- Skin lesions
- CN V, IX, X, XI deficits (30%)

Physical examination should include inspection of the pinna, EAC, and middle ear for ulcers, mass lesions, soft tissue swelling or induration, old scars (*e.g.*, previously excised skin cancers may have been forgotten by the patient), and otorrhoea. Perform a thorough CN examination. Close inspection for facial weakness is crucial. Perform audiometry if hearing loss is suspected and a complete head and neck examination. The patient's general medical condition should also be evaluated because it may have a great impact on treatment options and outcome.

Presenting features of posterior skull base lesions

Unilateral hearing loss is overwhelmingly the most common symptom present at the time of diagnosis and is generally the symptom that leads to diagnosis. Consider any unilateral sensorineural hearing loss as an acoustic neuroma until proven otherwise. The tumor can produce hearing loss through at least 2 mechanisms, direct injury to the cochlear nerve or interruption of the cochlear blood supply. Progressive injury to cochlear fibers probably accounts for slowly progressive sensorineural hearing loss observed in a significant number of patients with acoustic neuromas. Sudden and fluctuating hearing losses are more easily explained on the basis of disruption of cochlear blood supply.

Consistent with direct injury to cranial nerve VIII, a significant number of individuals with acoustic neuroma have speech discrimination scores reduced out of proportion to the average pure-tone; a feature deemed typical for retrocochlear lesions. Such marked reductions in speech discrimination scores (often the teens or twenties) are not invariable. However, a normal speech discrimination score does not rule out an acoustic tumor. A significant number of patients with acoustic tumors have normal or near-normal hearing or speech discrimination scores.

Hearing loss associated with acoustic neuroma can be sudden or fluctuating in 5-15% of patients. Such hearing loss may improve spontaneously or in response to steroid therapy. Consequently, an acoustic tumor should be considered in anybody with a sudden or fluctuating loss even if hearing returns to normal.

Patients with acoustic neuroma have normal hearing at the time of diagnosis in 3-5% of cases. Surprisingly, patients with medium and large tumors are nearly as likely to have normal hearing as patients with very small tumors. Not surprisingly, the discovery of acoustic neuromas in persons with normal hearing has been increasing as gadolinium-enhanced MRI is becoming more common. The presence of unilateral tinnitus alone is a sufficient reason to evaluate an individual for acoustic tumor. Although tinnitus is the most common manifestation of hearing loss, a few individuals with acoustic tumors (around 10%) seek treatment for unilateral tinnitus without associated subjective hearing loss.

Vertigo and dysequilibrium are uncommon presenting symptoms among patients with acoustic tumors. Rotational vertigo (the illusion of movement or falling) is much more common when tumors are small. In Samii's series of 16 patients with intracanalicular tumors, 75% of patients presented with vertigo. This is an atypically high percentage even for small tumors. Dysequilibrium (a sense of unsteadiness or imbalance), on the other hand, appears to be more common in larger tumors. Overall, if carefully questioned, approximately 40-50% of patients with acoustic tumors report some balance disturbance. However, balance disturbance is the presenting symptom in less than 10% of patients. The destruction of vestibular fibers apparently is sufficiently slow as to permit seamless compensation.

Headaches are present in 50-60% of patients at the time of diagnosis, but fewer than 10% of patients have headache as their presenting symptom. Headache appears to become more common as tumor size increases and is a prominent feature in patients who develop obstructive hydrocephalus associated with a very large tumor.

Facial numbness occurs in about 25% of patients and is more common at the time of presentation than facial weakness (about 10% of patients). The motor fibers in the facial nerve can accommodate very substantial stretching as long as it occurs slowly, and they seem much more resistant to injury than sensory fibers. Objective hypoesthesia involving the teeth, buccal mucosa, or skin of the face is associated with larger tumors, but a subjective reduction in sensation that cannot be documented on objective examination occurs commonly with medium-sized and small tumors. Decrease in the corneal reflex generally occurs earlier and more commonly than objective facial hypoesthesia. Even though approximately 50-70% of individuals with large tumors have objectively demonstrable facial hypoesthesia, they are often unaware of it, and it is uncommonly the presenting symptom.

Facial weakness is uncommon (5-10% of patients) and if it is associated with a small or medium-size tumor should raise suspicion that it is not an acoustic neuroma. Entertain other diagnosis, such as facial neuroma, meningioma, granuloma, arteriovenous malformation (AVM), or lipoma. Large tumors (>4.0 cm) can obstruct the flow of spinal fluid through the ventricular system by distorting and obstructing the fourth ventricle. In the early decades of this century, 75% of patients with acoustic neuroma presented with hydrocephalus.

Table 4.1	
Sign/Symptoms	**Cause**
Ocular gaze palsy Facial Numbness	Involvement of CN III IV or VI at superior Orbital fissure or within cavernous sinus
	Involvement of CNV

5

Imaging Studies for Skull Base Lesions

CT AND MRI SCAN FOR SKULL BASE LESIONS

CT scan and MRI provide important and complementary information. A CT scan better depicts the remodelling or erosion of the bony skull base. An MRI better depicts the soft-tissue planes (including the interface of the tumor and soft tissue) and the presence of perineural and perivascular tumor. Both CT scan with contrast and MRI can be used to ascertain the relationship of the tumor to the internal carotid artery (ICA.) (Fig. 5.1 & 5.2).

MR angiography (MRA) and CT angiography (CTA) are invasive tests that demonstrate the arterial anatomy of the ITF and brain. Digital Substraction Angiography is preferred over MRA and CTA when preoperative embolization of the tumor is indicated (*e.g.*, juvenile nasopharyngeal angiofibromas [JNA], paragangliomas). Angiography identifies the vascularity of the tumor and its relationship to the ICA and demonstrates the cerebral circulation and its collateral vasculature. Neither of these anatomical tests, however, predicts the adequacy of the intracranial collateral blood supply after sacrifice of the ICA.

Collateral blood supply is better evaluated using single-photon emission computed tomography (SPECT) with balloon occlusion, transcranial Doppler, or angiography and

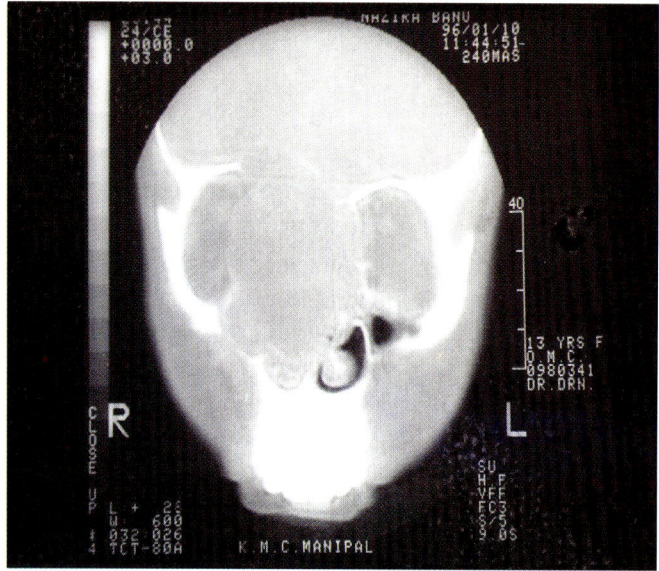

Fig. 5.1 CT scan showing soft tissue mass involving nasal cavity right maxillary sinus and bilateral ethmoids and also breaching the cribriform plate

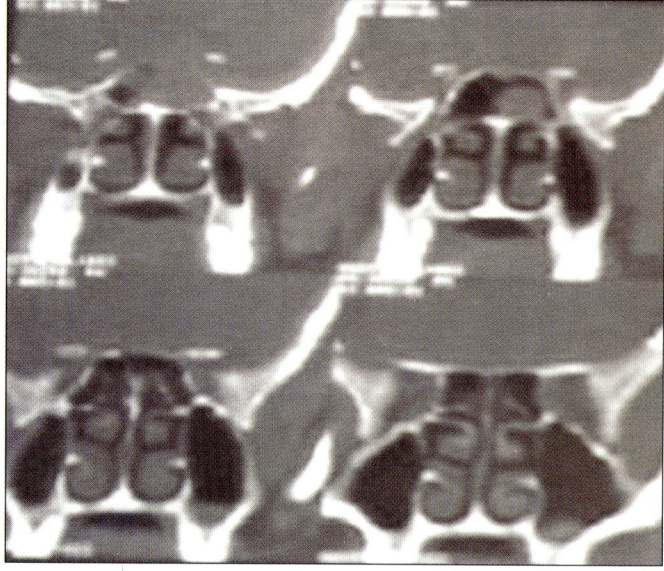

Fig. 5.2 CT scan showing the sphenoid mass with no suprasellar extension

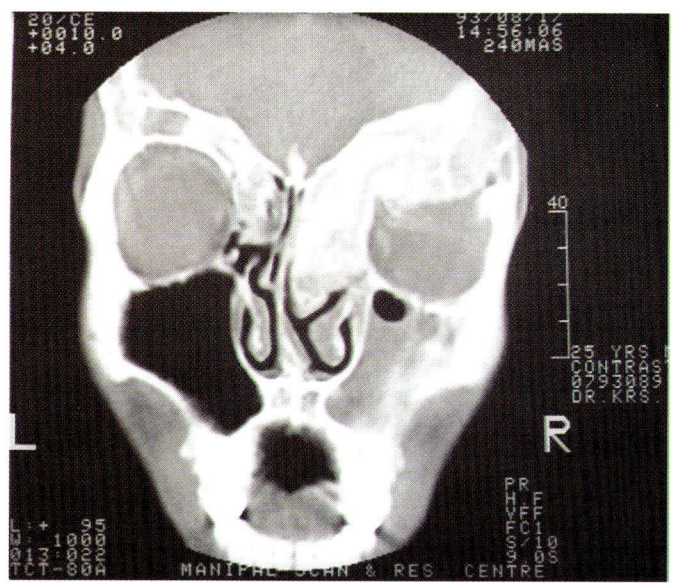

Fig. 5.3a CT scan showing the fibro-ossious lesion involving left ethmoid and frontal sinus with right maxillary sinus opacity

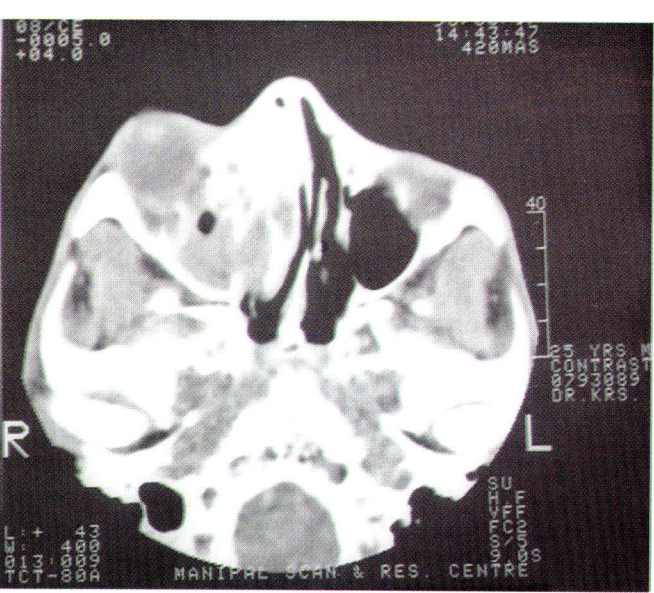

Fig. 5.3b Axial cut of the same patient

balloon occlusion with xenon-enhanced computed tomography (ABOX-CT) scan. These tests predict the probability of ischemia when the ipsilateral ICA is sacrificed and, therefore, are indicated when the risk for injury or the need for sacrifice of the ICA is high. Although technically and logistically, the ABOX-CT scan is more complex than other alternative tests, however the ABOX-CT scan is preferred due to its superior sensitivity and specificity.

During the ABOX-CT scan, a catheter with a nondetachable balloon is inserted into the ICA via the femoral artery. The balloon is inflated for 15 minutes, while

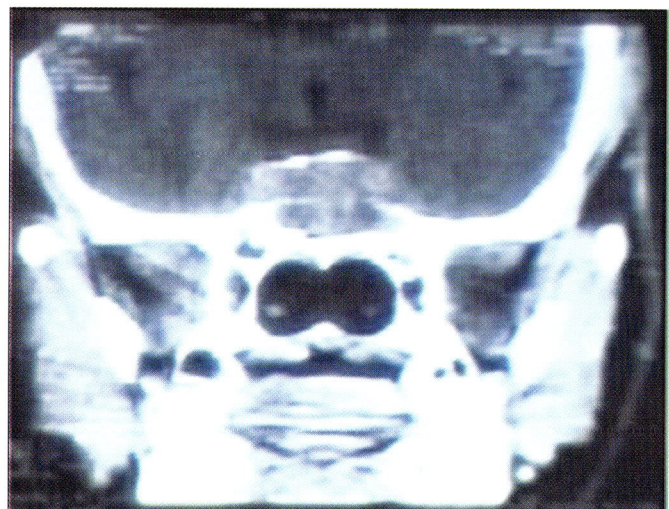

Fig. 5.4 CT scan showing the sphenoidal mass with suprasellar extension

the awake patient is monitored for any neurological deficit. Any neurological deficit warrants test cessation and classification of the patient in a high-risk category.

If no deficits develop, the balloon is deflated, and the patient is transferred to a CT scan suite. A mixture of 32% xenon and 68% oxygen is administered via facial mask for 4 minutes. CT scan demonstrates the cerebral distribution of xenon, which reflects the blood flow and, thus, provides a quantitative assessment measured as cubic centimeters (cm^3) of blood flow per minute per 100 grams of brain tissue ($cm^3/min/100$ g).

The process then is repeated after the ICA is occluded by inflation of the balloon. Special software calculates the differential of the xenon diffusion in the brain before and after balloon inflation. Using this information, it can identify those patients at risk for an ischemic injury after sacrifice of the ipsilateral ICA.

However, the patient can suffer from a stroke due to embolic phenomena or a loss of collateral vessels in the watershed areas that are not assessed by balloon occlusion testing. In addition, the ABOX-CT scan is performed under ideal and controlled circumstances and does not account for possible episodes of hypoxia, hypotension, or electrolyte- or acid-base disturbances, which may alter brain hemodynamics. Some have advocated the use of hypotension to increase the sensitivity of the test. In any event, preservation of the ICA is a preferred option.

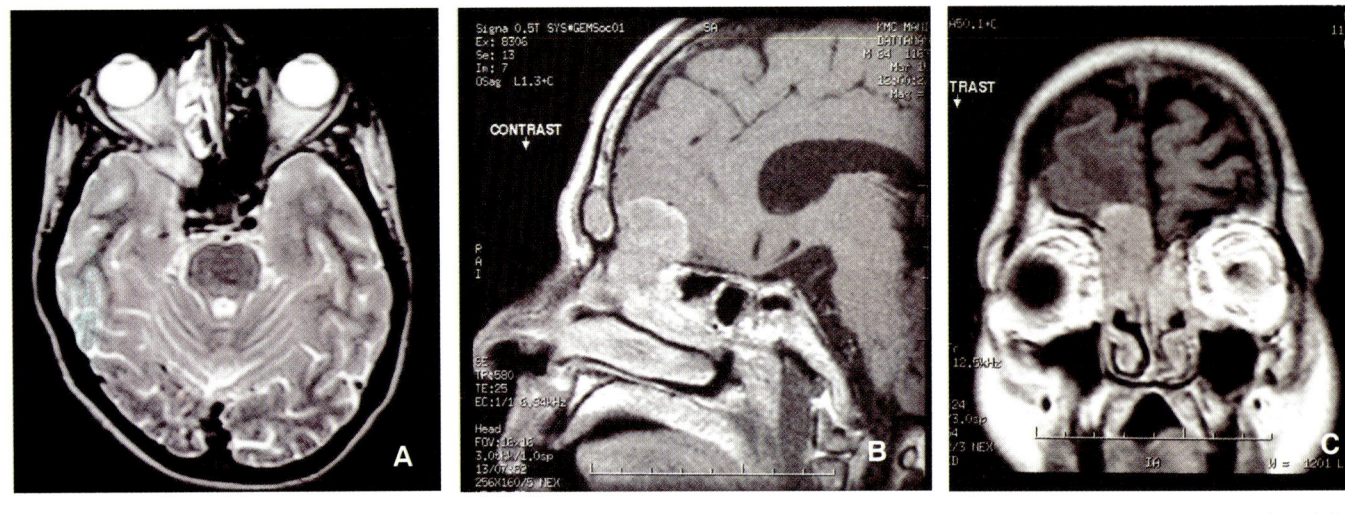

Fig. 5.5A MRI showing the axial cut of soft tissue mass involving the ethmoids **B.** Coronal cut showing the mass involving ethmoids and frontal sinus with extradural extension of the lesion **C.** Sagittal cut of the same patient.

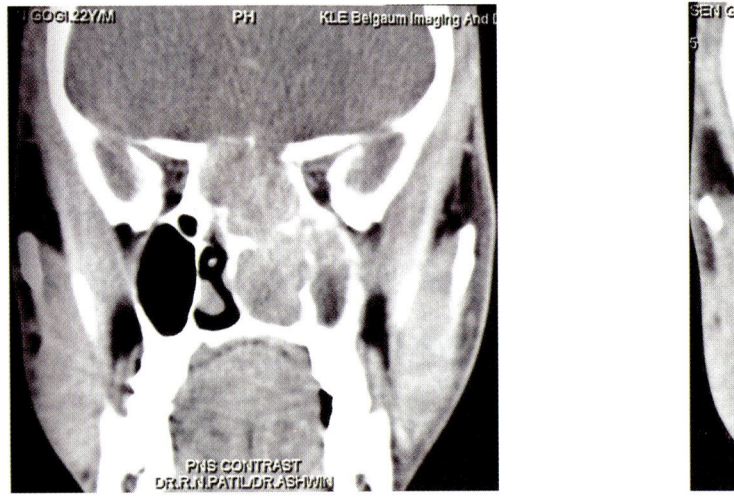
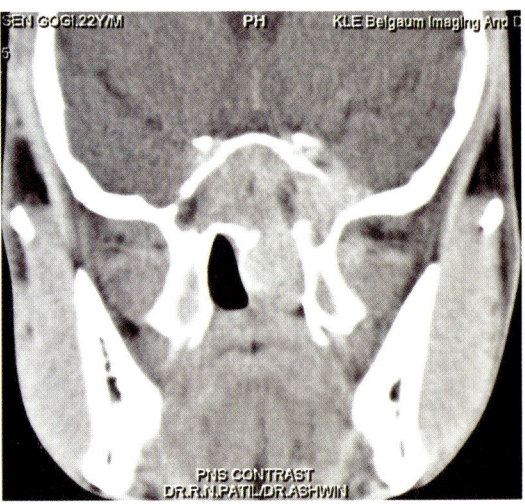

Fig 5.6 CT scan showing angiofibroma extendes to sphenoid and crosia sphenoid roof

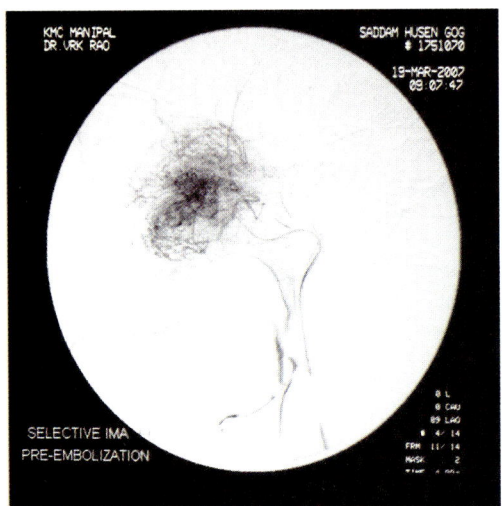
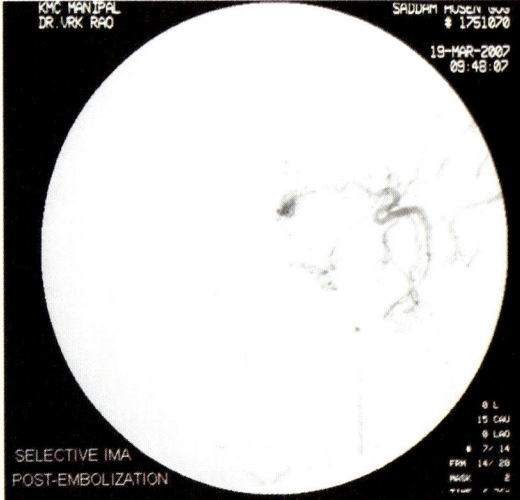

Fig 5.7 Pre embolization and post embolization of the same patient

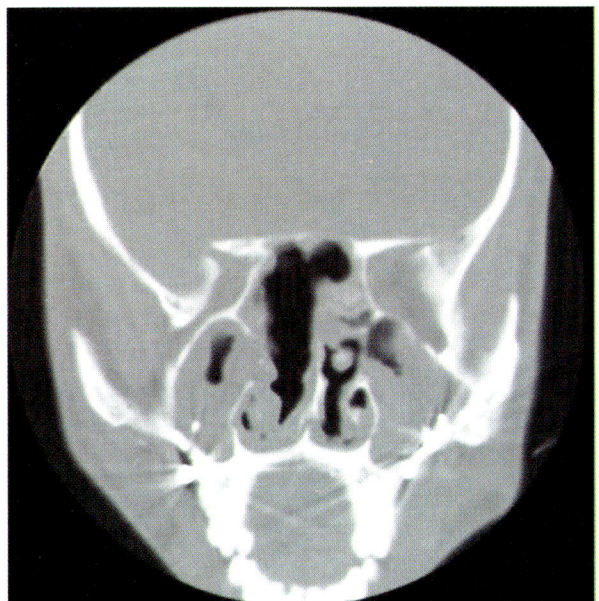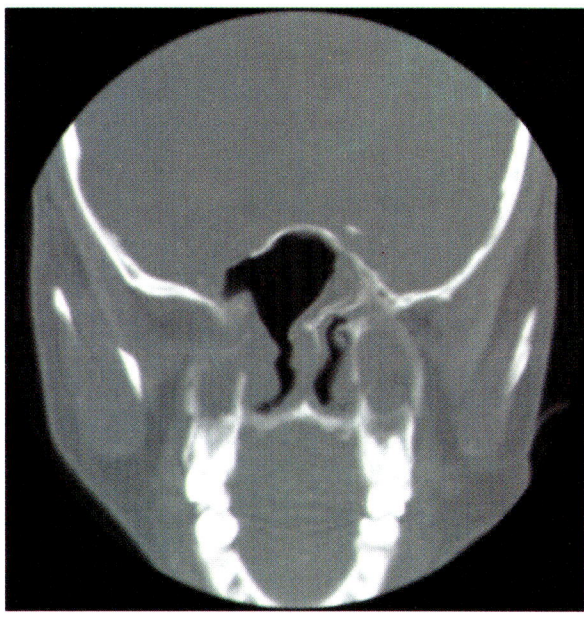

Fig 5.8 Post operation CT showing complete tumor removal

6

Anaesthesia in Skull Base Surgery

The surgical approach to the skull base has evolved tremendously in a relatively short period of time. As the field of skull base and craniofacial surgery has evolved, new approaches to the skull base have been described. With these new surgical approaches, as well as the technical advances in intraoperative monitoring and anesthetic care, the anesthesiologist has assumed more responsibility for the perioperative management of the patient. Lesions that were considered inoperable because of the location and the risk to other juxtaposed vital structures are in many instances curable and can be surgically corrected without long-term morbidity for the patient.

For the anesthesiologist, some of the knowledge and problems are new, while others have not changed much from the past. The initial challenges that come with anesthetizing a patient for any surgical procedure begin with an understanding of the patient's basic physical and mental health as well as the primary type of tumor and risks involved with inducing general anesthesia.

Most skull base neoplasms are benign slow-growing tumors and patients do not present with early symptoms. An exception to this is the neurosecretory glomus tumors which may manifest nonspecific systemic symptoms early in the disease process. It is also important for the anesthesiologist to know the primary type of tumor, its location within the skull base, the proximity of vital structures, and the skull base approach that is being used. This knowledge will be helpful in preparing for proper patient positioning and assessment of potential or general neurological dysfunction. Anesthetic management for these complex skull base approaches has some important concerns and risks that influence patient outcome. The following represent some of the primary concerns of the anesthesiologist when considering the intraoperative management of a patient undergoing a skull base surgical resection:

1. Airway
2. Patient positioning
3. Blood loss
4. Management of the carotid artery
5. Blood glucose concentration
6. Hypothermia
7. Antibiotics
8. Decompression of dura
9. Others

1. Airway

In most scenarios, the airway is not shared with the surgeons and the concerns of the anesthesiologist center on airway anatomy and the possibility of a difficult intubation. With the transcaninal, transmandibular, or the transmaxillary approaches to the skull base, the airway is shared with the surgeon and a decision must be made to determine whether oro tracheal intubation will facilitate the surgical approach or if the patient will require a tracheostomy. Most often the decision to intubate or perform a tracheostomy is made after discussion with the surgeon to obtain an estimate of the amount of upper airway edema that may occur postoperatively. If excessive edema is expected, a tracheostomy should be done to assure a controlled and stable airway in the postoperative period. Thus airway management for these particular approaches will be predictated on postoperative airway edema and the need for airway protection.

2. Patient positioning

Operative positioning has been found to influence complication rates. Patient positioning for skull base tumor resection can be complex and the procedures may be prolonged. Meticulous care with positioning is important because it is extremely difficult to reposition a patient once the surgery begins.

- Bony protuberances should be padded with foam, and in some instances the elbows must be wrapped completely to avoid ulnar neuropathy from pressure point contact at the ulnar groove.

- Metal edges should be isolated from the patient and abnormal flexion or extension of extremities checked to avoid diminished perfusion or nerve plexus injury.

- Padding should also be placed under the heels and buttock area.

- A pillow should be placed behind the knees to reduce tension on the back, especially during procedures in which the patient is supine for a long duration

It is well recognized that head-above-heart positioning (i.e., sitting or "park bench" positions) offers better surgical exposure and the potential advantages of improved hemostasis. However, as has been well described, these "head-elevated" positions carry with them a higher incidence of VAE (venous air embolism) and pneumocephalus. Open sinuses, noncollapsable bone like sinuses and large veins like the jugular vein can contribute to an increased risk for VAE. Also, increased risk of quadriplegia, paraplegia, peripheral nerve injuries, and facial and glossal edema have been reported when patients are placed in the sitting position. Venous air embolism can occur in all types of tumor surgery and should be a consideration when the surgical field is higher than the heart. The incidence of neurosurgical skull base VAE in any head-elevated position has been noted to be 28% for sitting craniotomies compared with 5% for supine and prone positions. With the transtemporal and transcochlear approaches to the skull base, the patient is supine and the surgical field is neutral to the heart. Prophylactic measures to monitor and protect against VAE are not used.

3. Blood loss and maintenance of intravascular volume

More studies are needed to discern the morbidity rates resulting from blood loss during complex skull base surgeries. Iso-molar crystalloid are sufficient to replace urine output and insensible losses on a one-to-one basis. As a general rule hyposmolar solutions and those containing dextrose are avoided. Extreme fluid restriction can result in hypervolemia, hypotension, and possible ischemia from hypoperfusion. The overall goal of the anesthesiologist is to maintain normal intravascular volume. Usual practice is to replace obligatory losses slowly with supplement.

Lesion characteristics such as size, location, and histological type should be considered in planning for blood loss. Meningiomas have been shown to produce a tissue plasminogen activator that leads to significant changes in fibrinolytic parameters and increased blood loss during tumor resections.

Strategies implemented to guard against significant intraoperative blood loss include:

- Hypotensive anesthetic techniques.

- Surgical control of major vessels.

- Preoperative tumor embolization.

4. Management of the carotid artery

Another concern of the anesthesiologist during skull base tumor resection is management of the CA. Some tumors either surround portions of major vessels or directly invade the external capsule. Resection of these tumors may necessitate complete occlusion or sacrifice of the involved artery or vein. If temporary occlusion of the CA is contemplated, the anesthesiologist should be informed early so that a plan may be developed to protect the brain intraoperatively.

Some of the options that could be used to reduce neurological injury include:

- Support of blood pressure to increase perfusion through the circle of Willis and collateral circulation.

- Infusions of vasoactive agents such as neosynephrine.

- Increasing blood pressure with crystalloid therapy could increase perfusion while simultaneously reducing viscosity to improve blood flow to the ischemic area. Blood pressure is targeted at 10 to 15% above awake-patient values whereas the hematocrit level is preferentially titrated to approximately 30%.

5. Blood glucose concentration

Blood glucose concentration is also important during episodes of ischemia. It is postulated that hyperglycemia, in the presence of hypoxia, will increase intracellular acidosis. Insulin has a direct protective effect on ischemic neural tissue. Not only does it reduce blood glucose levels, it stimulates $Na^+ K^+$ adenosine triphosphatase, which enhances Na^+ extrusion with K^+ entry into the cell. Insulin also protects mitochondria and modulates synaptic transmission. Insulin and glucose infusions should be used to titrate the patient to a near-normoglycemic level. Administration of steroids, although necessary to reduce cerebral edema, may be detrimental during periods of incomplete forebrain ischemia because of the associated hyperglycemia. Insulin infusions should be used to reduce blood glucose to normoglycemic levels if carotid artery occlusion is anticipated.

6. Hypothermia

Hypothermia can also be used to provide neuroprotection during episodes of diminished cerebral blood flow. Prior to the anticipated CA occlusion, the patient's body temperature can be lowered by passive convective cooling in the operating room. Temperatures can be easily reduced to 34°C, which has been found to decrease cerebral metabolism by 10 to 15% from normothermic levels. It has also been demonstrated in animal studies that significant reductions in excitatory amino acid release have occurred after forebrain ischemia with moderate hypothermia. Transmembrane ion flux is also reduced and basal energy expenditure is diminished providing a neuron-sparing effect.

7. Others

Other protective measures available to the anesthesiologist include the use of hypnotic agents to reduce cerebral metabolic activity.

Barbiturates are the most extensively studied cerebroprotective agents.

- They reduce cerebral metabolism in a dose-dependent fashion, with reductions as high as 50% at levels titrated to EEG electrical silence.

- Barbiturates are also thought to enhance gamma aminobutyric acid activity and antagonize the *N*-methyl-D-aspartate receptor, which reduces ischemic excitotoxicity.

- Propofol, like other barbiturates, will induce burst suppression in a dose-dependent fashion. Furthermore it is metabolized quickly and therefore does not accumulate, providing a more predictable wake-up time for the patient.

Volatile anesthetics can also be used to reduce cerebral metabolism but their universal ability to dilate the arterioles and reduce blood pressure make them a less than optimal choice when attempting to maintain cerebral perfusion to ischemic areas.

Other agents such as *N*-methyl-D-aspartate receptor antagonists, Ca^{++} channel blockers, free radical scavengers, and ion transport inhibitors have been administered in human trial studies with minimal success.

The local anesthetic lidocaine may provide some added benefit through its ability to block the Na^+ channel, reduce $Na^+ K^+$ transmembrane flux, and decrease basal energy expenditures. Usually 1 to 2 mg/kg of lidocaine may be given as an intravenous bolus immediately prior to the ischemic event.

8. Antibiotics

Preoperative intravenous antibiotic agents are administered during induction of general anesthesia to provide broad-spectrum coverage during the procedure. The aim is to provide prophylaxis against gram-positive and gram-negative bacteria as well as *Bacteroides*. Intravenous antibiotic administration is continued through the postoperative period as long as the pack is in place.

9. Decompression of the dura at the onset of the procedure

- Do not use anesthetic agents that may increase the intracranial pressure.
- Rapidly infuse mannitol.
- With the patient in the lateral decubitus position, a lumbar puncture (lumbar subarachnoid tap with an 18- gauge spinal needle) is performed and an intrathecal catheter placed for intra- and postoperative CSF drainage. Intra-operatively, the anesthesiologist drains 10 ml of CSF until adequate brain relaxation is achieved to minimize handling and retraction of the brain. Generally, 30 to 60 ml of CSF is drained for a standard anterior CFR.
- Ensure slight hyperventilation to reduce the PCO_2.

Choice of anesthetic agent and technique depends on:

- The extent of intracranial dissection
- The potential for brain or vascular injury
- Systemic hemodynamics

- The need for monitoring of cortical and brainstem functions (*e.g.*, brainstem-evoked response, SSEP, EEG)

- The need for CN monitoring (i.e., CNS VII, X-XII).

The endotracheal tube is secured with a circumdental or circummandibular wire ligature (*e.g.*, #26 stainless steel wire). Spinal drain is inserted when intradural dissection is anticipated.

Preoperative preparation of the patient

- The scalp and facial hair (except the eyebrows) is shaved (in case of males), in case of craniofacial resection.

- In a planned myocutaneous or free flap reconstruction, preparation of that particular area has to be done preoperatively.

- Anticipate the need for blood replacement. Preoperatively, type and cross match the patients blood for 2-6 units of packed red blood cells (PRBCs) according to the extent and nature of the tumor and surgery. Autologous blood banking is used when feasible, although it is frequently impractical. A cell-saver or auto-transfusion device may be used during the resection of benign vascular tumors.

- Administer wide-spectrum perioperative antibiotic prophylaxis with good penetration of the blood-brain barrier before the surgery, and continue it for 48 hours postoperatively.

- Bowel preparation can be done the previous night of surgery in order to prevent any post operative complication.

- Written and informed consent: patient has to be explained about the procedure and its complications.

- Various skin sensitivity tests like xylocaine sensitivity, BIPP sensitivity etc has to be done prior to surgery.

- **Preexisting lower cranial neuropathies** (*e.g.*, CNS IX-XII) are common in patients with tumors at the parapharyngeal space, tumors that extend to the jugular foramen, or both. These patients present with hypernasal or slurred speech, nasal regurgitation, dysphagia, aspiration, and dysphonia (CNs X and XII). Lower cranial neuropathies presenting with aspiration have life-threatening consequences. Patients with a proximal vagal paralysis may benefit from a medialization laryngoplasty and an arytenoid adduction procedure with speech and language and swallowing therapy.

- **A tracheostomy** to facilitate tracheal toilet and **a gastrostomy tube** to facilitate postoperative feeding and to decrease the risk of prandial aspiration.

- Preoperatively evaluate corneal sensation and protective mechanisms.

Somatosensory evoked potential (SSEP) monitoring of the median nerve proximity to nerves. Facial nerve monitoring is routinely used for transparotid or transtemporal approaches.

7

Anterior Skull Base Approaches

Anterior Skull Base Approaches consists of three components: **approach, definitive resection and reconstruction.**

The Three main approaches are
- Transfacial approach
- Craniofacial approach
- Endoscopic approach

Trans Facial approaches include

a. Transnasal Transantral approach
   - Lateral rhinotomy (Moure's)
   - Extended lateral rhinotomy
   - Midfacial degloving
   - LeForte type I osteotomy
   - Medial maxillectomy
   - Total maxillectomy
   - Barbosa's modified approach
b. Facial translocation approach
c. Midfacial split
d. Wilson's transpalatal approach
e. Biller's midline transmandibular oropharyngeal approach
f. Transcervical approach
g. Trans nasal endoscopic approach

TRANSNASAL TRANSANTRAL APPROACH

This approach was designed to remove benign well circumscribed mass, angiofibroma being a classical example. However extensive angiofibromas can also be removed by modified weber Ferguson or midfacial degloving approach.

Advantages of Transnasal transantral approaches

- Removal of antral extension.
- Posterior antral wall can be assessed for any destruction.
- If posterior antral wall is eroded, pterygopalatine fossa can be opened and extension tackled.
- Sublabial incision can be extended as far as necessary to remove cheek extensions.

  If still not sure of complete removal then modified Weber Fergusson approach can be used as a radical measure.

LATERAL RHINOTOMY (MOURE'S)

- It is an incision along the side of the nose.
- The incision can be extended to provide wide access to interior of nose or the paranasal sinuses.
- Extensions of lateral rhinotomy.

Incision

- From just beneath the medial aspect of brow, it extends down and forwards to within 5 mm of inner canthus extended along the side of nose midway between dorsum and nasomaxillary crease. Incision terminates at level of ala (Fig. 7.1).

Indications

- Lateral rhinotomy with medial maxillectomy is the gold standard for the removal of inverted papilloma.
- It was originally intended for the removal of frontoethmoidal tumors.
- Malignancy confined to the nasal cavity. Malignant

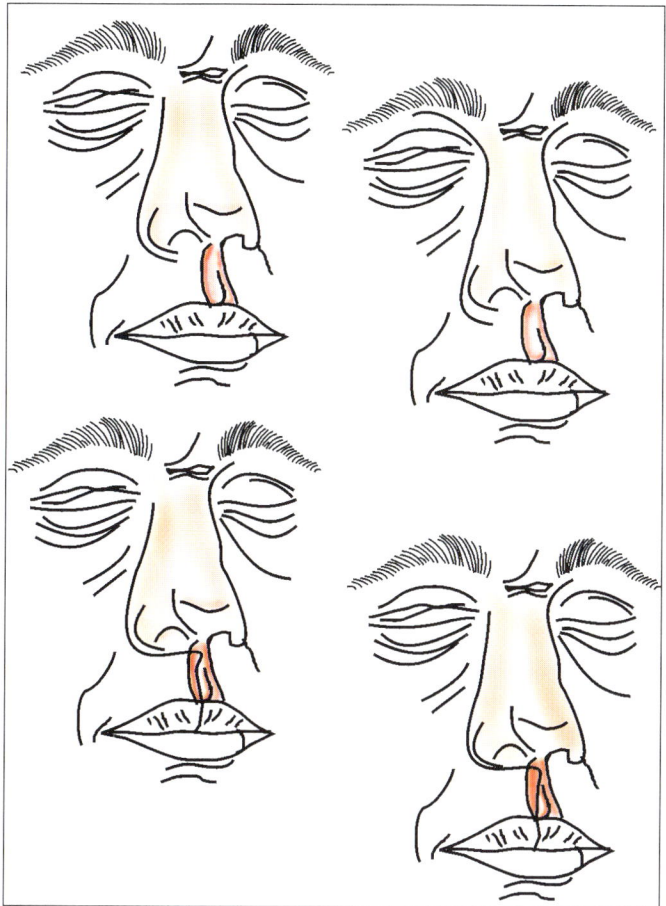

Fig. 7.1 Showing various modifications of lateral rhinotomy

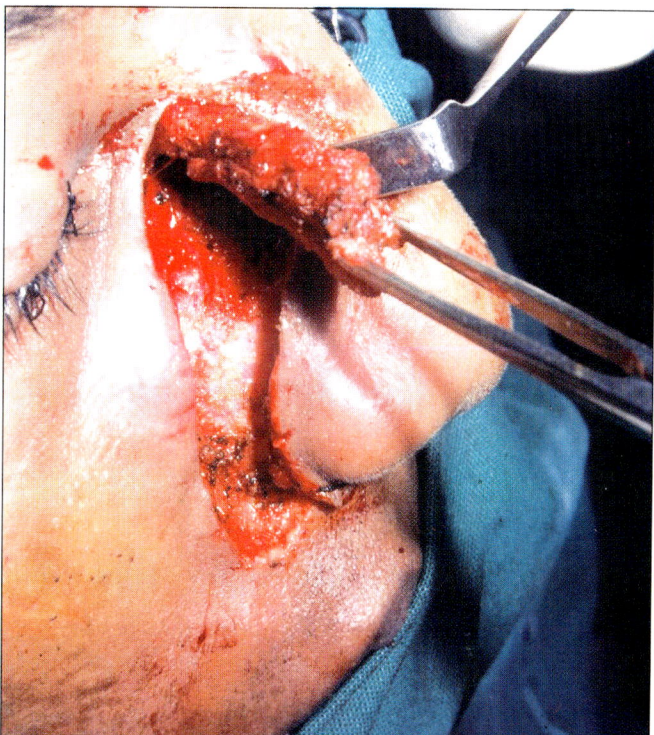

Fig. 7.2 Flap being raised

melanoma and benign neoplasms arising within the nasal cavity medial maxilla, ethmoids, pterygomaxillary region and nasopharynx. Angiofibroma, inverted papilloma, osteoma, neurofibroma are also approached through this approach.

Surgical technique (Fig. 7.2)

- The procedure consists of a incision beginning in the medial aspect of the eyebrow, between the medial canthus and nasal dorsum along the nasomaxillary junction along the alar crease and into the nasal vestibule.

- After the skin incision the periosteum is incised and elevated over the nasal bone and the fronto-nasal process medially and laterally to the orbital rim and to the face of the maxilla as far as the inferior orbital foramen.

- The medial canthal ligament can be detached from the lacrimal crest.

- The lacrimal sac is mobilized from its fossa and the lacrimal duct is transected.

- The orbital periosteum is freed from the lamina papyracea.

- The anterior ethmoidal vessels can be cauterised and divided to improve access

- The medial orbital periosteum is elevated and the orbit is retracted laterally.

- Osteotomies for medial maxillectomy are then performed.

- The first bone cut is vertically made through the anterior aspect of the medial wall of the maxillary sinus.

- Second cut is made horizontally along the inferior aspect of the medial maxillary sinus wall.

- Third cut extends through the medial wall of the orbit just inferior to the fronto ethmoidal suture line.

- Fourth osteotomy travels through the orbital floor just medial through the intra orbital canal.

- Final cut are made posteriorly, usually with a heavy curved scissors through the posterior aspect of the medial maxillary wall at the pterygomaxillary fissure.

Advantages

- It provides excellent exposure of the interior of the nose, the paranasal sinus and nasopharynx with minimum postoperative deformity.

- The safety and effectiveness of lateral rhinotomy is superior to transnasal, transpalatal and transantral approach.

Contraindication

- Any lesion which appears to have compromised the cribriform plate or an orbital apex.

Complications of lateral rhinotomy

Early complications

- Hemorrhage
- Blepharitis
- Lid edema
- Wound infection
- CSF leak
- Meningitis

Late complications

- Crusting
- Alar lift
- Epiphora
- Facial paresthesia
- Diplopia
- Frontonasal recess obstruction
- Telecanthus with secondary mucocele
- Vestibular stenosis

EXTENDED LATERAL RHINOTOMY APPROACH

Indications

- Access to nose, nasopharynx, pterygopalatine and infratemporal fossae, paranasal sinuses.

Extension of incision in case of extranasopharyngeal spread of tumors

- From the alar end incision is extended down around the base of nose to the base of columella and down towards the center of philtrum of upper lip. Incision over the mucosal surface of lip is in Z fashion, then incision is carried down to gingivobuccal sulcus continued in the sulcus upto maxillary tuberosity. Upper end of the incision can be extended upto forehead (Lynch extension).

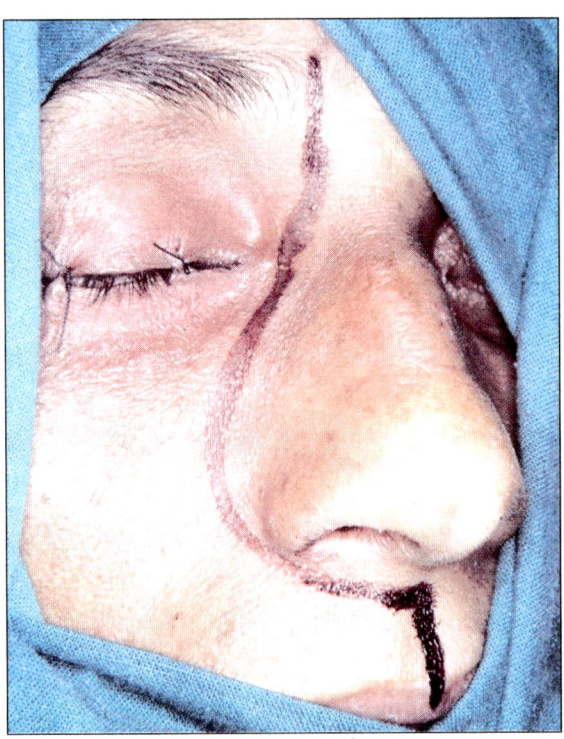

Fig. 7.3 Lateral rhinotomy with lynch extension to forehead and from alar end incision is extended around the base of the nose down towards the centre of the philthrum

Steps

- Facial flap is elevated off the maxilla. Nasal bones, frontal process of maxilla and anterior surface of maxilla are removed. Small fragment of bone is preserved around infraorbital foramen. Through the antrum is visualised anterior bowing of posterior maxillary wall.

- Posterior wall is removed, internal maxillary artery or its branches can be identified and ligated.

- Tumour can now be dissected from pterygopalatine, infratemporal fossae by pushing medially with packing.

- Inferior turbinate is divided posteriorly, middle turbinate may be divided anterior to the portion involved with tumour mass. The turbinates and middle meatus can be retracted to expose posterior nasal cavity and choana.

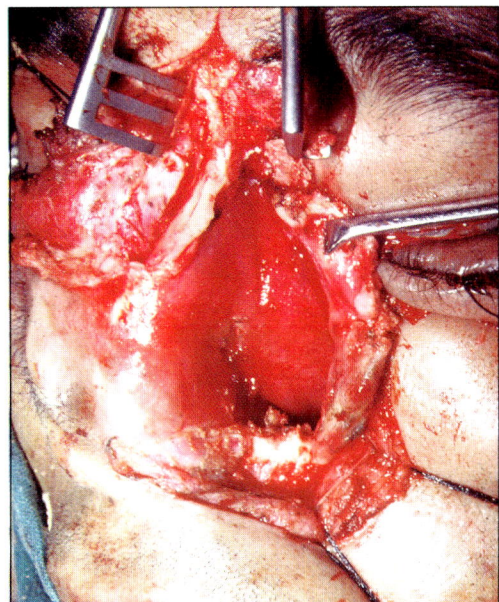

Fig. 7.4 Tumor exposed after extended lateral rhinotomy approach

- Orbital periosteum is elevated to inspect for tumour invasion into orbit amina papyracea and lacrimal bone are removed to inspect ethmoids. Anterior and posterior ethmoid cells are removed to inspect sphenoid sinus involvement. If involved, tumour is removed by packing the sinus and pushing the tumour downwards and outwards.

- Once tumour is removed, cavity is packed with BIPP for 1 week.

- Wound closed in layers.

Complications

Early

- Hemorrhage
- Blepharitis and lid oedema
- Infraorbital nerve anaesthesia
- CSF leak
- Meningitis

Late

- Epiphora - Due to inadvertant transection of nasolacrimal duct.
- Cosmetic - Alar lift, Vestibular stenosis, Webbing of incision, Columellar retraction, Saddling.
- Diplopia - As the superior extent of incision affects the trochlea.

- Telecanthus - If medial canthus is not reapproximated.
- Mucocele formation due to obstruction of frontonasal duct.
- Nasocutaneous fistula.

MID FACIAL DEGLOVING

This technique allows the exposure of the structures of the middle 1/3rd of the face without an external skin incision.

Indications

- For benign lesions such as osteomas and fibromas.
- Adequate exposure of the anterior skull base tumors such as inverted papilloma, angiofibroma and ameloblastoma.
- Malignant tumors most commonly squamous cell carcinoma.
- Resections such as medial maxillectomy, total maxillectomy and maxillectomy with orbital exenteration can be done without external skin incision.
- Septodermoplasty and repair of large septal perforation.
- Mid-facial fracture correction.
- Mid-facial osteotomies.
- Mid-facial bone grafting for counter restoration.
- Selected malignant tumors, which can be adequately encompassed by the exposure.

Surgical technique

- General anaesthesia is administered via an oral endotracheal tube.
- Lidocaine 1% with adrenaline 1:2,00,000 is then infiltrated in the maxillary gingivobuccal sulcus, canine fossae, and the greater palatine foramina bilaterally. The nose is injected in a fashion similar to that for septorhinoplasty.

Four incisions are made

1. Bilateral Inter-cartilaginous incisions. (Fig 7.5)
2. Septo-columellar- complete transfixation incision (Fig. 7.6)
3. Bilateral sublabial incisions from one maxillary tuberosity to the other (Fig 7.8)
4. Bilateral piriform aperture incisions extending to the vestibule.

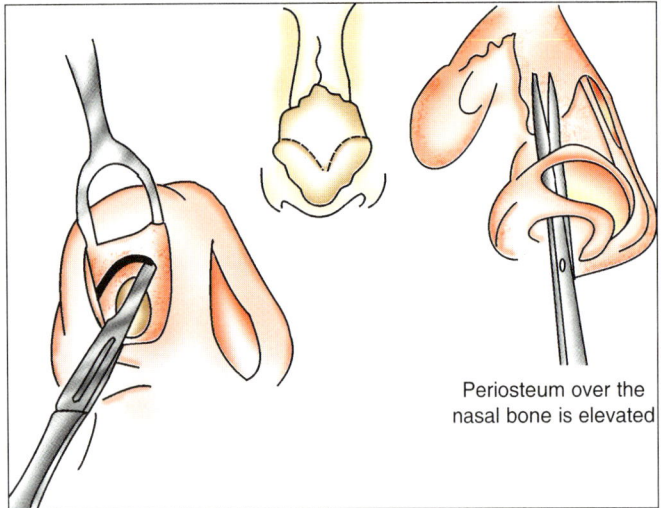

Periosteum over the nasal bone is elevated

Fig. 7.5 Bilateral Inter-cartilaginous incisions

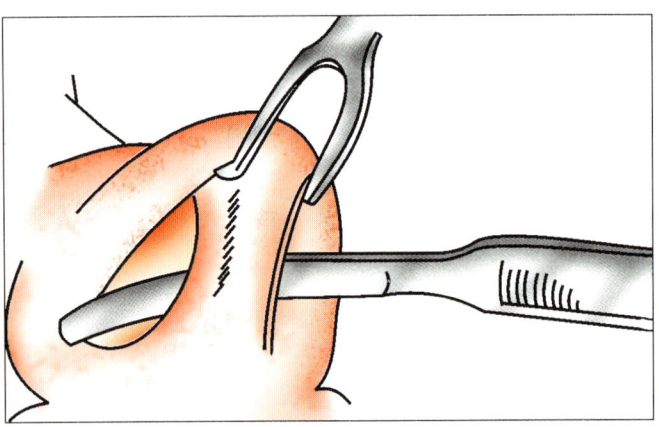

Fig. 7.6 Septo-columellar- complete transfixation incision

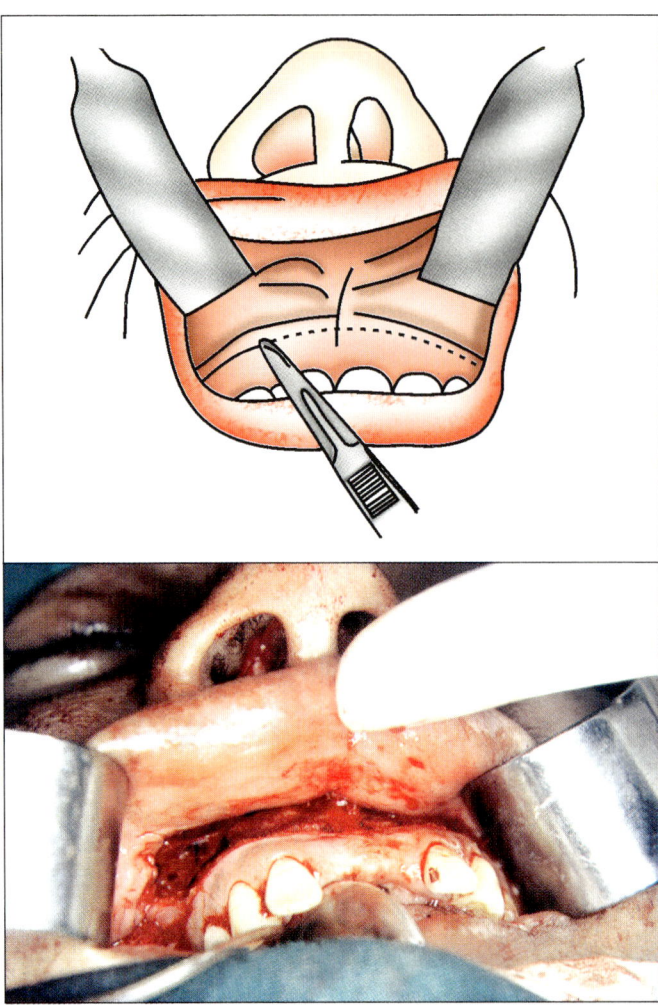

Fig 7.8 Bilateral sublabial incisions from one maxillary tuberosity to the other

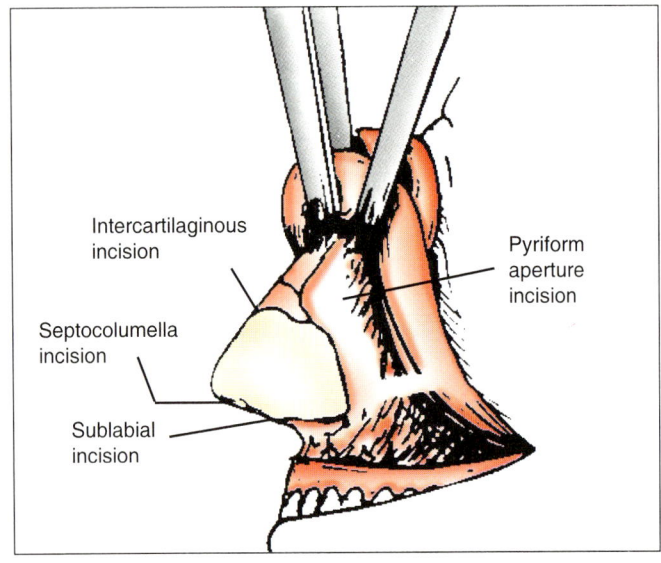

Intercartilaginous incision

Septocolumella incision

Sublabial incision

Pyriform aperture incision

Fig. 7.7 Showing sites of all the four incisions

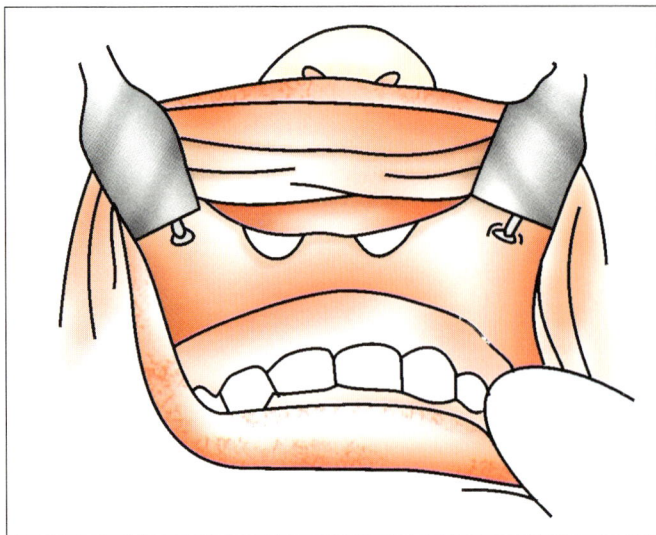

Fig 7.9 Shows periosteum over the anterior face of maxilla is raised upto infra orbital nerve.

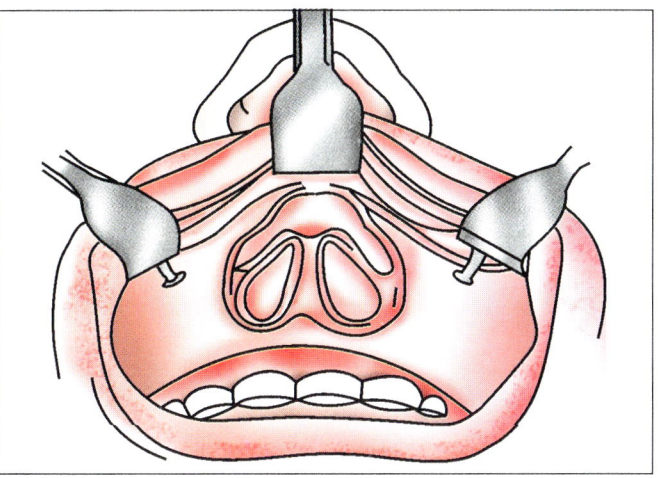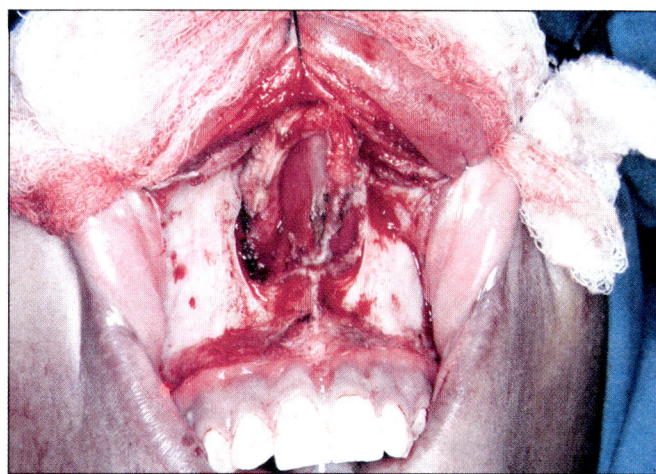

Fig 7.10 Shows skin of the middle one third of the face is degloved from the skull superiorly to the frontonasal suture line and infraorbital rim.

Procedure

- The sublabial incision is carried straight down to the level of bone and laterally extended out to the maxillary tuberosity on both sides.

- The periosteum over the anterior face of maxilla is raised with the soft tissue bilaterally taking care to identify and preserve the infraorbital nerve.

- Routine rhinoplasty intercartilagenous incisions are made.

- The periosteum overlying the nasal bones is elevated as far laterally as possible and superiorly to the root of the nose.

- A transfixion incision is then performed along the dorsal and caudal end of the cartilaginous septum.

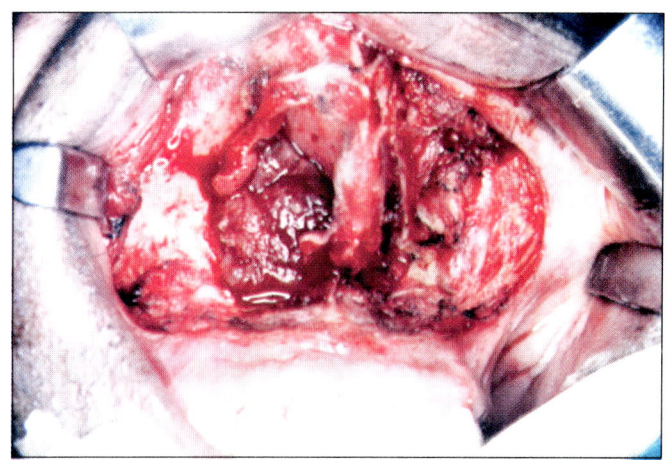

Fig 7.12 Tumor seen in right nasal cavity

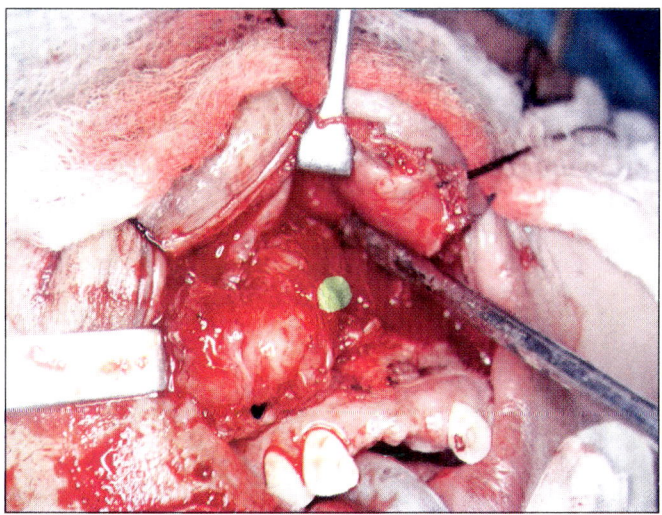

Fig 7.11 Excission of the tumor

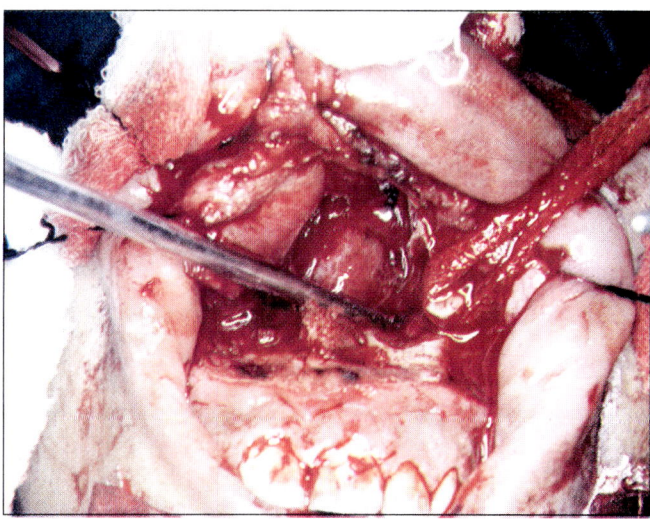

Fig 7.13 Tumor being exposed by midfacial deglowing

- This incision is further extended across the floor of the nose to the lateral aspect of the piriform fossa connecting it with the inter-cartilagenous incision to complete a circumvestibular release.

- The skin of the middle third of the face can now be degloved from the skull all the way superiorly to the frontonasal suture line, infraorbital rim and zygomatic process.

- It is now possible to gain excellent access to the nasal cavities, nasal septum, and enter the maxillary sinus anteriorly in usual way.

- Exposure of the nasopharynx can be obtained by removal of the anterior and posterior wall of the maxilla, control of the internal maxillary artery, removal of the lateral wall of the nose, including the perpendicular process of palatine bone.

- The whole nasal septum is accessible and can be removed if necessary upto the level of the cribriform plate.

- The posterior wall of the sphenoidal sinus, pterygoid muscles and plates and the base of sphenoid are the posterior limits of the resection.

- The cribriform plate and the anterior cranial fossa are the superior limits.

- Lateral limit is the coronoid process of the mandible.

- The inferior boundary is the palate.

Advantages

- No facial skin incisions and results in minimal functional impairment.

- There is no facial scar.

- It is particularly appropriate for excision of JNA as excellent exposure of the lesion and direct control of the internal maxillary artery.

- It offers excellent bilateral exposure of the nasal cavities. Middle third of face and central skull base.

- Allows adequate modification and extension.

- Minimal post-operative complications.

- Successful control of wide variety of diseases.

- Good patient tolerance.

Contraindication

In extensive lesions of the skull base involving the frontal sinus, orbit and cribriform plate.

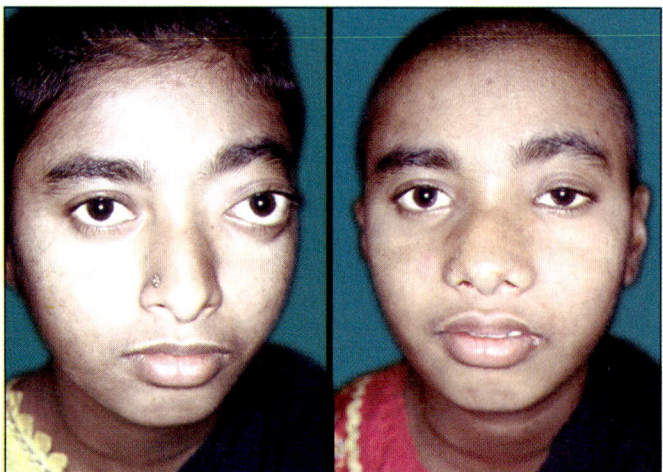

Fig. 7.14 Pre and post operative pictures of midfacial degloving. Note the absence of any facial scar, no poroptosis

Disadvantages

Occasional occurrence of nasal vestibular stenosis.

Complications

1. *Sensory loss:* The most frequent complaint reported by patients following this approach is sensory loss in the distribution of the infraorbital nerve.

   In performing this approach, care is taken to identify and preserve the infraorbital nerve by staying in the subperiosteal plane of dissection.

2. Facial bruising

3. Malar paraesthesia

4. Vestibular stenosis

5. Crusting of nasal cavity

6. Telecanthus.

LEFORTE TYPE I OSTEOTOMY APPROACH

It is a fracture made that extends from the nasal pyramid to each of the pterygoid plates resulting in detachment of the upper jaw from the cranial base.

Indications

1. LeFort I osteotomy is usually reserved for treatment of large tumors like resection of JNA.

2. Removal of extensive central skull base and paranasal sinuses tumors.

3. Removal of benign tumors of the pterygopalatine fossa.

4. Cosmetic benefits especially in long face patients.

5. Inferior repositioning of the maxilla and widening of the maxilla are also possible.

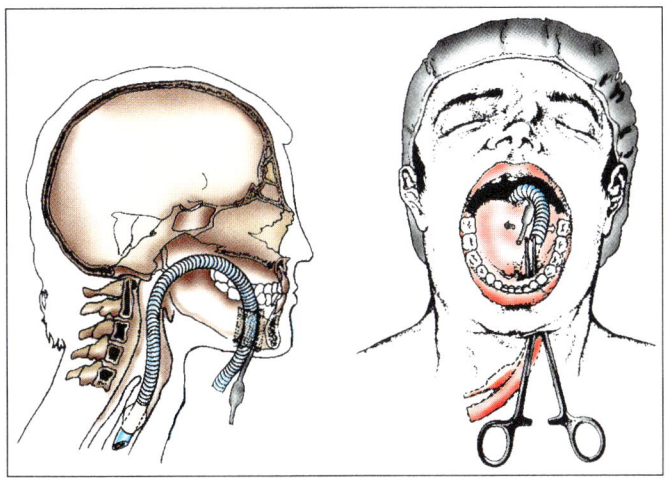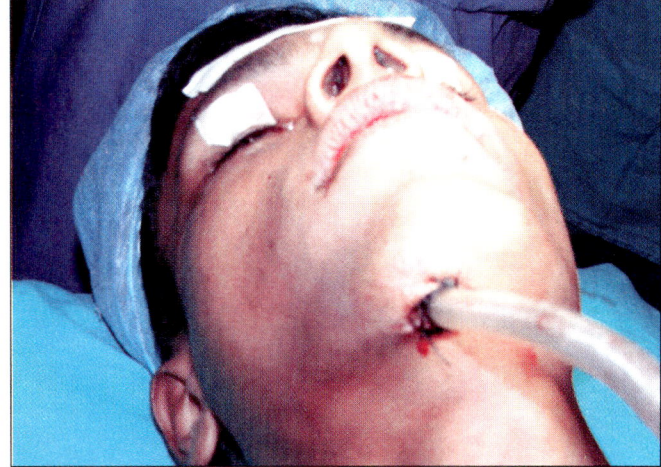

Fig 7.15 Showing submental intubation for le-fort Type I osteotomy to achieve good occlusion by intermaxillary fixation

Surgical Technique

- This is done under general anaesthesia through nasal intubation or submental route of endotracheal intubation. (Fig. 7.11).

- Patient is placed in the supine position with varying degrees of tilt for access.

- Nasal cavity is decongested and infiltration is given using 2% xylocaine with 1:200,000 adrenaline over the sublabial mucosa and nasal mucosa is done.

- Horizontal incision is made through gingivobuccal sulcus between the 2nd maxillary premolars.

- Mucoperiosteal flap is elevated to expose the piriform aperture, nasal spine, floor of nasal cavity and anterior wall of maxillary sinus. (Fig. 7.12).

- LeFort I osteotomy is done by using a microdrill bilaterally extending from piriform aperture to the posterior maxilla. (Fig. 7.13).

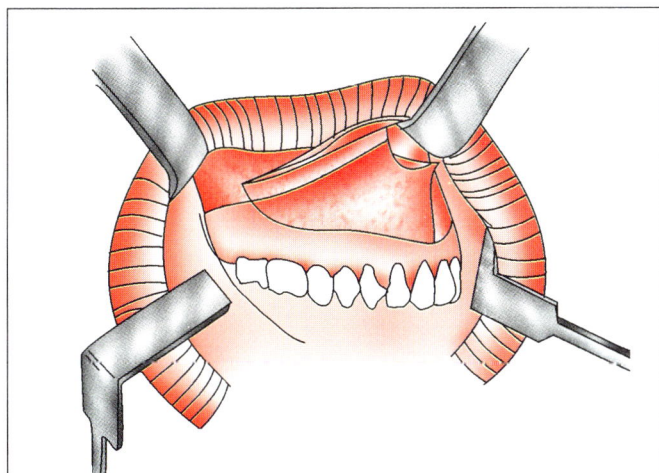

Fig. 7.16 Exposure required

- A curved chisel is used to complete the pterygomaxillary dysjunction. (Fig. 7.15)

- Nasal septum and vomer are detached from the maxillary crest with a straight chisel. (Fig 7.16)

- The maxilla is downfractured with the help of two Rowers clamps exposing the maxillary sinus and nasopharynx. (Fig. 7.17)

- A modified Dingman's gag can be inserted to keep the mucosa and maxillary segment retracted which opens a clear view of the surgical site.

- To gain further access posteriorly, we can excise the posterior ends of the inferior turbinate and septum. This added exposure allows us to employ a nasal endoscope and an operating microscope.

- Once the tumor is removed the maxilla is replaced and plated. The predrilled holes help achieve good alignment. (Fig. 7.18)

- The nasal cavity is packed with wollen soaked in BIPP, which is removed the following morning.

- The mucosa is closed with a continuous absorbable suture. The patient is allowed fluids after 24 hours and can progress to a soft diet.

Advantages

- In contrast to a palatal splitting technique, downward displacement of maxilla gives a direct line of sight for tumors removed that is not hindered by the soft palate.

- By avoiding an external facial scar this approach affords excellent cosmetic results.

- Disruption of facial growth is unlikely because the osteotomy does not pass through the growth centers.

- LeFort type I approach is suited for large skull base

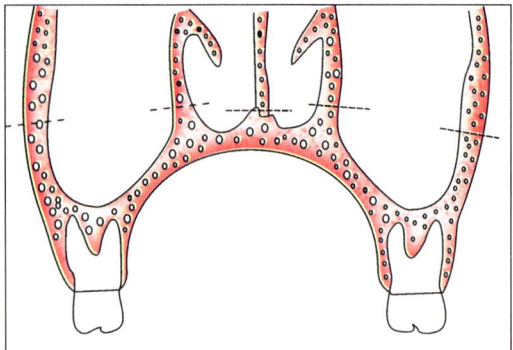

Fig 7.17 Coronal cut showing the level of bone cuts

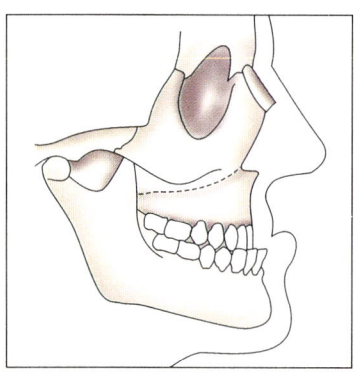

Fig 7.18 Showing incision line

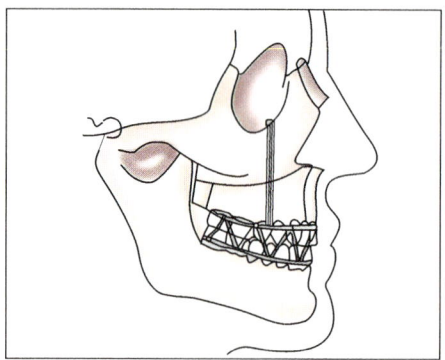

Fig 7.19 Intermaxillary fixation done before osteotomy to maintain good occlusion

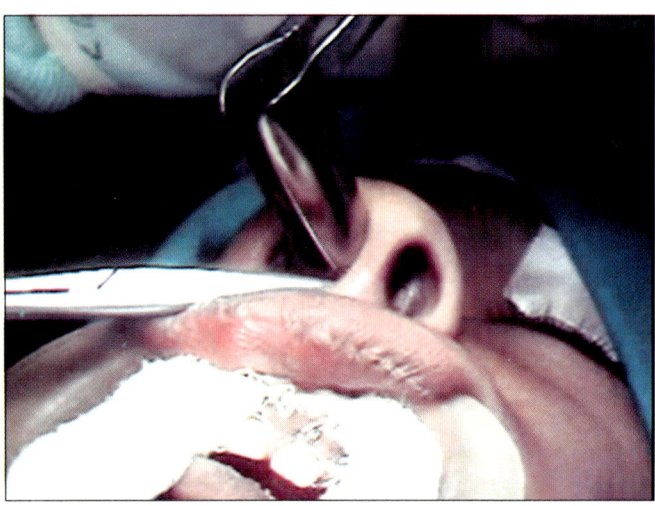

Fig. 7.20 Intercartilagenous incision

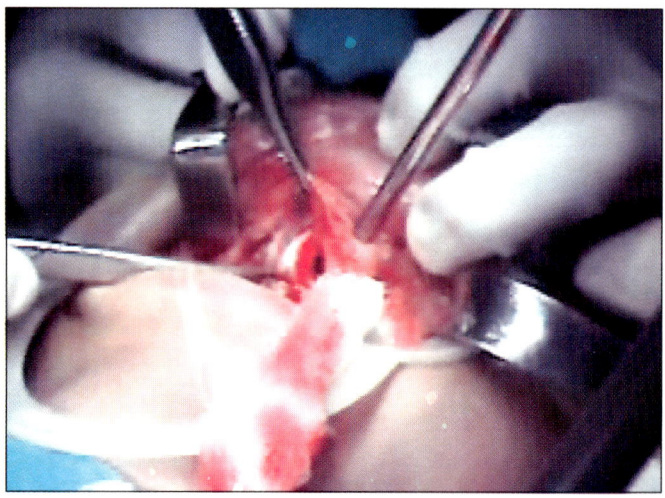

Fig. 7.21 Midlle one third of face is degloved

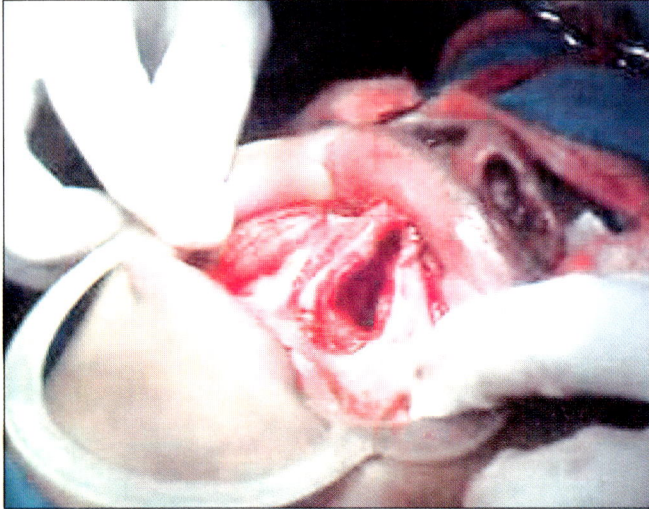

Fig. 7.22 Piriform aperture, nasal spine floor of the nasal cavity and anterior wall of maxillary sinus is exposed

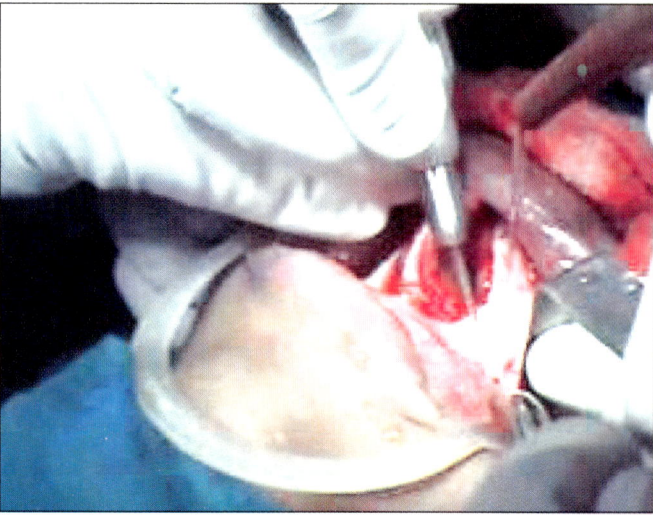

Fig. 7.23 Le-fort I osteotomy is being done by using a microdrill bilaterally extending from piriform aperture to the posterior maxilla

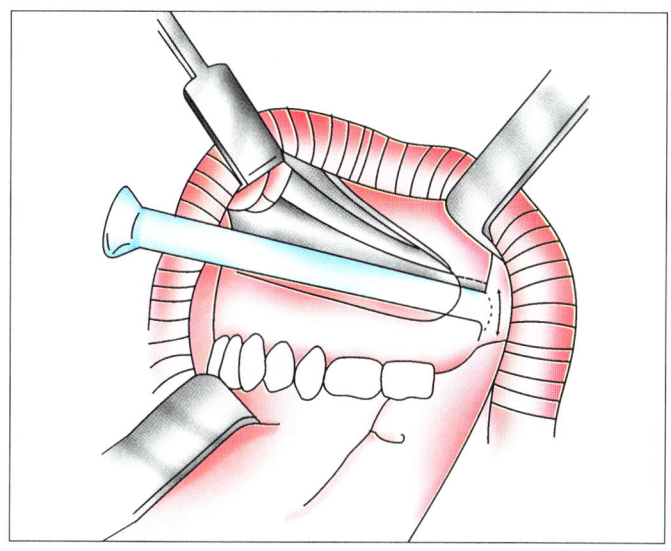

Fig 7.24 Showing separation of pterygoid plates

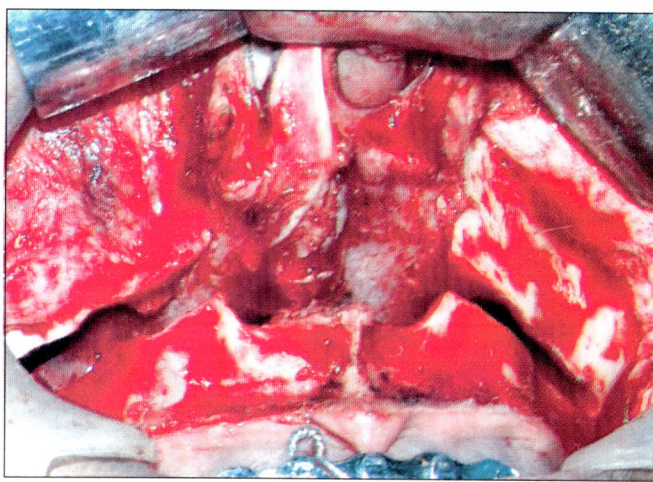

Fig 7.26 The maxilla is down fractured

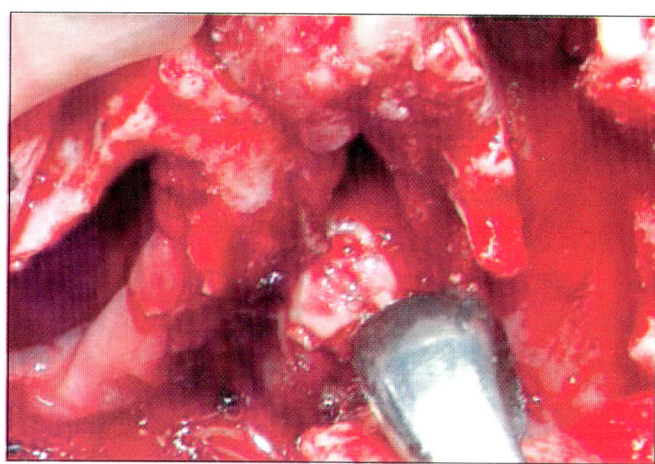

Fig 7.27 Tumor exposed after Le-fort osteotomy

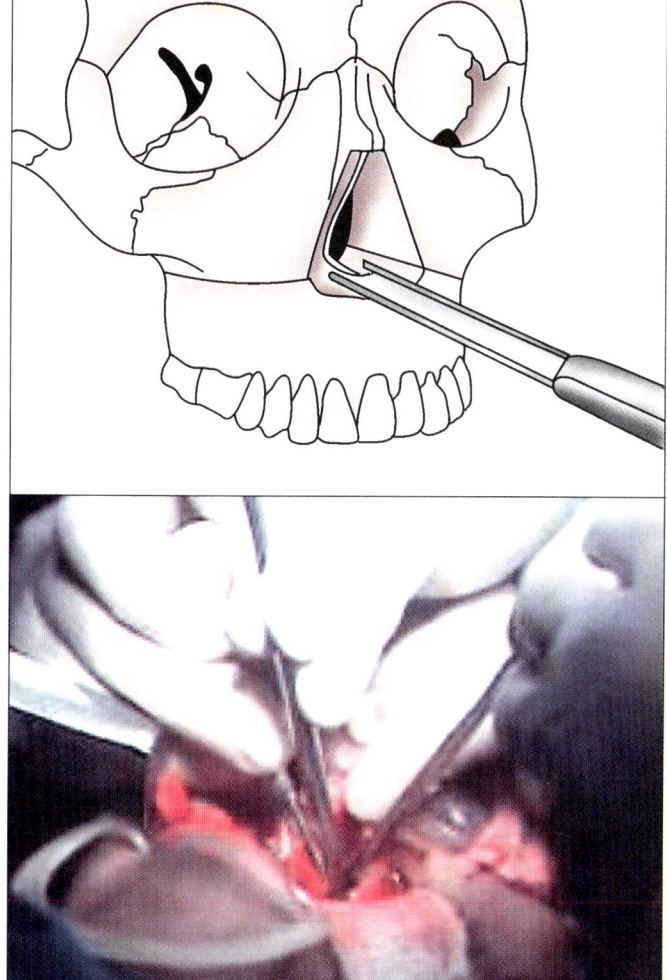

Fig 7.25 Nasal septum and vomer are detached from maxillary crest with straight cheisel

lesions especially if the pterygomaxillary space, the sphenoid sinus and the clival region are involved.

- In a transpalatal approach, palate dehiscence can occur.

- The transpalatal technique is limited to tumors from the nasopharynx, nasal cavity and sphenoidal sinus.

- LeFort I approach is a safe technique both in terms of surgical aspects and neoplasm control.

- The surgery is performed with relative ease and minimal bleeding.

- The procedure offers wide surgical exposure with good access to voluminous tumors including those with intracranial extension.

- Preferred approach for JNA resection, as with resection of the posterior wall of the maxillary sinus it allows a direct access to the vascular pedicle of the JNA.

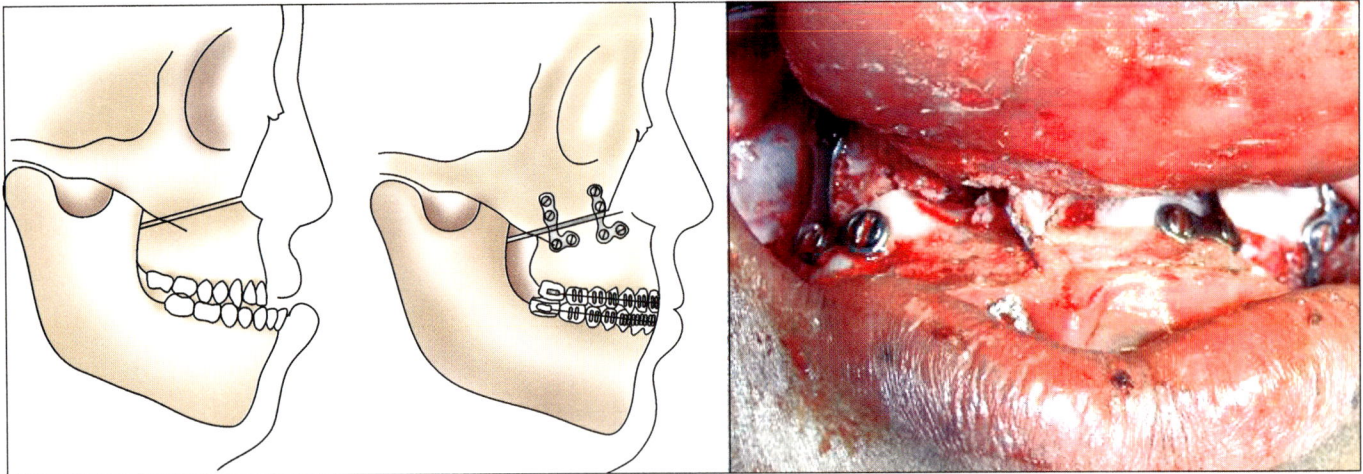

Fig 7.28 Maxilla is replaced and plated

Complications

- Delayed union or non union following maxillary osteotomies is not uncommon and is usually manifested by maxillary mobility beyond the normal 6 week period.

- Development of oronasal fistula.

- Nasal airway obstruction due to edema of the nasal walls, septum and turbinates.

- Obstructive sleep apnea syndrome.

- Infraorbital paresthesia.

- Intraoperative hemorrhage during maxillary osteotomy. The vessel commonly involved in the descending palatine artery.

- Pseudo aneurysms of the sphenopalatine artery during maxillary osteotomies tends to present as epistaxis within the first 2 weeks after surgery.

- Maxillary avascular necrosis resulting in loss of vitality of one or more teeth due to sequestration of major segments of bone and teeth.

- TM Joint complications like anterior meniscal displacement and perforation.

MEDIAL MAXILLECTOMY

Medial maxillectomy through lateral rhinotomy incision is the gold standard for the removal of an inverted papilloma. It has the advantages of excellent exposure of the lateral nasal wall and paranasal sinuses. The success is related to the en bloc resection of the lateral nasal wall, ethmoid labyrinth, and medial portion of the maxilla, which are the sites of formation and extension of this tumor.

This is a procedure that allows visualization of the tumor margins while allowing preservation of the orbital rim, the eye and its attachments, the lacrimal apparatus, the nasal pyramid, and the palate. The medial maxillectomy allows an en bloc removal of the ethmoidal labyrinth and the medial aspect of the maxilla from the cribriform plate superiorly to the floor of the nose inferiorly; and from the anterior extent of the ethmoidal cells back to the area of the optic nerve. The lamina papyracea is included in the tissue block. This technique can be expanded to involve the removal of the cribriform plate when combined with an intracranial approach.

A lateral rhinotomy incision is made beginning in the medial aspect of the eyebrow, angling around to midway up the lateral wall of the nose and into the alar groove. A notch can be made in the medial canthal area to prevent webbing. The exposure should be adequate without cutting the lip, which also gives a better final cosmesis. A subperiosteal dissection is performed exposing the anterior wall of the maxillary sinus. The infraorbital nerve is identified and protected. The medial wall of the orbit is dissected exposing the anterior and posterior ethmoid arteries which will be the superior most aspect of the dissection. The lacrimal sac is dissected out of its sulcus and divided at its most distal aspect. An antrostomy into the maxillary sinus is performed and then the remainder of the maxillary sinus is removed taking care to preserve the infraorbital nerve.

Various osteotomies in medial maxillectomy

1. A lateral osteotomy of the nasal bone is performed to give better visual exposure.

2. The first major cut is along the floor of the sinus. This cut is made in the inferior meatus from the anterior tip of the inferior turbinate to the most posterior aspect.

3. The second bone cut entails the medial most part of the orbital rim, which is drilled down using a cutting burr until on the floor of the orbit. This aspect may be omitted but it gives better visual access with minimal structural defect.

4. The third cut is made along the anterior aspect of the maxillary sinus involving the lacrimal fossa, anterior to the middle turbinate and into the ethmoid cells. The anterior bony rim forming the piriform aperture and the nasal rim is left intact.

   If the lacrimal duct is left in place the cut is made posterior to it. It is usually cut and marked for stenting later in the operation.

5. The fourth cut involves retracting the orbital contents to expose the frontoethmoidal suture line and the anterior ethmoid artery. A small osteotome is used to perforate the ethmoidal cells and the nasal cavity is entered inferior to the suture line, beginning anteriorly in the lacrimal fossa and extending posteriorly. The suture line and the ethmoidal arteries establish the position of the cribriform plate. If more posterior dissection is needed the anterior ethmoidal artery may be ligated.

6. The fifth cut involves freeing the posterior and lateral aspect of the lamina papyracea. The cut is extended along the posterior part of the lamina with a curved mayo scissors and goes along the inferior part of the orbit along the rim just medial to the infraorbital nerve. This will then join with the drilled incision through the rim. The remaining bony attachment of the lateral nasal wall is that portion of the palatine bone that is anterior to the pterygoid process of the sphenoid bone. This attachment extends from the nasal floor up to the superior turbinate. The en bloc specimen is gently rocked bimanual to reveal the remaining attachments. Thus using a right-angled scissors starting interiorly through the nose and placing the lateral blade in the maxillary sinus while the medial blade lies in the inferior meatus, a cut just anterior to the pterygoid plate is made which is the posterior aspect of the inferior and middle turbinates. The superior aspect of the incision is technically impossible to perform using the scissors.

A bimanual maneuver using one index finger placed in the maxillary sinus and the other in the nose the bone is used to fracture this area. The attached mucosa must then be cut. The en bloc specimen is delivered through the nasal aperture. Bony spicules should be smoothened by the burr and all sinuses should be opened widely into one large cavity, which allows for easy postoperative examinations.

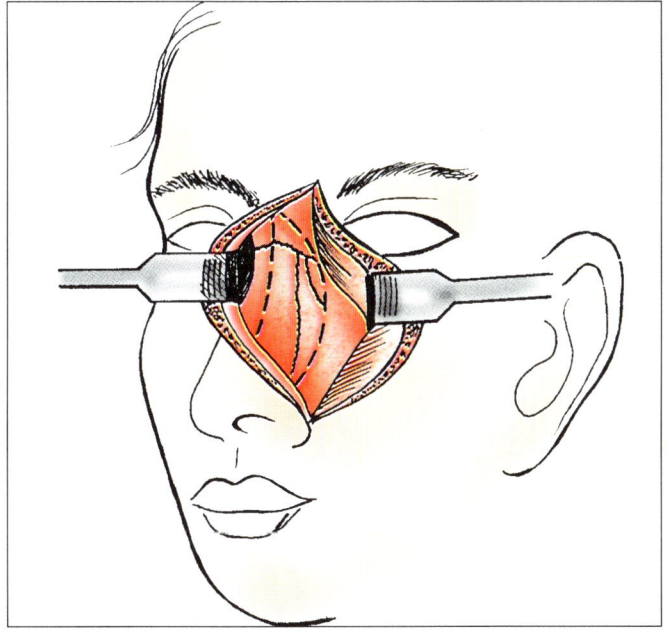
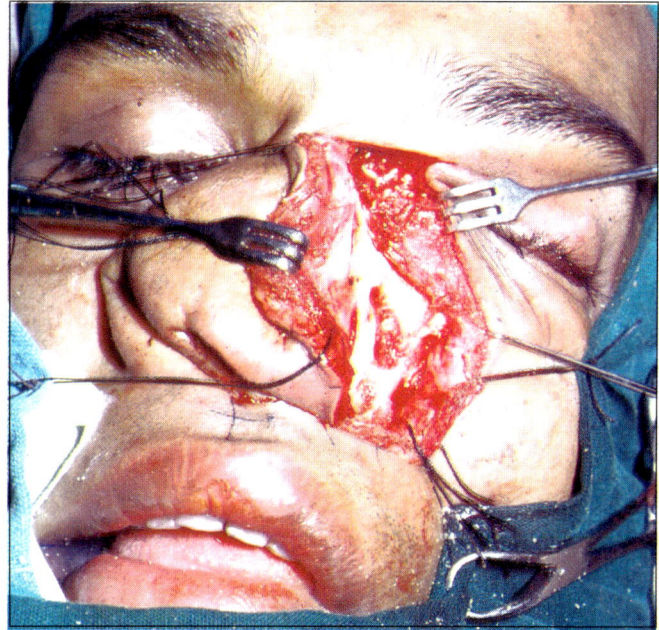

Fig. 7.29 Showing markings for preliminary 'rhinoplasty' type osteotomies of the nasal bones

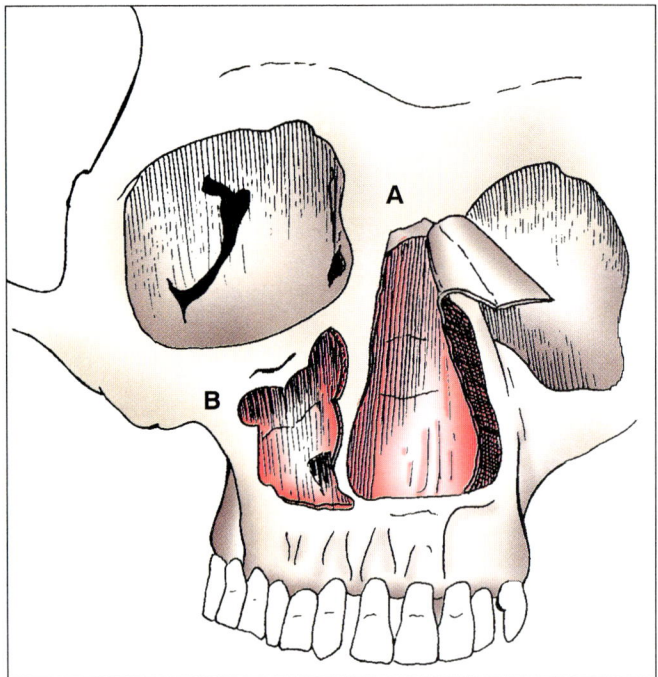

Fig. 7.30 A. Rhinoplasty type cuts are made to allow reflection and preservation of the nasal bone thus minimizing postoperative deformity. **B.** Creation of defect in anterior maxilla

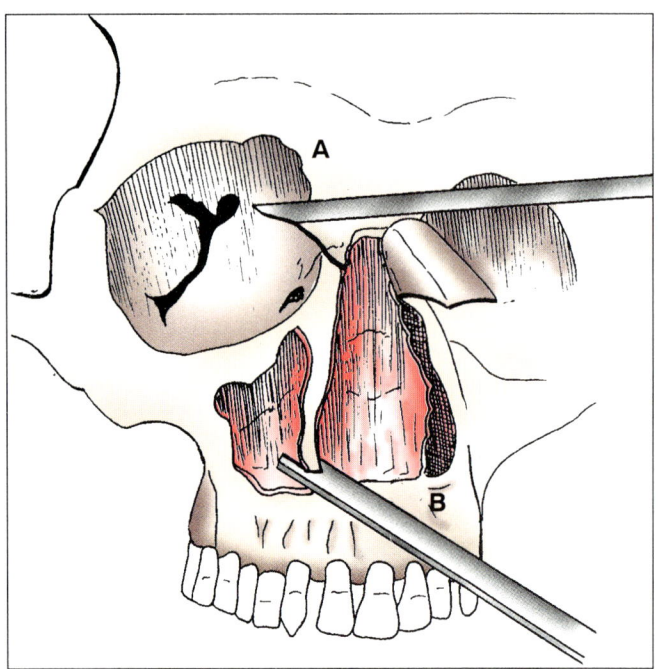

Fig. 7.31 A. Superior osteotomy cut is placed just below the fronto ethmoid suture and extend to the region of posterior ethmoidal artery. Note - The optic nerve will be 6-10 mm posterior to this. B. Cut along the floor of the nose and maxillary aetrum, extending back to the level of posterior antral wall i.e. region of pterygoid plates.

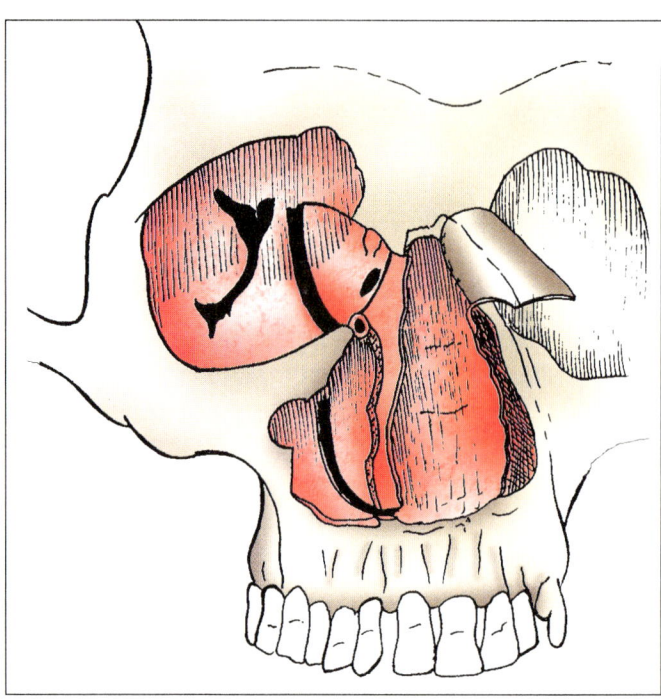

Fig. 7.32 Medial infraorbital rim is linked supramedially with the posterior end of the upper osteotomy.

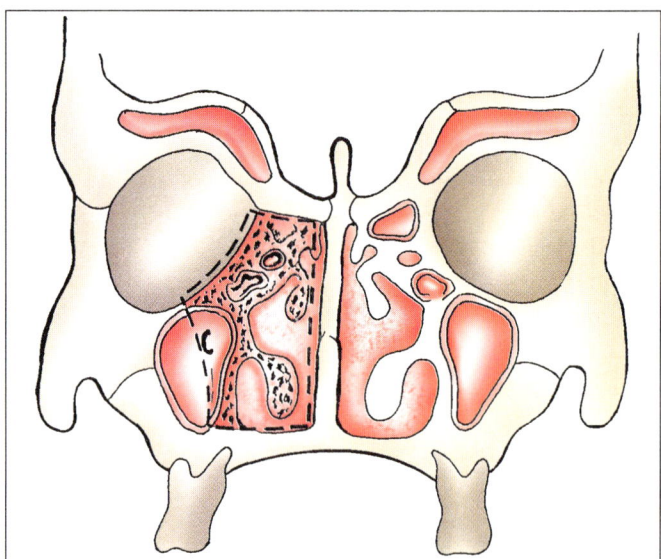

Fig. 7.33 Schematic coronal view of skull showing standard osteotomies of medial maxillectomy

Antibiotic coated gauze is used to pack the nose. The nasal bone is returned and secured. The lacrimal drainage is restored by placing silastic tubing into the sac and securing this with a purse string suture. This will be left in place for 6 weeks to form a mucosalized lining to secure adequate drainage. The medial canthal ligament and periosteum is secured in its proper position.

Complications

The most common complication found is epiphora. The amount of epiphora has improved with DCR management of the lacrimal sac at the time of surgery. Other complications discribed are transient diplopia, mucocele, CSF leakage, epistaxis, and scar formation.

TOTAL MAXILLECTOMY

Total maxillectomy is indicated for treatment of malignant tumors of the maxillary antrum. The Weber-Fergusson incision has been considered to be the standard approach for a total maxillectomy.

There are advantages of using the extended lateral rhinotomy instead of the classic Weber-Fergusson incision in patients undergoing total maxillectomy. First, by avoiding a sub ciliary incision it eliminates any disruption to the lower lid skin-muscle-tarsus complex. This minimizes lower eyelid complications, particularly ectropion and prolonged eyelid edema. Additionally, its postoperative cosmetic appearance is superior to that of the Weber-Fergusson incision. Another advantage of the extended lateral rhinotomy incision is that it avoids a trifurcation or an acute angle at the medial canthal region. This reduces the frequency of skin break- down and cheek flap tip necrosis at the medial canthal area. This is especially important for previously irradiated patients, who are more prone to develop medial canthal dehiscence. Similarly, because the vascularity of the thin lower eyelid skin is not affected by the lateral rhinotomy incision, patients who undergo orbital floor reconstruction with implants such as titanium mesh or porous polyethylene (Medpore) have less chance of developing implant exposure.

The extended lateral rhinotomy incision has several functional and cosmetic advantages and provides an adequate approach for a safe oncologic resection. Extension of the lateral rhinotomy incision beneath the medial eyebrow shifts the fulcrum of rotation of the soft tissue flap superiorly and laterally, which enhances lateral exposure. In fact, the lateral extent of the exposure obtained by the extended lateral rhinotomy is not different from that obtained with a classic Weber-Fergusson incision.

Whichever incision is used, elevation of the facial flap is usually done in the subperiosteal plane. However, if the tumor has invaded the anterior wall of the maxillary antrum, a supraperiosteal plane is used. Occasionally, if it is involved with tumor, the skin overlying the maxilla is included with the specimen. The globe is protected, a temporary tarsorrhaphy stitch. The periorbital is dissected along the medial, inferior, and lateral orbital walls.

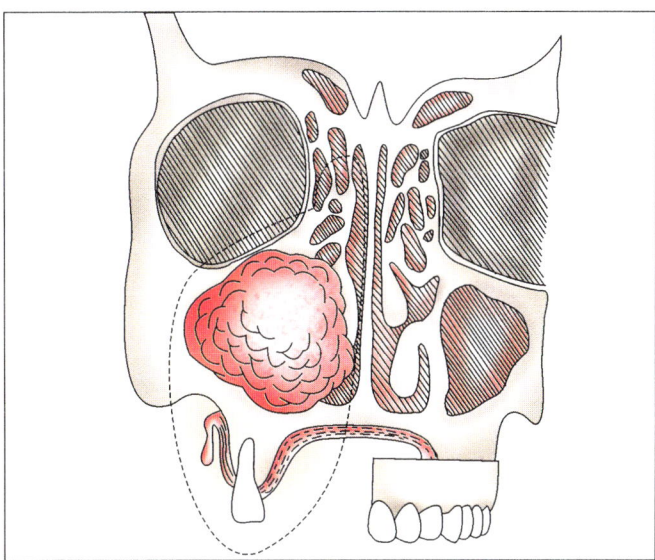

Fig. 7.34 Showing extent of dissection in total maxillectomy

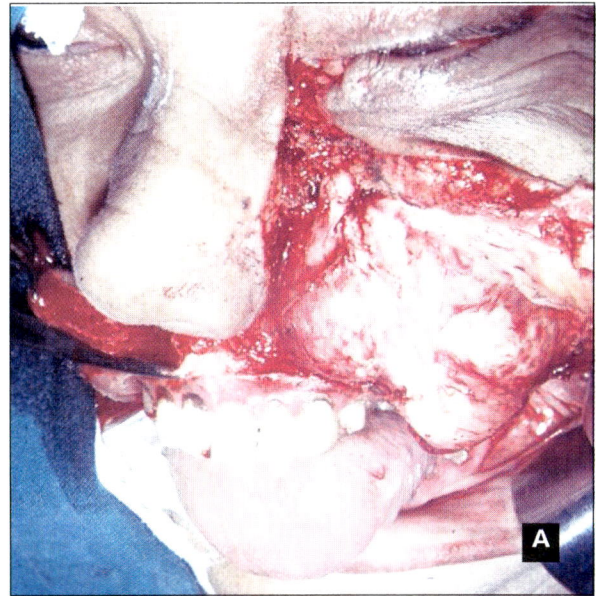

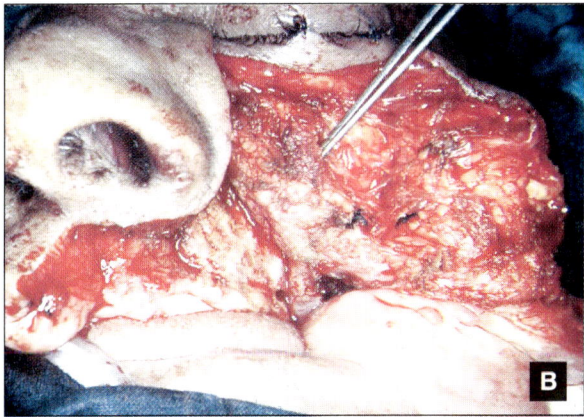

Fig. 7.35 A & B showing extent of dissection in total maxillectomy with Weber fergusson incision

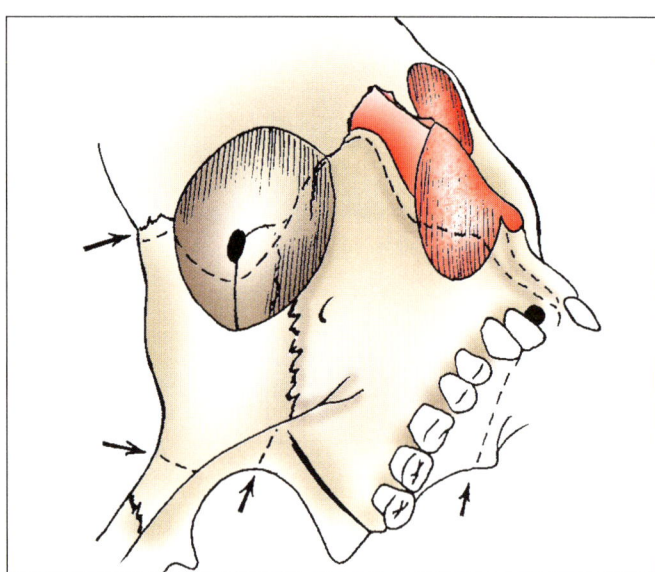

Fig. 7.36 Maxillectomy: Sites of division of bony struts

Lateral osteotomies are performed along the frontal and temporal processes of the zygoma. Osteotomies are done along the frontal process of the maxilla and along the medial orbital wall just inferior. The ipsilateral central incisor should be preserved, if possible, to enhance prosthesis retention. Finally, after the internal maxillary artery has been identified, ligated and transected, at its entrance through the pterygomaxillary fissure a posterior osteotomy is done to disarticulate the maxilla from the pterygoid plates. The maxilla is delivered by anteroinferior traction, while the remaining soft tissue attachments are cut with a curved heavy scissors. Bleeding is usually encountered at this point and is controlled by temporary packing of the cavity, followed by electrocoagulation of bleeding mucosal surfaces or ligature of bleeding points.

The pterygoid plexus of veins may be a source of persistent bleeding and can be managed by hemostatic 'figure-of-8' sutures and Surgical packing. Bleeding is usually minimized if the internal maxillary artery is ligated before; the posterior osteotomy is done along the pterygomaxillary fissure.

Any remnants of bone and mucosa of the ethmoid air cells are removed, and a wide sphenoidotomy is performed. The pterygoid plates are then removed with a burr or bone rongeurs. The pterygoid musculature is then sewn over the bony remnants of the pterygoid plates. The surgical defect is lined with a split-thickness skin graft covering the periorbital, pterygoid musculature, and deep aspect of the cheek flap. This minimizes the formation of granulation tissue in the surgical cavity, prepares the surgical defect to receive an obturator, and reduces soft tissue contracture of

the overlying cheek. A bolster formed of iodoform (Xeroform) gauze is used to pack the cavity, aiding in hemostasis and skin graft immobilization. A preformed surgical prosthesis is then wired or screwed to the remaining contralateral maxilla. Alternatively, it can be wired to the remaining dentition. The obturator helps in stabilizing the bolster, as well as in promoting early postoperative speech and swallowing rehabilitation.

As an alternative to a prosthetic obturator, the palatal and maxillary defects may be reconstructed with the use of microvascular free flaps. Reconstruction of the orbital floor may be necessary to provide adequate support of the eye, especially if the periorbital has been resected. The indications and pros and cons of the various reconstructive options are discussed later under Reconstruction and Rehabilitation. The medial canthal ligament is reattached to the nasal bone in its anatomic position to prevent telecanthus. Closure of the facial incisions is done in a meticulous multilayered fashion. The temporary tarsorrhaphy stitch is removed at the end of surgery.

MODIFIED BARBOSA APPROACH

The Barbosa approach was modified by adding a lateral incision in the mandibular gingivobuccal fold from the canine tooth to the retromolar area. This technique is especially useful for tumors in the pterygopalatine fossa extending into the maxillary sinus.

Contraindications

- Poor physical condition.
- Spread of the tumor into the nasopharynx.
- Involvement of the 6th, 9th, 10th or 12th cranial nerves, or radiologic evidence of destruction of the lesser wing of the sphenoid or invasion of the middle cranial fossa.

Inaccessible metastasis

Incision

The first incision divides the upper lip in the midline, passes under the nasal pyramid, and extends laterally, reaching the level of the temporomandibular joint. An incision is then made along the maxillary buccogingival fold on the involved side, running from the midline to the retromolar area. Another incision is made along the mandibular buccogingival fold on the involved side, running from canine to retromolar area (Fig. 7.37).

Steps

- Flap is reflected to expose the anterior aspect of

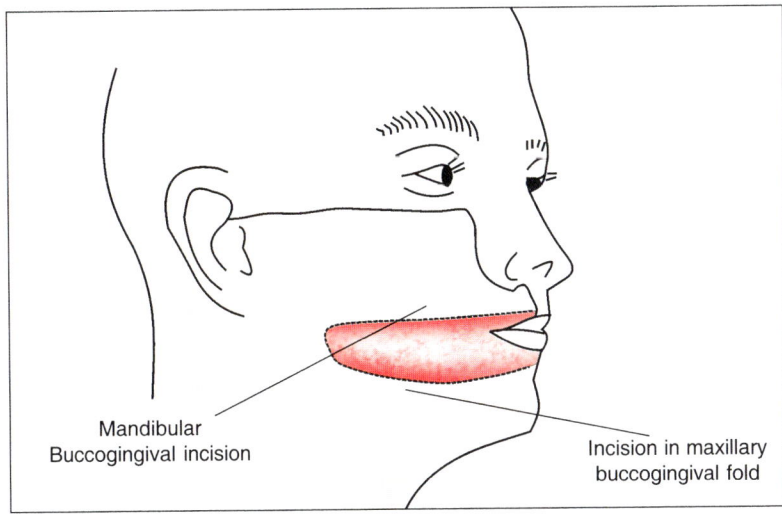

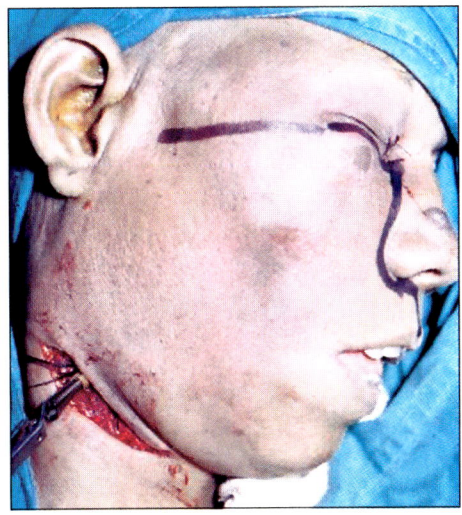

Fig. 7.37 Showing the skin marking for the incision

maxilla, inferior half of the orbital rim, the inferior portion of the temporalis, zygomatic bone and zygomatic arch, external aspect of temporomandibular joint, and masseter and the mandibular ramus (Fig.7.38).

- Mandible is retracted anteriorly, parotid gland retracted posteriorly, a space is thus created to isolate internal maxillary artery, which is tied and divided.

- Masseter is sectioned just below zygomatic arch, temporalis muscle is sectioned just above zygomatic

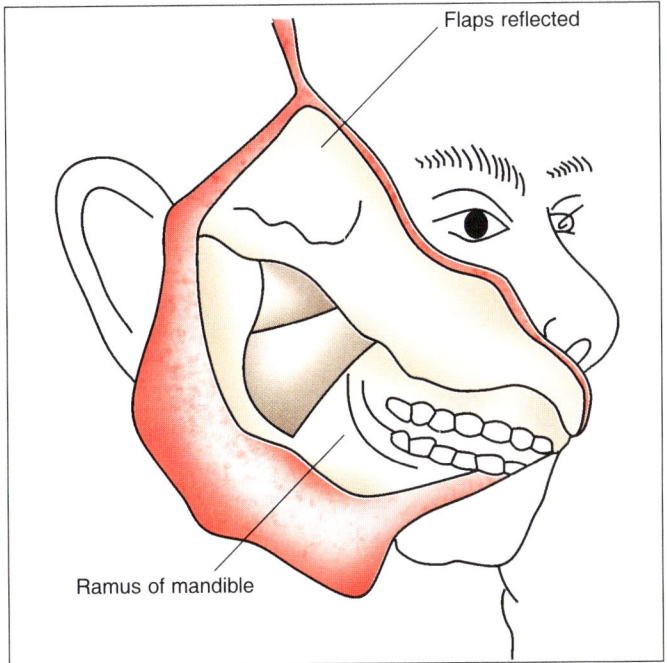

Fig. 7.38 Showing exposure of anterior aspect of maxilla, orbital rim, zygomatic process, inferior portion of temporalis, TMJ and mandibular ramus

arch, zygomatic arch is cut at both ends but not removed.

- Mandibular ramus is sectioned transversely above the angle of the mandible and temporomandibular joint is disarticulated (Fig. 7.39a).

- Lateral pterygoid muscle is raised to expose external aspect of tumor, inferior part of temporal fossa, external aspect of orbit, lateral surface of lateral pterygoid process, pterygopalatine fossa and the lateral surface of medial pterygoid muscle to achieve adequate margin at posterior limit of the tumour.

- Central incisor tooth on involved side is removed. Incision on the hard palate is carried from this point upto the hard - soft palate junction, then laterally to meet the previous incision on buccogingival sulcus.

- Nasal process of maxilla is divided; nasal cartilages are separated from the maxilla.

- Orbital contents elevated by blunt subperiosteal dissection to expose inferior orbital palate.

- Lateral edge or orbit is divided just above zygoma.

- Aleveolus and hard palate are divided just away from the midline.

- Fibers of medial pterygoid muscle attached to the pterygoid processes are cut of remove the specimen (Fig. 7.39b).

- Few remaining soft tissue attachments are divided and entire specimen is out.

Advantages

- Less bleeding
- Adequate margins obtained

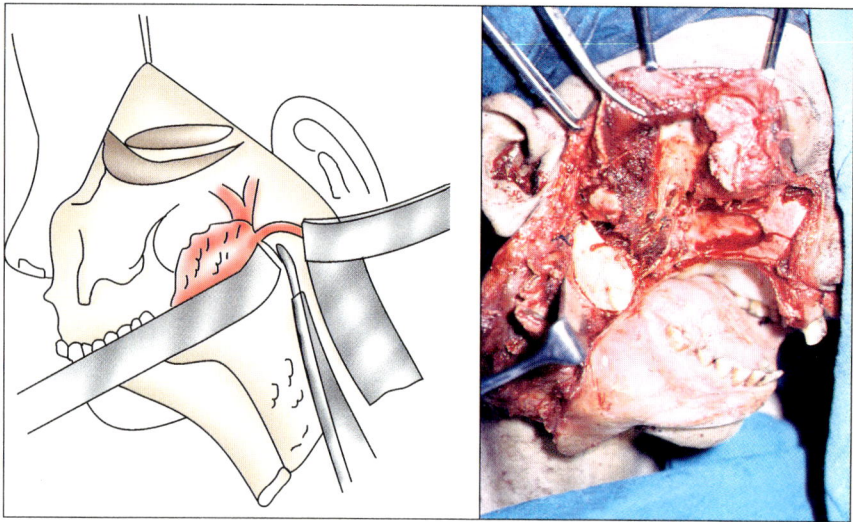

Fig. 7.39a Showing isolation of maxillary artery and its ligation and division

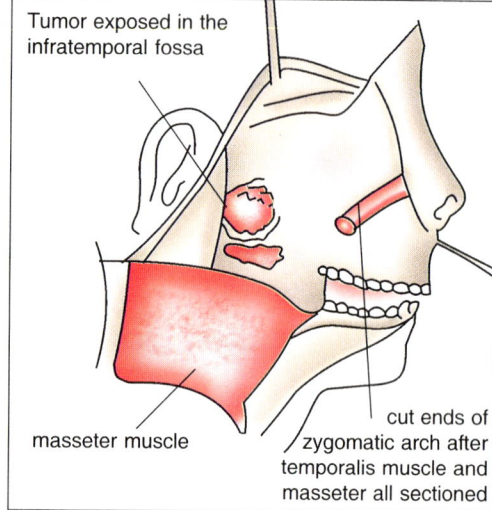

Fig. 7.39b Tumor exposed in the infratemporal fossa

FACIAL TRANSLOCATION APPROACH

Indications

For extensive tumors involving the pterygopalatine fossa, infratemporal fossa spreading superiorly through infraorbital fossa, orbital apex, supraorbital fissure into the middle cranial fossa adjacent to cavernous sinus.

Surgical technique (Fig. 7.40)

- Hemicoronal incision.
- Lateral rhinotomy with lip splitting incision.
- Pre-auricular incision.
- The horizontal incision connects the lateral rhinotomy incision with the hemicoronal incision to create superior and inferior soft tissue flaps.
- At this stage the frontal branch of the facial nerve is identified and tagged and divided to be reconnected later on.
- The horizontal incision, which transects the lower lid fornix through the conjunctiva, and lateral canthus meet the vertical, horizontal and pre-auricular incisions.
- The cheek flap is reflected inferiorly to the level of hard palate after the elevation of maxillary periosteum (Fig. 7.41)
- The fronto temporal scalp flap is reflected towards midline.
- The craniofacial skeleton is exposed from the midline (forehead, nasion, nasal process of maxilla, superior, lateral and inferior orbital rims, maxilla and zygomatic arch.

- Osteotomies of the orbito-maxillary skeleton are performed to free the anterior face of maxilla, malar eminence, zygomatic arch, inferior and lateral orbital rims, as well as the orbital floor (Fig. 7.42).
- An oblique subperiosteal osteotomy at the base of coronoid process of mandible helps to translocate the temporalis muscle, inferiorly, which is used to augment the orbital floor
- Nasopharynx and Pterygoid plates are exposed (Fig. 7.43)
- Craniotomy can be performed, to provide additional access to the intracranial extension of the tumour (Fig. 7.44)

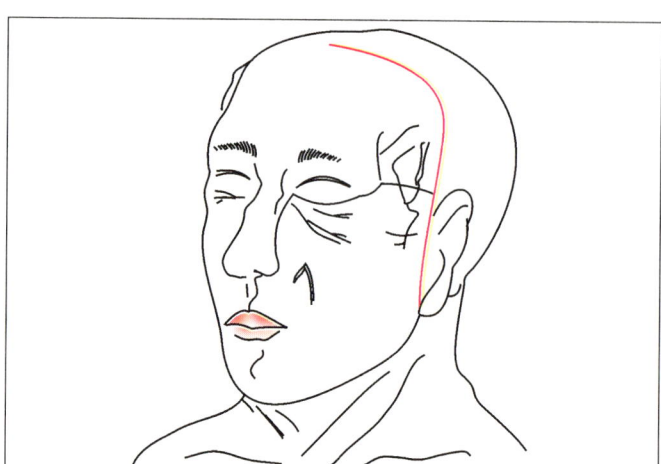

Fig. 7.40 Incision for facial translocation

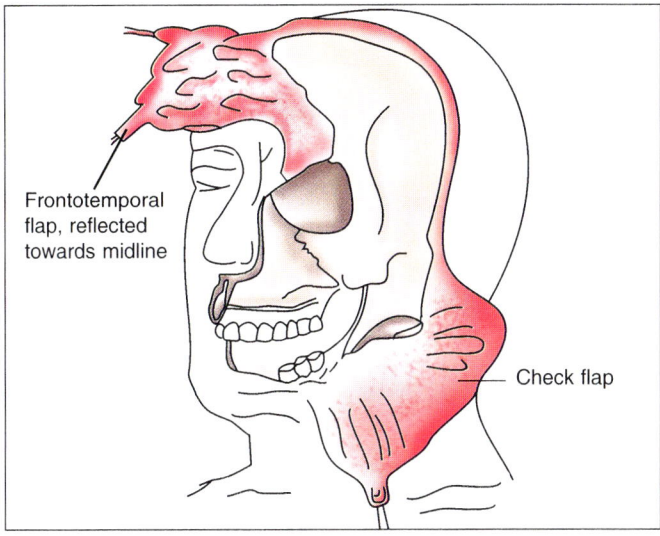

Fig. 7.41 Facial flap been elevated to expose facial skeleton

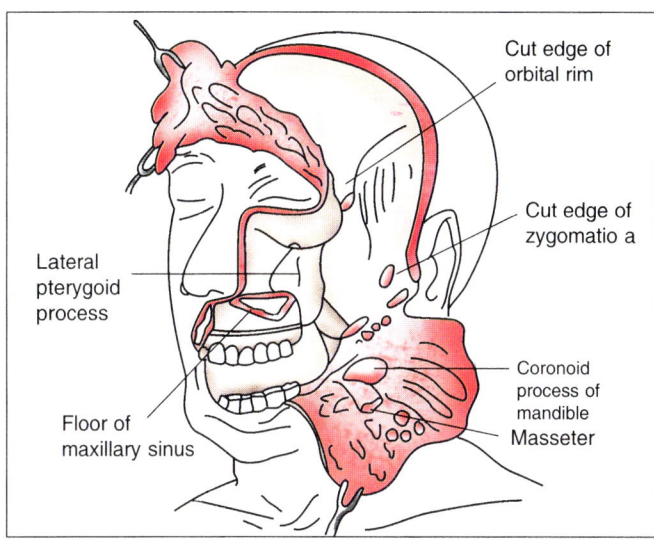

Fig. 7.43 Bone is removed and nasopharyngo and pterygoid plates have been exposed

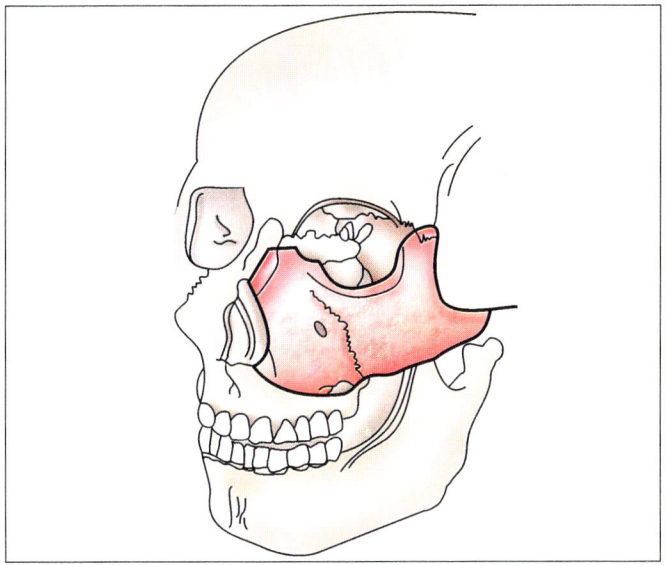

Fig. 7.42 Marked area shows region of bone removed as single unit

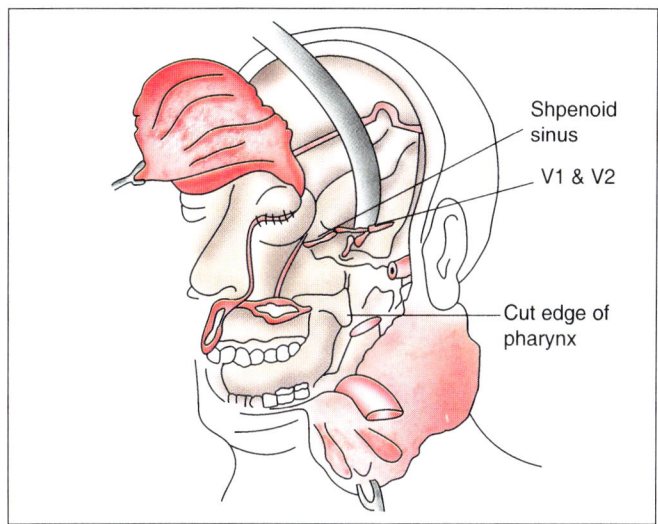

Fig. 7.44 Craniotomy been performed to provide access to intracranial space

- The internal maxillary artery is ligated before manipulating the tumor mass.
- Intra cranial part of the tumour is operated by the neurosurgeon under an operating microscope.
- After tumour removal, the temporalis fascia is placed below the orbit to give support as it also occludes part of infra-temporal fossa.
- The zygomatico-orbital maxillary skeletal complex removed during the procedure is replaced back and fixed with mini-plates.
- The conjunctiva of the lower fornix is sutured.
- The facial nerve is reconnected and sutured.

Advantages

- The infratemporal fossa, nasal cavity, nasopharynx, sphenoid, pharyngo-palatine fossa and clivus may all be reached clinically within a single surgical field, which may be modified to suit the individual lesion.
- The facial translocation approach is superior to any other **approach to antero lateral skull base,** which extends from the contralateral Eustachian tube, along the posterior pharynx, clivus, as well as the anterior wall of sphenoid sinus, through the ipsilateral pterygopalatine fossa, infra temporal fossa up to the geniculate ganglion.

Easy access for complete tumour removal as well as visualization of practically all surgical margins of the tumour.

- The procedure is considered as an excellent approach to completely excenterate angiofibroma, extending to the nasopharynx, superior oblique fissure, cavernous sinus, infra temporal fossa and pterygopalatine fossa.

Disadvantages

- Reconstruction of the naso lacrimal system is necessary.
- Horizontal scar across the temple is unavoidable.
- Anastomosis of the forehead branch of the facial nerve is required.
- There is anaesthesia of the cheek due to resection of the inferior orbital nerve.
- There is a need to perform temporary lateral tarsorraphy.

Complications

- Bone graft necrosis in patient with post-operative radiotherapy.
- Facial hematoma
- Delayed facial cellulitis
- Aspiration pneumonia
- Local recurrence

MIDFACIAL SPLIT APPROACH

Used for very extensive tumors involving central compartment and extending into clivus, craniovertebral junction or infratemporal fossa, and parapharyngeal space (lateral compartment). Incision are made as described in Fig. 7.45, following which facial soft tissue flaps are reflected laterally to expose orbitonasomaxillary skeleton.

Horizontal incision across the nasion for access to upper orbits.

Midline nasal incision separating upper and lower lateral cartilages to expose the septum. Carried inferiorly along one side of philtrum splitting the upper lip.

Gingivobuccal incision as shown in figure by dotted line gives bilateral maxillary exposure.

- Osteotomies may be made to include hard palate to provide access to clivus, nasopharynx and oropharynx.
- Tumour is separated from surrounding attachment and delivered.

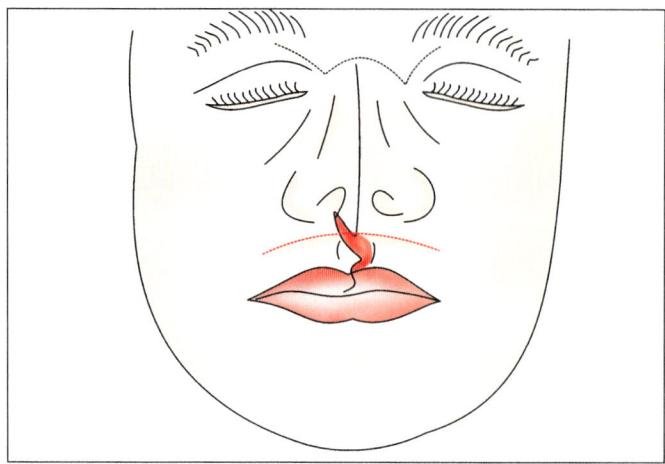

Fig. 7.45 Showing incisions for midfacial split

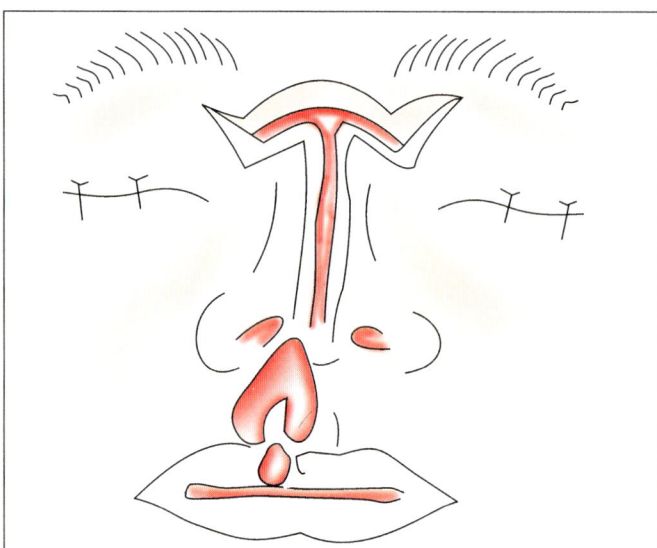

Fig. 7.46 Partially developed facial soft tissue flap with attached nasal cartilage

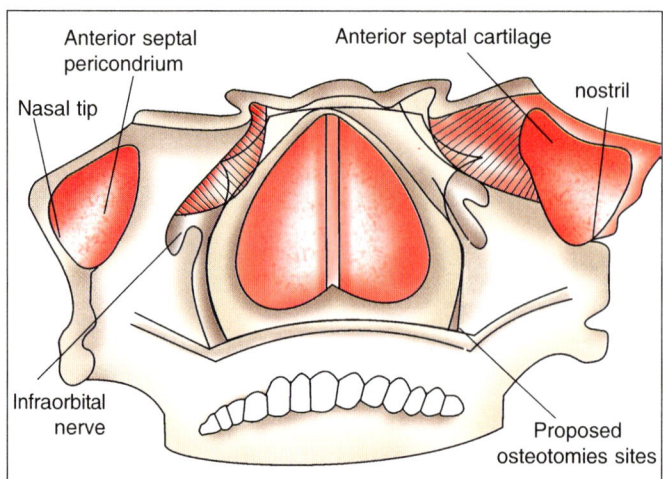

Fig. 7.47 Facial soft tissue flaps are reflected laterally to expose orbitonaso-maxillary skeleton.

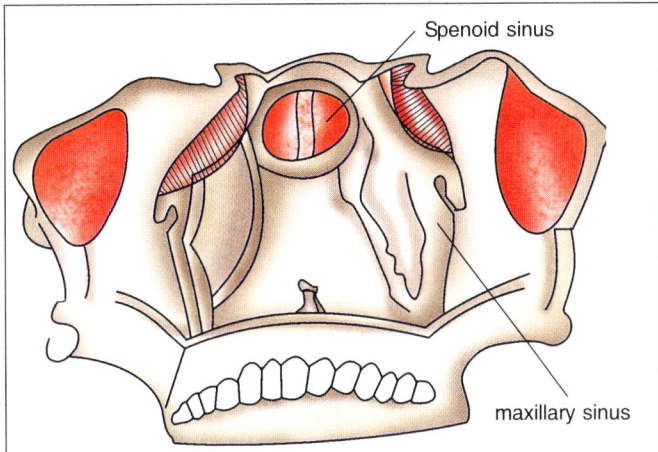

Fig. 7.48 Osteotomies are made and midfacial exposure achieved after removal of bilateral anterior walls of maxilla, nasal bones, medial and inferior orbital walls.

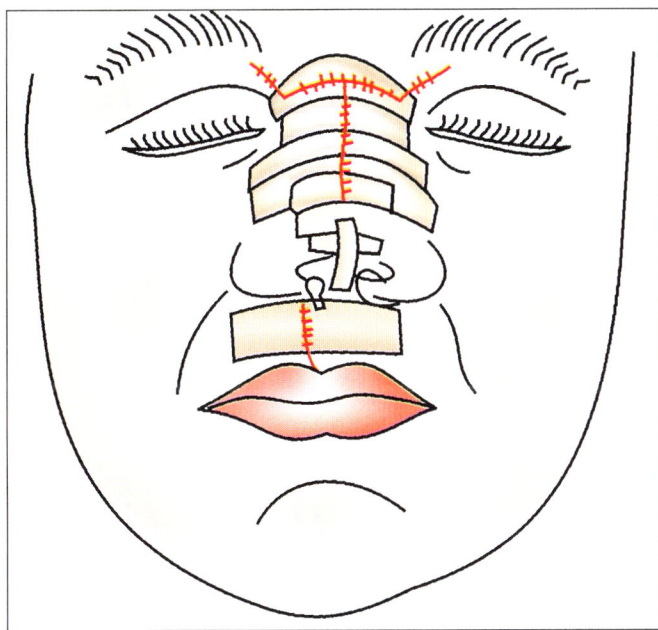

Fig. 7.49 Showing final closure. Orbitonasomaxillary bone segments are replaced

- Orbitonasomaxillary bone segments are replaced and secured with microplates (Fig.7.49).

- Soft tissue closure done and closure of wound in 2 layers is done.

- Adhesive strips are applied and nasal stents (silastic) are used for 1 week postoperatively.

These extended transantral approaches i.e. lateral rhinotomy, Weber Fergusson, can be used for extensive lesions with extranasopharyngeal spread.

DENKER AND KAHLER APPROACH

Extended Caldwel-Luc procedure

Combine transpalatal with transantral approach. Bone is dissected from face of maxillary pyriform aperture, ascending process of maxilla with removal of the lateral nasal wall to give wide exposure.

TRANSPALATAL APPROACHES

WILSON'S TRANSPALATAL APPROACH

Indication

- Tumors
  - **Nasopharyngeal:** Angiofibroma, Lipoma, Dermoids, Teratoma
  - **Others: Chordoma**, Sphenoid tumors, Chonal Atresia, Vidian neurectomy, Inflammatory lesions, Sphenoiditis, Mycotic infections, Nasopharyngeal strictures.

SARDANA'S APPROACH (Bhatia Sardana)

Angiofibroma without intracranial extension is the ideal lesion for removal by transpalatal route. For lateral extensions of the tumour into pterygopalatine and infratemporal fossa and extensions into cheek, this approach can be combined by sublabial approach, Sardana's approach 1965. In which the cheek mass is approached sublabially and nasopharyngeal, infratemporal, pterygopalatine fossae extensions by transpalatal or transantral routes with Sardana's separate sublabial incision for cheek extension extended to retromolar trigone area to access pterygo maxillary and buccal spaces.

Disadvantage

Bleeding from pterygoid plexus resulting in unpleasant postoperative cheek hematoma.

MISHRA AND BHATIA'S MODIFICATION OF TRANSPALATAL APPROACH (1964)

Transpalatal incision can be extended in sublabial plane curving around the maxillary tuberosity. This gives a good exposure and easier dissection of tumour from areas of cheek and infratemporal fossa after the pterygoid plates are removed.

Technique

Position: Supine with neck hyperextended. GA by orotracheal tube.

Dingman self-retaining oral retractor applied for maximum view of palate and oropharynx. 'U' shaped incision begun at level of 2nd to 3rd molar carried along alveolar edge keeping anterior and lateral to greater palatine artery (Fig. 7.50).

Flap is elevated using freer dissector. Posterior hard palate is removed with rongeurs as much as necessary for exposure. Posterior nasal septum may be removed if desired (Fig. 7.51).

- For posterolateral exposure bone of greater palatine foramen posterior to greater palatine artery is removed and one or both greater palatine arteries divided.

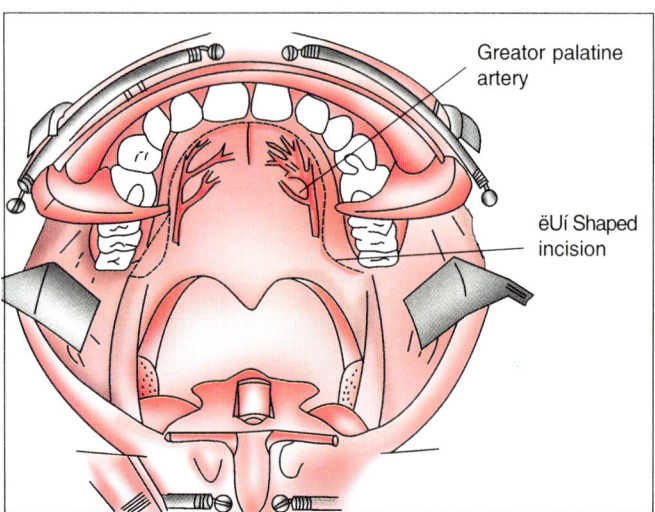

Fig. 7.50 U shape incision for preservation of palatal length

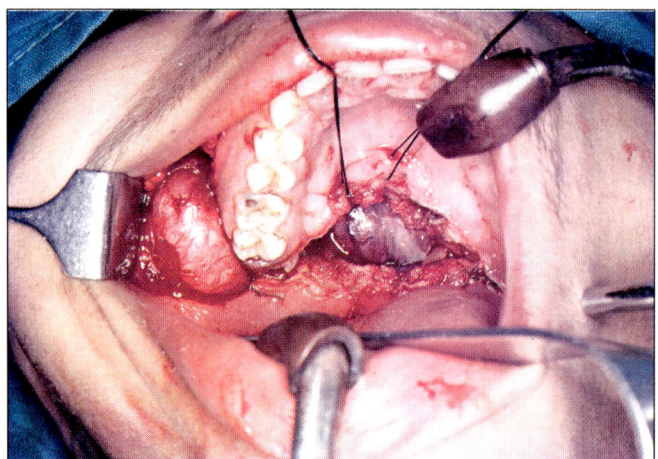

Fig. 7.51 Nasopharyngeal angiofibroma seen behind the soft palate

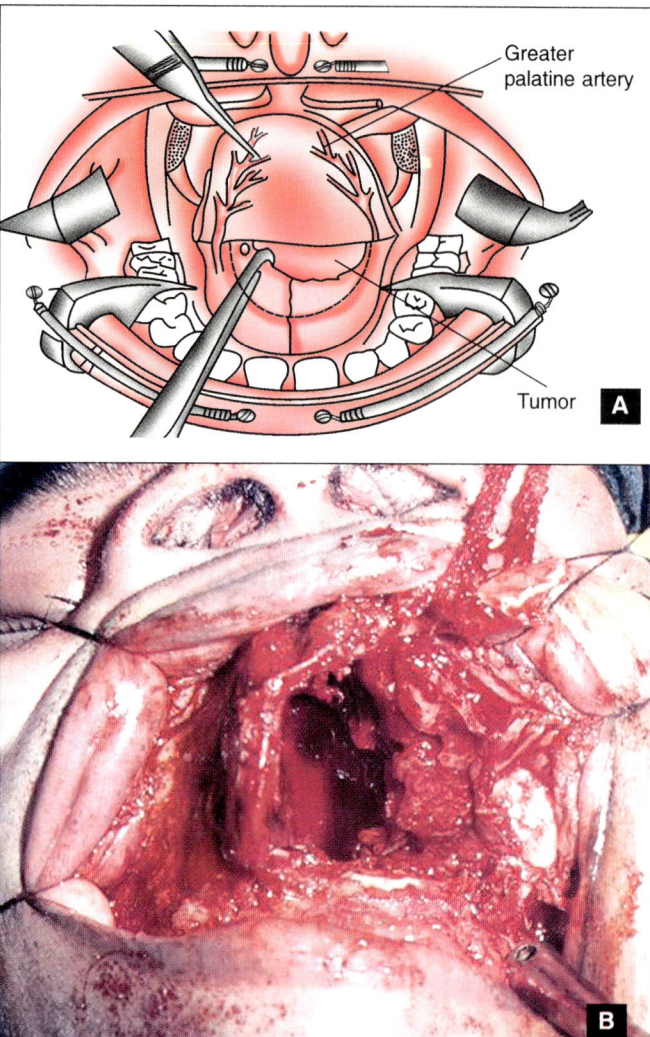

Fig. 7.52 Posterior hard plate is resected to expose the nasopharyngeal tumor

- Further exposure may also be sought by extending incision into gingivobuccal sulcus into expose posterolateral aspects, (Bhatia and Mishra) pterygoid plates are removed for further exposure of lateral extension.

- Nasopharynx can be packed with BIPP once tumour is out and hemostasis is achieved.

- Mucoperiosteal flap replaced (Fig. 7.53).

Variations of transpalatal incisions

- Midline palatal incision devised by Dibble, King and Alonso et al. can lead to palatal shortening velopharyngeal insufficiency

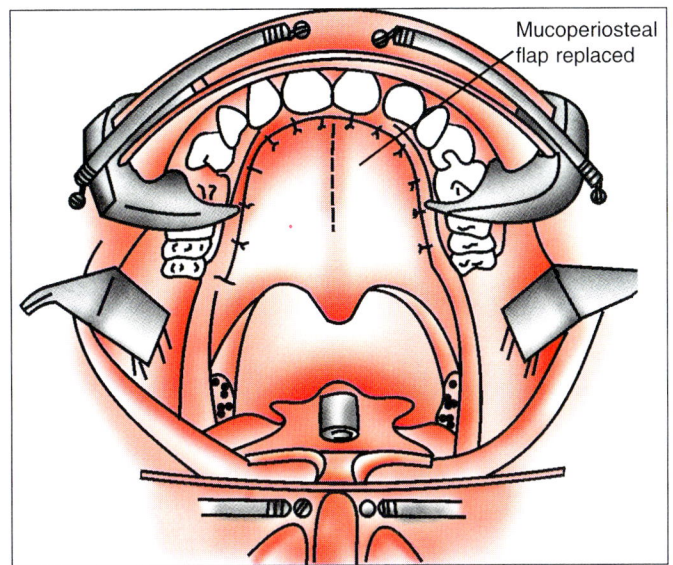

Fig. 7.53 Showing final closure. Mucoperiosteal flap replaced and sutured

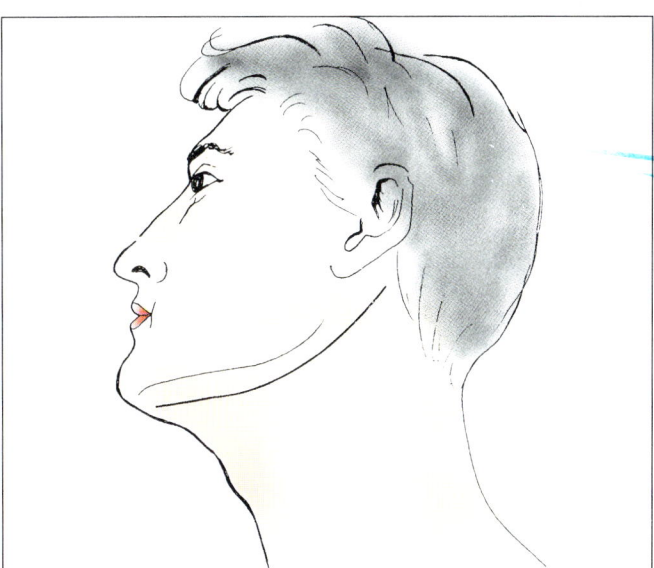

Fig. 7.54 The incision for the inferior approach

- U-shaped incision as described earlier although preserves palatal length, the exposure is limited.
- S-shaped incision avoids palatal shortening and also gives excellent exposure.
- However, closure is difficult due to increased thickness of lateral soft palate and greater incisional length.

Complications

1. Palatal fistula: Scar contracture leading to palatal shortening and velopharyngeal insufficiency, patient develops.
2. Hypernasality of speech.
3. CSF leak and meningitis in case of inadvertent dural breach.

TRANS CERVICAL APPROACH

INFERIOR APPROACH

Indications

- Infra temporal fossa lesions
- Parapharyngeal space lesions

Incision

Horizontal incision just above the level of hyoid bone extending from midline up to the posterior border of sternocleidomastoid muscle (7.54).

Steps

- Submandibular gland is exercised. Part of tumour extension of parapharyngeal space is approached and plane of separation created by blunt dissection between the tumour on one hand and inner aspect of medial pterygoid muscle and deep lobe of parotid on the other.
- Much of the procedure is blind as upper part of tumour is largely out of view. To enhance exposure of infra temporal fossa, medial pterygoid muscle is divided at its insertion into the mandible.
- Medially and anteromedially tumour is separated from superior constrictor muscle.
- Division of horizontal ramus of mandible can be done to give exposure to upper part of infratemporal fossa. In this process inferior alveolar artery can be damaged and hemostasis has to be achieved.
- After division of mandible, ascending ramus is everted upward and laterally. Tumour is delivered out with blunt dissection. Mandible is rewired and wound closed in layers with suction drain in site.

Disadvantages

- Restricted access to the superior part of infratemporal fossa due to long distance between submandibular triangle and skull base.

Complications

- Damage to mandibular branch of facial nerve during removal of submandibular gland or due to excessive traction on upper flap.

- Permanent mental anaesthesia.
- Instability due to improper fixation of mandibular fragments.
- Approaches to pterygopalatine fossa.

BILLER'S MIDLINE TRANSMANDIBULAR OROPHARYNGEAL APPROACH (MANDIBULAR SWING)

Indications

- Lesions of lateral compartment of skull base that is involving nasopharynx, parapharyngeal space, infratemporal fossa and pterygomaxillary space.
- Lesions of medial compartment of skull base that is sphenoid bone, clivus, occipital condyle, upper cervical vertebrae.
- Midline Mandibulotomy + Division of soft tissue of floor of mouth + Division of suprahyoid musculature provides exposure of infratemporal fossa, roof of parapharyngeal space, inferior surface of petrous temporal bone.
- Division of eustachian tube at bony-cartilagenous junction with attached muscles permits pharynx to be elevated in prevertebral space and retracted to contralateral side. This gives exposure to posterior nasal cavities, nasopharynx, sphenoid sinus, clivus and upper cervical vertebrae.
- Elevation of palate + Removal of pterygoid plates gives broad surgical exposure for resection of variety of lesions.

Steps

Preliminary tracheostomy and endotracheal anaesthesia.

Incision

- Starting from the midline of lower lip, extending in a staggered fashions from vermilion to submental crease extending downwards to hyoid bone and then horizontally backwards over the sternocleidomastoid and then superiorly to the mastoid.
- Lower lip divided. Inferior labial artery ligated.
- Neck incision deepened to deep fascia investing the submandibular gland taking care to avoid injury to mandibular branch of VII nerve.
- Digastric tendon is detached and mylohyoid muscle is divided and reflected superiorly along the submandibular gland (Fig. 7.55).

- Carotid sheath contents, hypoglossal and accessory nerves are identified.
- Periosteum over mandibular symphysis is elevated. Mandibular osteotomy done from central incisor teeth downward in a staircase fasion up to inferior border of mandible. Two burr holes made on either side of cut edges of bone for repair at the later stage.
- Soft tissue of floor of mouth is incised in midline between Wharton's ducts and incision is carried up to anterior tonsillar pillar (Fig. 7.55)

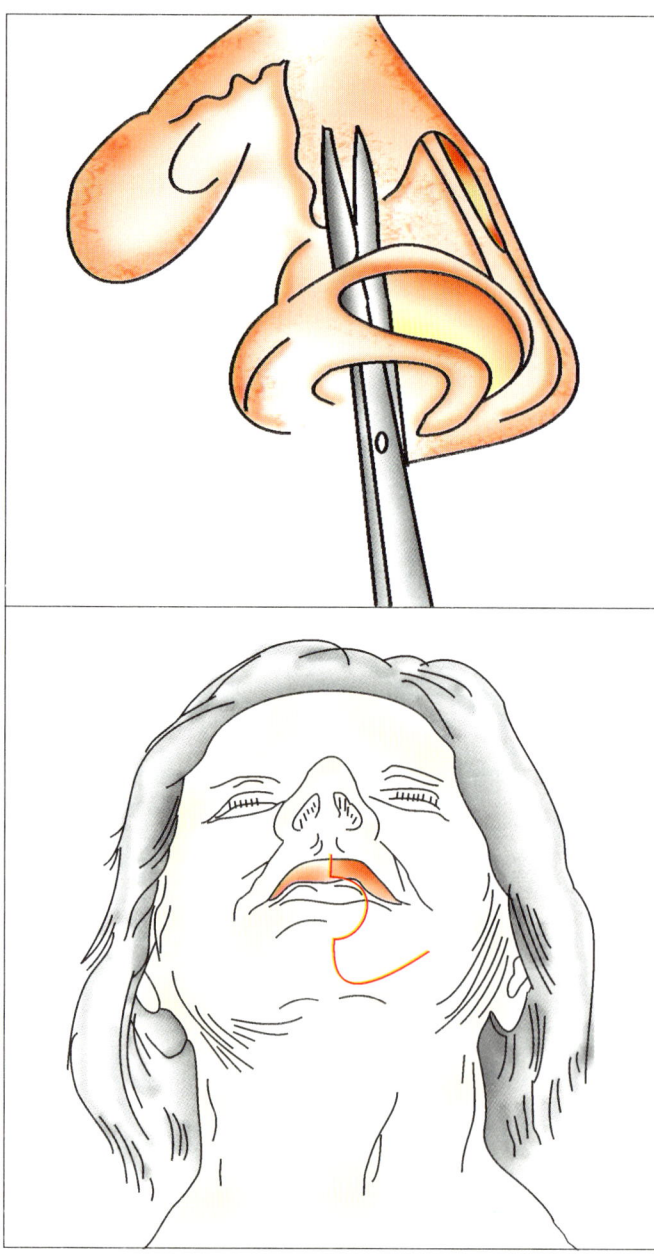

Fig. 7.55 Showing incison for Biller's approach

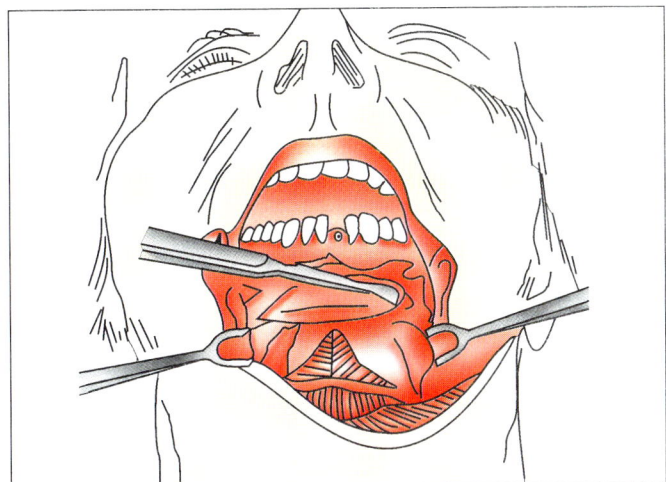

Fig. 7.56 Showing incison for Biller's approach

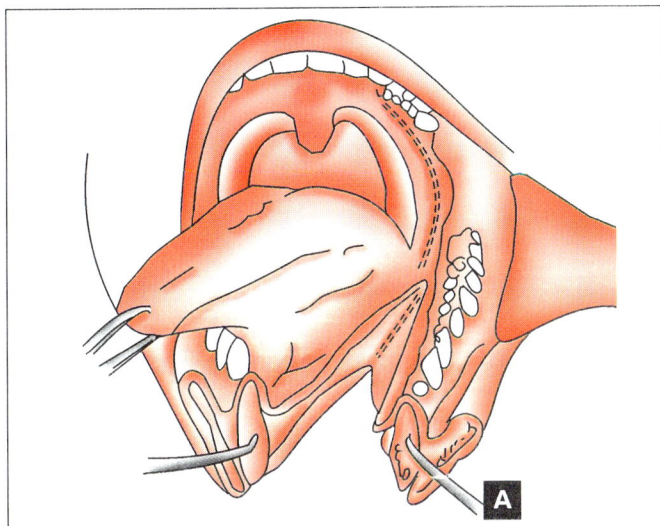

Fig. 7.57 A Soft tissue of floor of the mouth incised.

- Division of Wharton's duct and submandibular ganglion with preservation of lingual nerve and hypoglossal nerve facilitates lateral rotation of mandible. This provides access to infratemporal fossa and parapharyngeal space.

- ECA divided and ligated if remained.

- Styloid process identified. Its ligamentous and muscular attachments are sectioned. Dissection medial to styloid process exposes ICA, IJV and X, XI, XII cranial nerves. These are traced up to skull base.

- Intra oral incision extended up to tuberosity. Mucoperiosteum over hard plate elevated and posterior border of hard palate removed with rongeurs.

- Nasal mucosa elevated over medial pterygoid plate. Lingual nerve identified and traced superiorly. Foramen ovale identified.

- Medial pterygoid muscle divided close to its origin.

- Now cartilagenous Eustachian tube and its attached muscles are the only structures attaching pharynx to the skull base. Cartilaginous Eustachian tube and its attached muscles are divided and pharynx retracted to the opposite side to expose clivus and cervical vertebrae.

- Pterygoid plates removal plus Removal of mucosa between nasopharynx and posterior nasal cavity exposes sphenoid sinus.

- Extension of incision from maxillary tuberosity to maxillary vestibule and removal of lateral and posterior walls of maxillary sinus exposes pterygomaxillary space (Fig. 7.58).

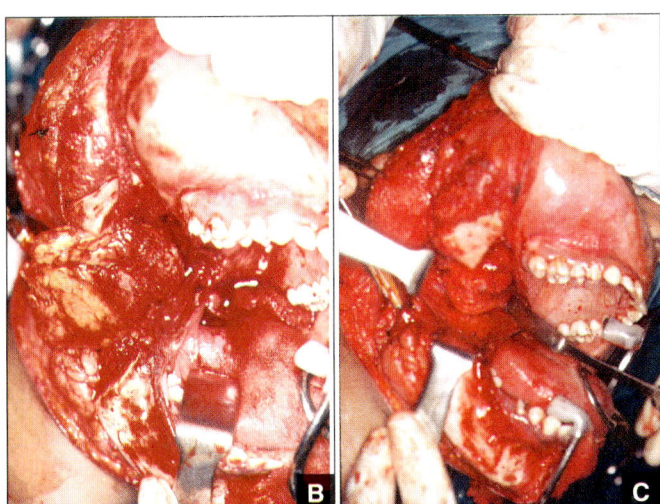

Fig. 7.57 B, C Operative photograph showing incison for Biller's approach to exposer in tumor

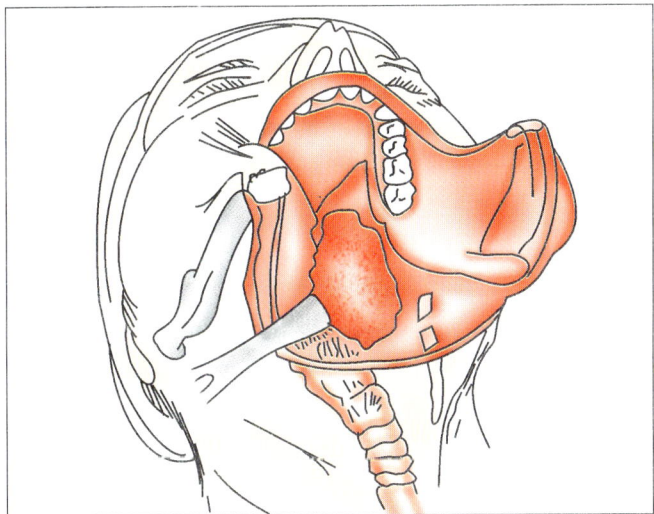

Fig. 7.58 Removal of the lateral and posterior sinus exposes pterygomaxillary space

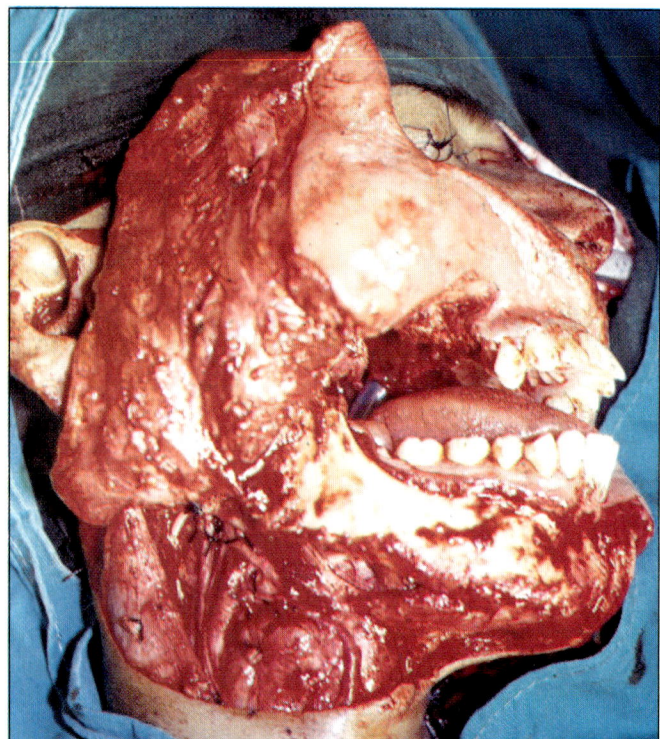

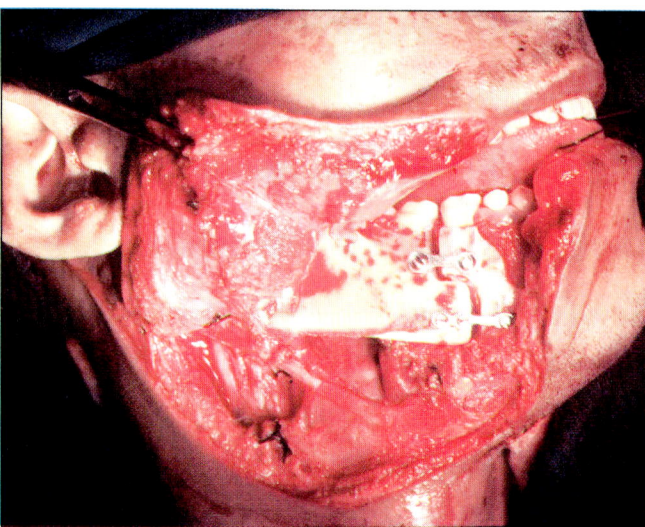

Fig. 7.59 Operative photograph showing fixation of the mandible after osteotomy

- After removal of the lesion, superior constrictor reattached to skull base.

- Posterior nasal pack placed.

- Palatal mucoperiosteal flap, floor of mouth mucosa, suprahyoid muscles and mandible repositioned and anchored with sutures.

- Lip closed in layers.

- Tracheostomy and Ryles tube inserted.

Complications

- Serous otitis media requiring myringotomy with placement of ventilation tube.
- Salivary fistula leading to infection of neck spaces.
- Meningitis
- Non-union rarely (in diabetic patients).

Advantages

- Wide exposure of both lateral and medial compartments of skull base.
- Better than lateral osteotomy approaches considering their functional and cosmetic deficits.
- A new surgical approach to extensive tumors in the pterygomaxillary fossa and the skull base.

ENDOSCOPIC APPROACHES TO SKULL BASE

Transnasal endoscopic approach for angiofibroma

It is used for limited lesions of angiofibroma arising from sphenopalatine foramen extending medially into posterior aspect of nasal cavity and laterally into pterygopalatine fossa stopping at pterygomaxillary fissure (Pre-operative embolization is a must).

Steps

- 0°4 mm nasal endoscope is used and the nasal cavity is packed with cotton pledges saturated with 1/1000 adrenaline solution and left in place for 10 minutes.

- The area anterior to the uncinate process and the anterior and posterior ends of the middle turbinate are infiltrated with 2% Xylocaine with adrenaline.

- Posterior part of the middle turbinate is carefully excised to visualize the neck of the tumour.

- Uncinate process is then incised and removed.

- Maxillary sinus ostium is identified at the bulla-uncinate angle posteriorly, and widened superiorly until the orbital floor, inferiorly until the inferior turbinate, posteriorly until the posterior wall of the maxillary sinus, to clearly visualize the posterior wall of the maxillary sinus (Fig. 7.60).

- The superior aspect of the posterior wall of the maxillary sinus is then removed from medial to lateral utilizing a large diamond burr on an angled hand piece.

- Periosteum of the pterygopalatine fossa and lateral extension of the tumour are accordingly exposed.

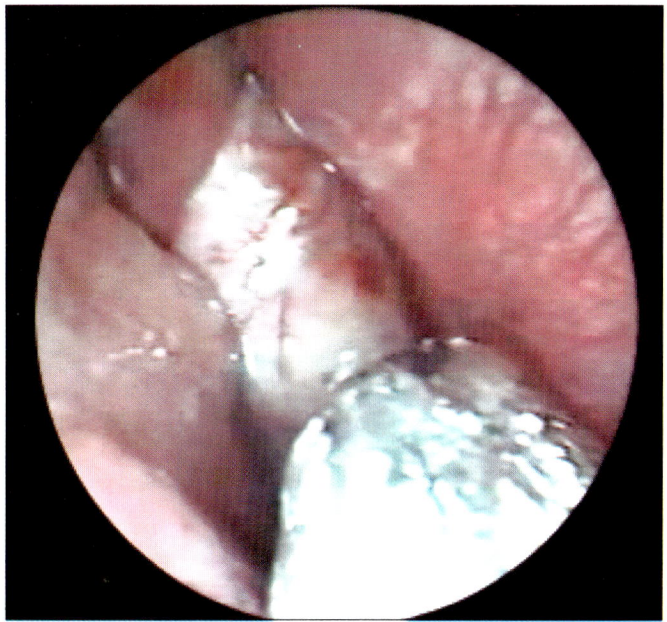 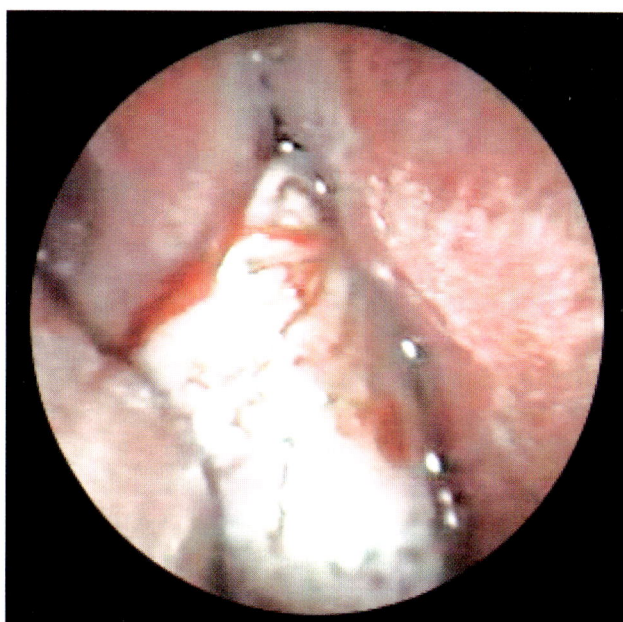

Fig. 7.60 Endoscopic view of angiofibroma

- Anterior rim of the sphenopalatine foramen is removed.

- Bipolar coagulation is used to secure bleeding points.

- Mucosa superior, posterior, medial and inferior to the tumour was cauterized a few millimetres from the attachment of the tumour.

- The mucosa was then incised and gently dissected towards the pedicle utilizing a sucker dissector. The tumour is dissected off the floor of the sphenoid sinus, he posterior margin of the nasal septum, medial pterygoid plate and perpendicular plate of the palatine bone. A bipolar cautery is then used to dissect the tumour from the periosteum of the pterygopalatine fossa. Meticulous endoscopic examination of the cavity insured complete removal of the tumour and all bleeding points are secured (Fig. 7.61).

Advantages

- Avoids external, palatal, sublabial incisions, less postoperative morbidity.

- Allows careful dissection of tumour from the medial as well as lateral extensions.

- Meticulous examination of the cavity at the end of the surgery for possibility of residual tumour and for control of bleeding points.

Disadvantages

- Done only for patients with limited lesions of Angiofibroma.

- High skill in intranasal endoscopic surgery is required.

- Surgeon, may have to resort to external approach under direct vision when access is limited during endoscopic surgery.

- Lengthy and technically difficult; needs a lot of patience (Fig. 7.62a & b).

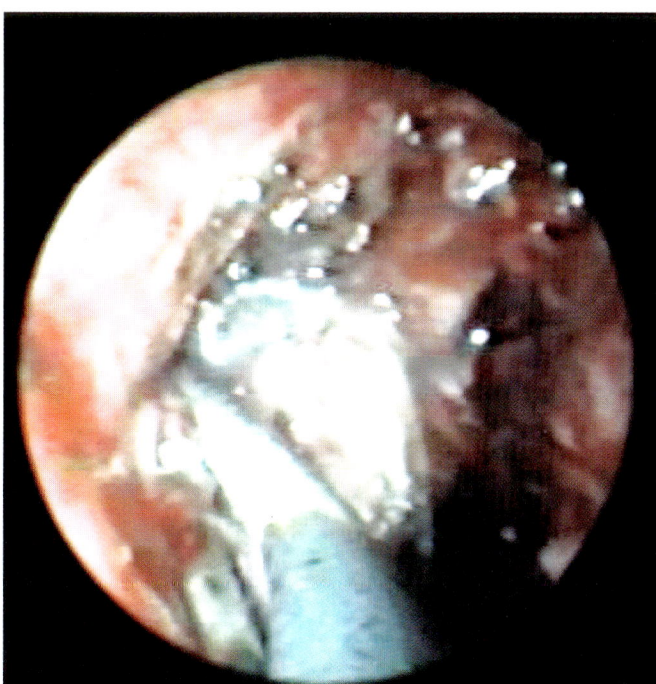

Fig. 7.61 Use of bipolar cautomy for tumor dissection

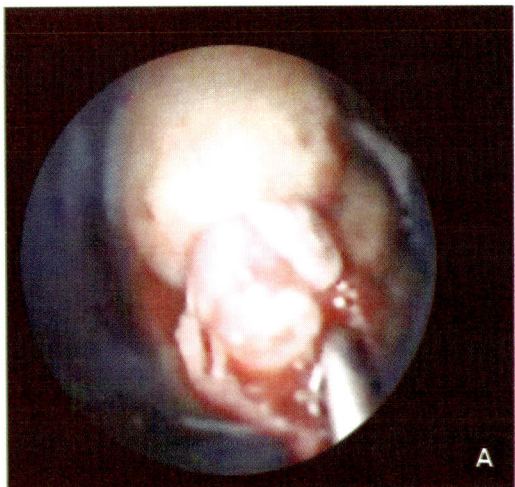

Fig. 7.62 A Endoscopic view showing tumor being pulled out from the nostril

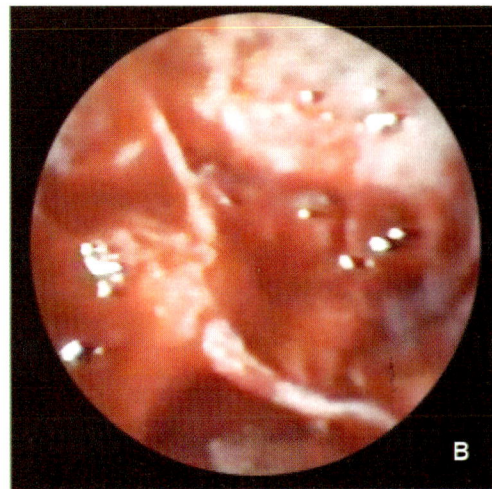

Fig. 7.62 B Endoscopic view of post operation cavities

TRANSSPHENOIDAL APPROACH TO THE PITUITARY GLAND

The two standard approaches to the sellar region are:

1. Craniotomy-subfrontal, pterional, bifrontal and supraorbital endoscopic key hole.

2. Transsphenoidal. Although there are modifications in this approach taken to reach the sellar region, the direct approach remains the safest. This can be accomplished with one of three methods:
   a. Endonasal : Microscopic, Endoscopic
   b. Sublabial
   c. Transseptal microscopic

ENDOSCOPIC ENDONASAL APPROACH

The Micro-Endoscopic Surgical Technique

Four important remarks should be recalled before proceeding with the description of the surgical technique in a step-by-step fashion:

1. Close teamwork between the otorhinolaryngologist and the neurosurgeon is advised.

2. Surgery is routinely carried out under general anesthesia and oral endotracheal intubation.

3. Septal structures are handled following the principles of Cottle's "maxilla-premaxilla" approach to the septum, with very few modifications.

4. A surgical microscope is used throughout the transseptal approach.

Indications

- Tumors
- Cysts
- Cerebrospinal fluid rhinorrhoea
- Chordomas
- Miscellaneous lesions

Preoperative Evaluation

1. Full pituitary profile/endocrinologist evaluation.

2. Full visual field study.

3. MRI with and without contrast medium enhancement.

4. CT with bone window (may be helpful in preoperative planning).

5. Angiogram/MRA if vascular lesion is suspected.

Anesthesia

1. General anesthesia with endotracheal intubation is almost always preferred.

2. Eyes should be protected with generous lubrication and gauze taped over them.

3. The patient is kept "dry" by anesthesia. This avoids a false-positive high urine output, which may be misinterpreted as diabetes insipidus.

Patient Preparation

1. A lumbar drain may be placed before positioning for larger lesions (>1.5 cm). Intraoperatively the anesthesiologist may need to inject 10 to 20 ml of air or saline to facilitate tumor delivery into the operative field.

2. The throat should be packed with ribbon gauze. This prevents blood draining into the stomach. A tap should be placed on the gauze for easy retrieval at the completion of surgery.

3. Both nares should be packed back to the sphenoid ostium with cottonoids soaked in oxymetazoline, cocaine or xylocaine with 1:2,00,000 adrenaline. These can remain in place while scrubbing (10 to 15 minutes).

4. Proper patient positioning can make this procedure technically safer, easier, and less stressful on the surgeon's spine.

5. The abdomen should be drepped at the navel for a possible fat graft.

6. The bracket for the scope holder should be placed on the table (opposite side of surgeon).

7. Patient should be placed same as used for endoscopic sinus surgery.

Surgical Technique

1. With the position a right-handed surgeon, the right naris is preferred unless the septum deviates too much to the ipsilateral side. The Afrin/cocaine-soaked cottonoids are removed and replaced with povidone-iodine (Betadine)-soaked cottonoids, which are left in for 5 minutes (while setting up the scope and surgical equipment) (Fig. 7.63).

2. A 22-gauge spinal needle is used to inject the middle turbinate and mucoperichondrium back to the sphenoid ostium. The endoscope or loupes can be used for this.

3. The middle turbinate is outfractured. The posterior nasal septum is scored and fractured to the opposite side so both sphenoid ostia are exposed (Fig. 7.64).

4. Mucous membrane of the anterior wall of the sphenoid is to be cauterized by bipolar cautery or by laser.

5. The endoscope holder can be used to fix the scope and free a hand.

6. A small osteotome, Jensen-Middleton rongeur, or 1- to 2-mm angled Kerrison rongeur can then be used to remove a portion of the sphenoid bone and intersinus septum. This should be at least 10 mm but preferably 15 mm wide. The sellar floor and carotid grooves should be identified (Fig 7.65).

7. A nasal speculum can then be used for retraction and exposure. The advantage is less trauma to the mucous membranes with the constant and repetitive

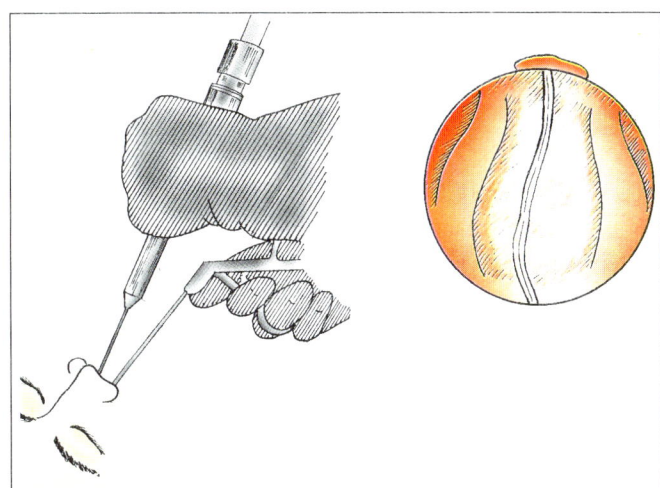

Fig. 7.63 Showing the position of the endoscope and instrument

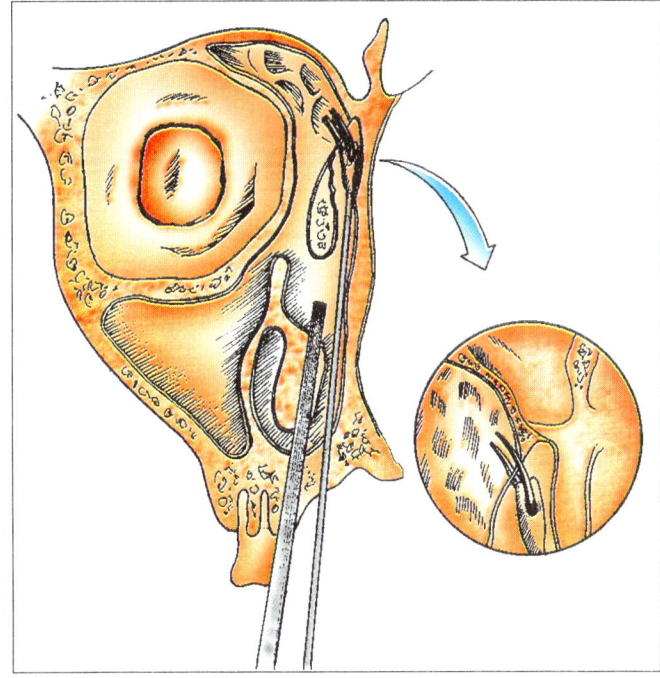

Fig. 7.64 Middle turbinate is outfractured

introduction of various instruments through the nasal passage. The disadvantage is that it limns maneuverability with instruments more so when using the endoscope.

8. A good set of bayonetted microinstruments is essential at this point. The sellar floor can be chipped away with a microcuret, drill, or Kerrison rongeur depending on its thickness. Before this, always confirm your position with the C-arm. This exposes the dura. A cruciate incision is made in the dura (Fig 7.66).

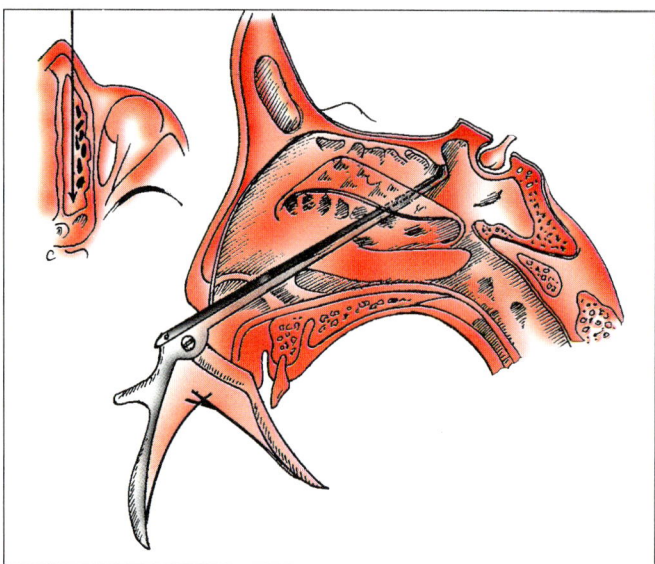

Fig. 7.65 Portion of sphenoid sinus and intersinus septum removed with Kerrison rongeur

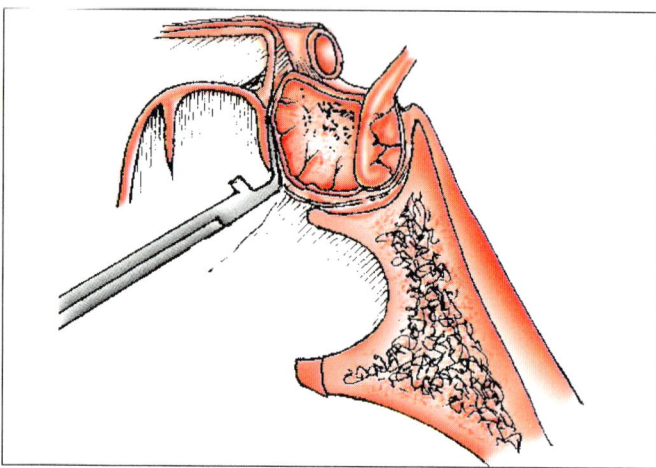

Fig. 7.67 Sellar floor removed with Kerrison rongeur

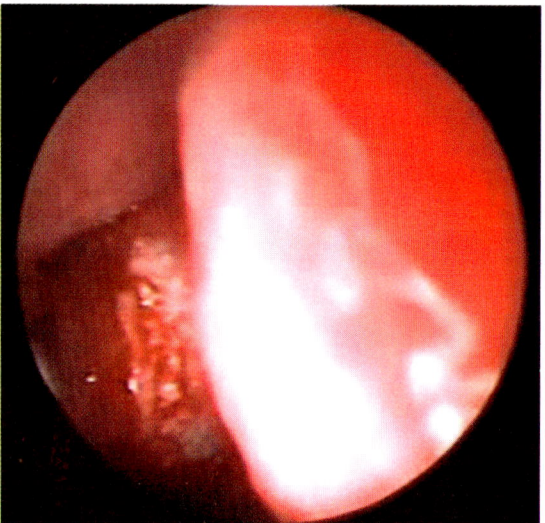

Fig. 7.66 Exposure of sphenoid via right nasal cavity endoscopic view

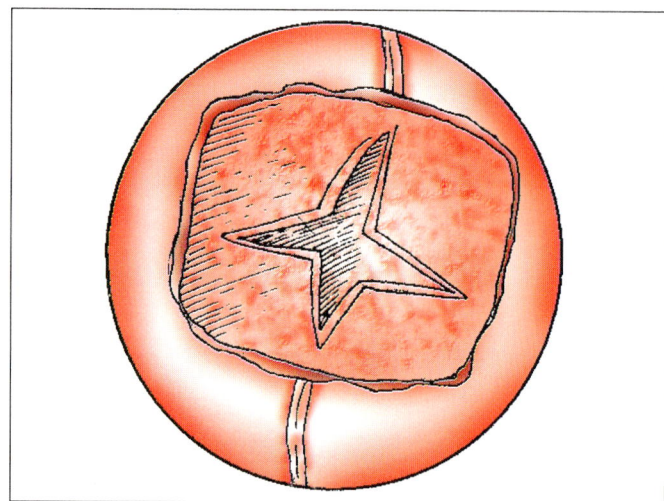

Fig. 7.68 Cruciate incision made in dura

9. For microadenomas the tumor may be encased in normal tissue and a linear incision in the normal gland is required. The sagittal view of the sella region seen with the 30-degree endoscope. The linear incision may lie placed laterally depending on the location of the lesion on preoperative imaging. The consistency of these tumors can vary from cystic fluid, a thick liquid (curdled milk), or firm with calcifications and attachments to normal structures such as the dura, optic apparatus, carotid arteries, cavernous sinus, and pituitary stalk. The firmer and larger the tumors are, the more difficult they are to remove.

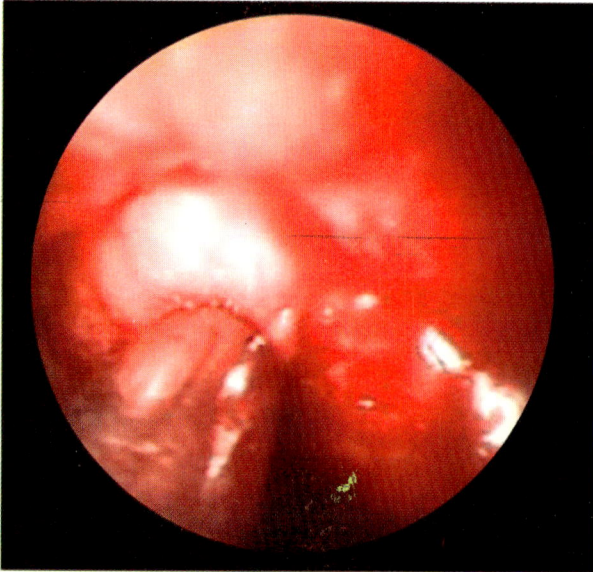

Fig. 7.69 Soft cystic pitutary tumor delivered through sphenoid

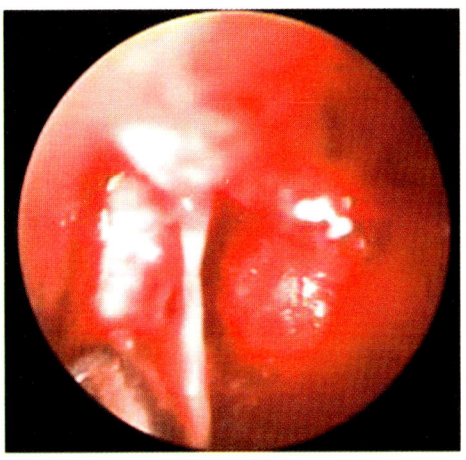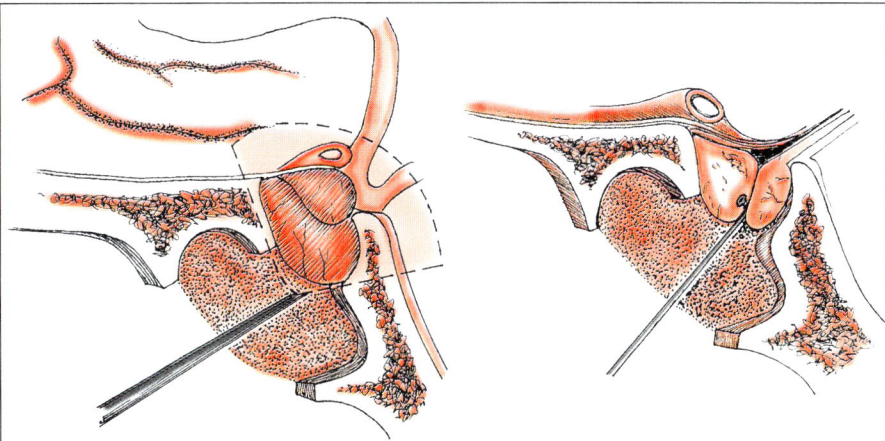

Fig. 7.70 Pituitary tumor removed in piece meal with curet

10. For tumor removal, variously sized and angled ring curets are the most helpful. A major portion of these resections is by feel. Two fingers on the curet with a gentle rubbing motion is the safest technique. Pituitary forceps can be used, but never pull or tear tissue you cannot see (Fig 7.70).

11. The straight and 30-degree angled endoscopes aid in visualization of the tumor cavity, optic chasm and cavernous structure. The author finds this superior to the microscope because it in effect allows you to "look around corners."

12. Once tumor removal is completed, hemostasis is checked and secured with single tip bipolar cautery, Celfoam, and/or Surgicel. With small tumors and no cerebrospinal fluid leak or bleeding (check with Valsalva maneuver) no packing of the sella is necessary. This can result in misleading or distorted postoperative imaging studies.

13. If the sellar floor requires reconstitution, then abdominal fat, Surgicel, Gelfoam, or a combination of these is usually required. Other more aggressive options include a bone strut wedged underneath the lips of the sellar floor. Allograft or resected sphenoid bone or septum can be used, Titanium craniotomy plates can also be used.

Postoperative Care

1. Care in the intensive care unit or neurologic observation unit is recommended for 24 hours.

2. Urine output is monitored closely for diabetes insipidus.

3. Cortisol and/or thyroid replacement therapy may be necessary.

4. Discharge is usually in 1 to 3 days after surgery in uncomplicated cases.

5. Follow-up should be arranged with an endocrinologist.

Complications

The following is a list of the more recognized complications of this procedure, but the list is by no means exhaustive. It is prudent to inform the patient of these complications.

- Cerebrospinal fluid leak
- Diabetes insipidus (permanent or temporary)
- Pituitary insufficiency (permanent or temporary)
- Infection (meningitis), abscess
- Hemorrhage or stroke (brain attack)
- Loss of vision
- Loss of smell and/or taste
- Vascular injury
- Cavernous sinus syndrome
- Brain damage and death

The endonasal approach is the least invasive and most direct. It avoids the unnecessary dissection of the upper gum and nasal septum. The sellar exposure is not sacrificed. This technique has come into favor in recent years with the advent of the endoscope. The endonasal approach can be utilized for almost all lesions involving the sella, with or without suprasellar or cavernous extension. With larger invasive lesions the surgeon should prepare the patient for a possible staged transcranial approach as well as possible adjuvant therapy.

Endoscopic Trans- Septal Approach (ETA) to Sellar and Para Sellar Region

Choice of the surgical approach

The choice of the surgical approach to the sellar region depends on the results of neuroradiologic studies. Magnetic-resonance imaging (MRI) of the sellar region and the sphenoid sinus is the most helpful exam in the neuroradiologic work-up of patients with sellar and parasellar tumors. MRI depicts the tumor's size, extent and characteristics, such as hemorrhagic and cystic changes. This exam also helps to delineate the tumor from the surrounding anatomical structures, and the position of the carotid artery is, in most instances, well depicted by coronal MRI . However, the relationship of the tumor to the osseous structures is best demonstrated by computed tomography (CT).

Basic criteria for patient selection

Two basic criteria for patient selection for trans-septal sphenoidal surgery must be considered:

1. All intrasellar pituitary tumors (and those with symmetrical, moderate suprasellar extension) can be operated via this approach. Initially conceived for the treatment of intrasellar tumors, the trans sphenoidal approach can be used in the surgery of some perisellar lesions (chordoma, craniopharyngioma) or in the debulking of lesions with suprasellar extension.

2. The sella turcica must be surgically accessible via an adequately pneumatized sphenoid sinus. There are three described anatomical varieties of sphenoid sinus: **conchal** (non-pneumatized), **presellar** and **sellar.** The sellar type is the most frequent and suitable for trans sphenoidal surgery.

Indications for the microscopic trans-septal approach

1. The excision of pituitary tumors.
2. The excision or debulking of non-pituitary skull base tumors.
3. Biopsy and culture of sphenoid sinus diseases.
4. Marsupialization of a sphenoid sinus mucocele.
5. Repair of CSF leakage into the sphenoid sinus.

Contraindications for the microscopic Trans-Septal Approach

1. Absolute contraindications
   Active sino-nasal infection
   Excessive tumoral extension
   Diffuse tumoral invasion by non-capsulated tumors

2. Relative contraindication
   A conchal or presellar type of sphenoid sinus

The surgical technique step by step

1. Once anesthetized, the patient is placed in a semi-recumbent position, the head reclined to the left and the face turned to the right, allowing a right-handed surgeon to stand in a sagittal plane without leaning over the patient's torso.

2. The surgeon or his assistant removes autograft muscle from the thigh or the upper lateral abdomen. Some fascia lata and fat can also be removed. The fascia can be used for reconstruction in the event of injury to the diaphragm sellae.

3. Draping is carried out after cleansing the skin with an antiseptic solution and protecting the eyes. The upper lips, nose, eyes and cheeks are left exposed. Some authors prefer to cover the face and leave uncovered only the nose.

4. Topical vasoconstriction of the nose with gauze strips soaked in saline solution (with 1 drop of 1:1000 adrenaline per ml of solution) is carried out.

5. The columella, floor of the nose and the caudal end of the septum are infiltrated with approximately 5 ml of 1 % lidocaine containing epinephrine (1:100,000).

6. The caudal end of the septum is exposed with a nasal speculum, a Cottle clamp or a blunt, double-ended hook.

7. A right hemitransfixion incision is made with a no. 15 blade and is made 2 mm behind the free border of the septal cartilage. It reaches from the floor of the nose to the septum and extends upward, parallel to the caudal margin, to a point near its junction with the major alar cartilage. The shape of the incision is that of an inverted "L" with its horizontal line pointing to the left of the surgeon. The soft tissues surrounding the incision, especially on the right side of the septum, are detached from the underlying surfaces to avoid unnecessary tension.

8. In women with small noses, the nostril may be enlarged by an incision at the base of the alar, which is later connected to the incision in the skin of the floor of the nasal cavity (lateral alotomy).

9. The superior lip is undermined for exposure of the maxilla and nasal spine.

10. The anterior nasal spine is dissected on both sides through the lower part of the hemitransfixion incision. The piriform crest of the nasal cavity is then dissected on both sides.

11. A right sub-mucoperichondrial dissection extending to the posterior area of the perpendicular plate of the ethmoid bone is performed. This dissection is carried out posteriorly using progressively longer nasal specula.

12. A left superior tunnel is created by dissecting the mucoperichondrium with scissors and a suction elevator.

13. A left inferior tunnel is created.

14. With sharp dissection along the chondro osseous junction of the septal cartilage with the vomer and premaxilla, the mucosa is progressively elevated from the posterior portion of the septum. Bony spines and crests are dissected carefully and removed, thus avoiding tearing of the mucosa and consequent bleeding and posterior scarring.

15. The cartilaginous septum is mobilized by luxating its lower part from its osseous groove on the nasal spine, premaxilla and vomer. This posterior attachment to the perpendicular plate of the ethmoid bone is separated. The premaxilla and the vomer may be shortened with a chisel, if necessary .

16. The posterior portion of septal bone, which obstructs access to the sphenoid rostrum, is resected with a sharp 4-mm chisel and the forceps. The mucosa is laterally elevated from the external surface of the sphenoid sinus.

17. A self-retaining speculum is introduced between the two separated layers of the septal mucosa, with the septal cartilage luxated to any side, according to the surgeon's preference. The speculum is pushed firmly but gently against the anterior wall of the sphenoid sinus. An imaginary line along the superior edge of the speculum blades must point to the tuberculum sellae if checked radiologically. At this level, operation microscope or endoscope can be used.

18. The rostrum of the sphenoid bone and sphenoid ostia are identified.

19. The anterior wall of the sphenoid sinus (which proceeds from the **superior ostial-orifice** level and is enlarged with **Kerrison forceps,** this foramina being the lateral landmark for the opening; is resected. This is done with flat chisels (4-5 mm) and a variety of punches. The septum of the sphenoid sinus is excised, and an adequate amount of sinus mucosa is removed. The sphenoid sinus is carefully inspected with 0° and 30° nasal telescopes, and some prominences can be noted, such as the carotid prominence, the bulge of the optic canal and the prominence formed by the maxillary nerve on the lateral wall of the sinus (Fig. 7.71).

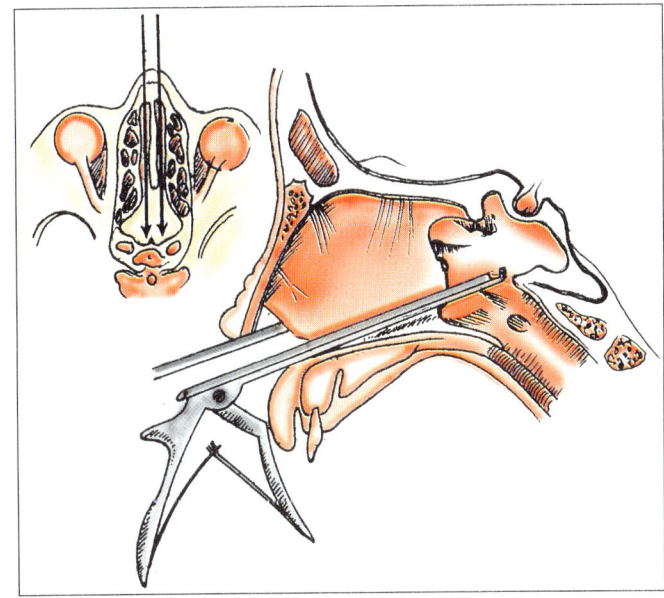

Fig. 7.71 Superior ostial orifice widen with Kerrison forcep

20. The frontobasal face of the sella is opened with a small, flat chisel or a micro-gauge and is removed) in a piecemeal fashion. The dura is carefully separated and exposed. The opening is made as large as possible, reaching the cavernous sinus on both sides and ending 1-2 mm below the inferior surface of the tuberculum sellae. The inferior edge of the opening lies on the horizontal part of the sellar floor. This step of the operation can also be controlled using televised fluoroscopy.

21. The exposed dura bulges out of the opening in the bony sellar floor in most cases. Careful hemostasis is done via coagulation with a bipolar forceps.

22. After a preliminary needle aspiration, the dura is opened by means of a cruciate incision made with a micro-sickle knife, and the flaps are elevated with right-angle hooks. The soft, gray-purple tumor tissue will then extrude through the opening if the tumor is a prolactinoma. Somatotroph adenomas are whitish in color, resembling cerebral white matter.

23. The adenoma tissue is removed with appropriate forceps, malleable ring curettes and spoons. Adequate suction is mandatory. An ultrasonic dissector is also used for the removal of the tumor. The adenoma tissue and a layer of normal pituitary tissue are both resected to ensure complete tumor extirpation. Tumor biopsy specimens are sent for histology, immunocyto-chemistry and ultrastructure examination. The complete removal of the sellar tumor is controlled by means of 0° and 30° nasal endoscopes.

24. Bleeding from the tumor bed usually stops after complete extirpation of the adenoma has been achieved. Some remaining oozing can be controlled by a 5-min application of cottonoids soaked in saline solution and monopolar coagulation of any remaining small vessels. Bleeding from the anterior intercavernous sinus is stopped by coagulation with bipolar, right-angled forceps and/or Surgicel.

25. Small pieces of muscle or fat tissue removed at the beginning of the operation from the thigh or abdominal fat soaked in gentamicin solution are placed in the tumor cavity to secure hemostasis and avoid CSF leakage. Overpacking must be avoided, because it may lead to optic-chiasma compression.

26. A piece of septal cartilage or bone is inserted between the margins of the bony sellar floor and the basal dura after packing the sella with muscle. The entire opening is sealed with a generous application of fibrin glue.

The sphenoid sinus can be filled completely if the diaphragma sellae has been damaged during the operation. The sphenoid sinus can be left with no filling at all. The speculum is removed.

27. The nasal structures are repositioned. The septal cartilage is returned to its correct midline position. Corrections of any remaining septal deformity that could impair the respiratory function of the nose are performed. Autologous cartilage can be reimplanted in the places from which septal cartilage has been resected, restoring the anatomy and consistency of this nasal structure, with all its functional implications. The mucosal incision in the right nasal antrum is closed with interrupted 3-gauge chromic catgut sutures. Thala, if incised basally, is closed with interrupted 5-gauge prolene or silk sutures.

28. Two plastic stents are placed on each side of the septum and fixed with 4-gauge prolene or silk sutures or a mattress suture or

29. The nasal cavities are packed with gauze strips soaked with antibiotic ointment, following the usual technique that begins on the floor of the nasal cavity and reaches the nasal cavity's roof.

30. The packing is removed on the third postoperative day. A nasal ointment is used for some days after retiring the packing, to prevent crusting.

31. The plastic stents are removed between the fifth day and the seventh day, depending on the amount of septal work performed.

CRANIOFACIAL APPROACH

It Combines a bifrontal craniotomy through a coronal approach with transfacial exposure of the nasal cavity, ethmoid, maxillary and orbital areas usually by modifications of lateral rhinotomy, midfacial degloving, or other transfacial approaches. The facial incisions can be modified to allow for orbital exenteration

Principle and aim of anterior craniofacial resection

Although techniques of anterior CFR have been evolving, key aspects of the procedure remain established. The goal of the operation is to obtain adequate exposure of the tumor and important structures in the vicinity, which can therefore be preserved to ensure good surgical margins around the tumor.

The CFR-related principles for malignant tumors include

- Adequate exposure of the tumor and adjacent vital structures;
- Minimal or no brain retraction: (intraoperative spinal drainage ± mannitol diuresis to maintain brain slack);
- Watertight dural repair by using dural patch (pericranium, fascia lata, bovine pericardium, cadaveric dura, or allograft) for large defects and direct suture for smaller ones; and reconstruction of the skull base defect by using galeal pericranial flap or free tissue transfer (rectus abdominis flap for large defects).

Indications

Based on the area involved

1. Cribriform plate and/or floor of the anterior cranial fossa.
2. Frontal sinus.
3. Ethmoid and antrum.
4. Anterior wall of the sphenoidal sinus (not the entire sphenoidal sinus)
5. Orbit and its contents
6. Nasal cavity (*e.g.*, extensive malignant tumors extending to the cribriform plate).
7. Meninges involving the anterior and possibly the base of the middle cranial fossa.

Based on types of tumors

Malignant

Neoplasms that originate in the sinonasal tract and invade the anterior cranial fossa floor, such as:

1. Squamous cell carcinoma.
2. Malignant tumors of the minor salivary glands (*e.g.* adenoid cystic carcinoma).
3. High-grade mucoepidermoid carcinoma arising from the mucosa of the paranasal sinuses, nasal cavity, or lacrimal apparatus.
4. Melanoma
5. Esthesioneuroblastoma
6. Chondrosarcoma
7. Invasive basal cell carcinoma of the skin involving the facial bones at the skull base.

8. Histiocytoma

Benign

Tumors That May Extend Through or Approach the Floor of the Anterior and/or Middle Cranial Fossa (Benign tumors invading the ethmoid complex and cribriform area) remaining outside the dura comprises the indication for anterior CFR in benign lesions

1. Olfactory meningioma
2. Fibrous dysplasia
3. Recurrent and invasive inverted papilloma (*e.g.* those that extend into the cribriform plate).
4. Congenital deformities (*e.g.*, orbital hypertelorism).
5. Fibromatosis

Contraindications

1. Tumor extension into the frontal lobes.
2. Beyond the posterior margin of cribriform plate.
3. Involvement of both the optic nerves.
4. Laterally outside the boundaries of fovea.
5. Old age and medically unfit for major surgery.

Types of craniofacial resections

1. Anterior craniofacial resection
2. Basal subfrontal resection
3. Frontal window craniotomy

1. Anterior craniofacial resection

Trans- facial approach with bifrontal craniotomy

This operation is performed in conjunction with a neurosurgeon and combines transfacial approach with a neurosurgical approach such as frontolateral craniotomy, to allow resection of extensive tumors.

The role of neurosurgeon in such procedures remains subject to discussion. The growth of skull base surgery as a sub speciality has exposed many otolaryngologists to various neurosurgical techniques and has obviated the need of immediate assistance of a neurosurgeon, but neurosurgical opinion should be sought in the preoperative workup. He may be able to offer significant help.

2. Basal subfrontal approach (Trans Basal -Derome)

Also called as trans basal approach. It is similar to anterior craniofacial resection operation except that the

1. Transfacial exposure is less extensive. Because the target area in this approach is more posterior (sphenoid and clivus) than in the anterior craniofacial resection (ethmoids and cribriform).
2. Craniotomy bone flap is generally somewhat larger.
3. Orbital bone cuts are broader.

Advantages

1. Wide exposure of the anterior skull base.
2. Minimal retraction of the brain.
3. Reconstruction of the whole skull base with galea. periosteum flap and bone.
4. Excellent cosmetic results with no visible skin scar.

Disadvantage

1. Loss of olfaction

Indications

1. Congenital abnormalities
2. CSF Fistula
3. Vascular lesions
4. Lesions of the midline that involve PNS, Anterior cranial fossa, Clivus, Sellar and suprasellar regions, lesions extending lateral to internal carotid artery and petroclival lesions.

Contraindications

1. High grade malignant tumors invading the cavernous sinus and internal carotid artery.

Steps

1. Begins with a bicoronal incision.
2. Orbital rims are exposed and periorbita is elevated from beneath the orbital roofs and medial wall.
3. The anterior and posterior ethmoidal arteries are identified as the land mark for osteotomies. They need not be divided because the axial ethmoid osteotomy can be made just above this level.
4. Bifrontal craniotomy is performed, dura is elevated from above the orbital roofs and cribriform area.
5. Orbital contents and brain is protected using malleable retractors. A reciprocating saw is used to create

osteotomies that result in a temporary removal of both orbital roofs and the supraorbital bar.

6. The coronal osteotomies along the posterior orbital roof should be made as far as possible to simplify reconstruction, by preserving the orbital contour and to prevent postoperative pulsatile exophthalmus. These orbital cuts can be made as far as back as the posterior ethmoid foramen but should be made under direct vision from intra and extra cranial perspectives. With the use of these osteotomies, a very broad and basal exposure of the entire cranial base is approached.
7. Working with the aid of the microscope, the approach is completed by using a ronger or drill to remove a small amount of bone remaining posteriorly to unroof the optic nerves, superior orbital fissures and sphenoid sinus.
8. Extirpation proceeds as required by tumor, followed by reconstruction which is similar to as that of anterior CFR.

3. Frontal window craniotomy

This procedure is essentially the original operation described in 1986 (Cheesman, Lund and Howard)

A lateral rhinotomy approach is used for anterior access and extended superiorly in a frown line to expose the frontal bone.

A small midline window craniotomy is made giving access to the floor of the anterior cranial fossa (Fig. 7.72)

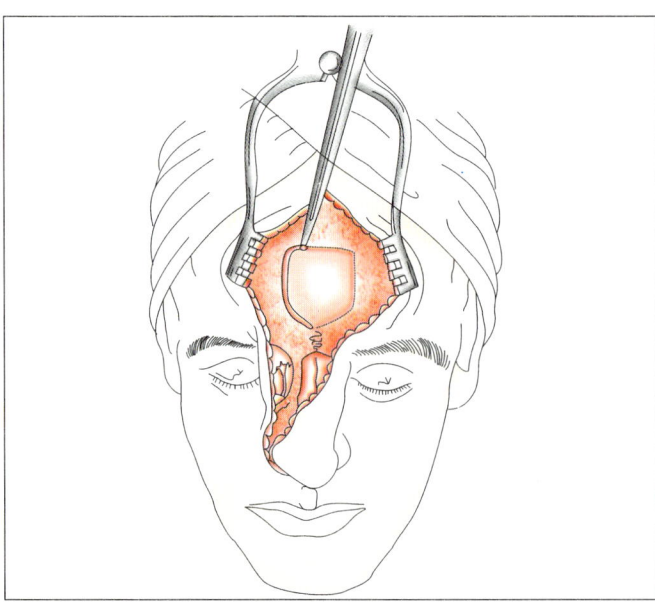

Fig. 7.72 Small midline window craniotomy being done

After shrinkage of the brain with controlled hyperventilation to reduce the end tidal pco2 to 22mmHg, the dura is elevated form the roof of the ethmoid and cribriform plate and the area is encompassed with a cranial steotomy (Fig. 7.73)

This osteotomy in conjunction with those of the lateral rhinotomy allows the en block resection of both ethmoid complexes. The involved dura can be excised and repaired with fascia lata (Fig. 7.74).

Involved brain can be excised but cure is unlikely at this stage, although palliation is excellent.

The window bone flap is replaced and refixed with mini plates (Fig and soft tissue is closed with remarkably little cosmetic defect (Fig. 7.75).

Combined approach gives a excellent visualization of the ethmoid region and allows for the extention of the resection in to the sphenoid, orbit, pterygopalatine fossa and the skull base centrally.

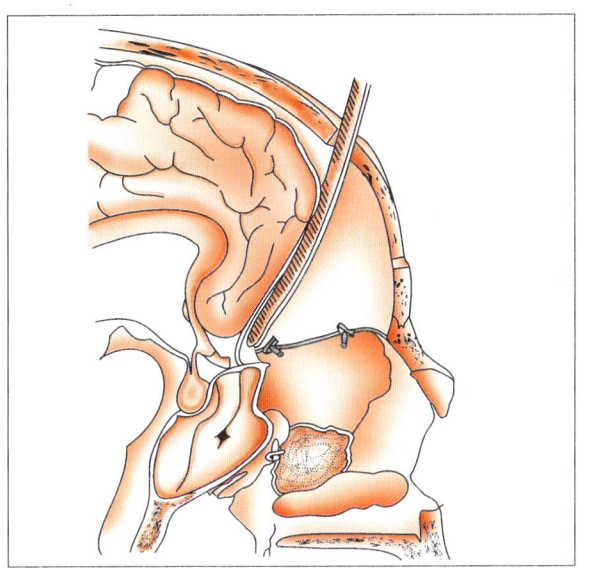

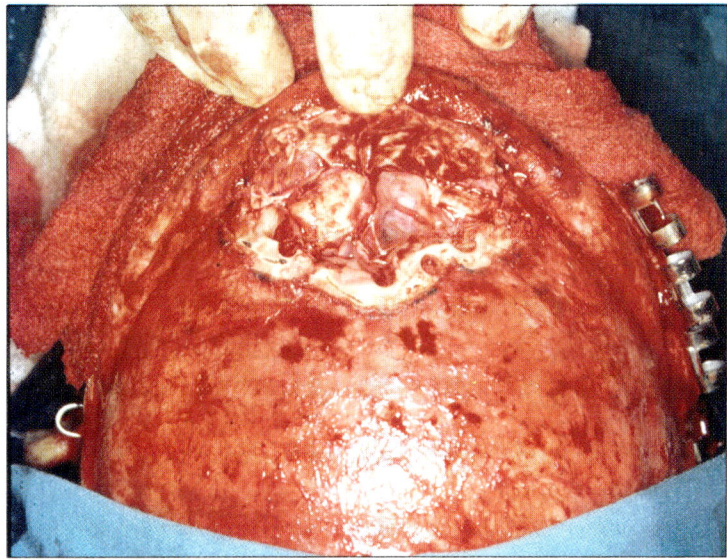

Fig. 7.73 Showing frontal lobe retraction with the malleable retract through the frontal bone window

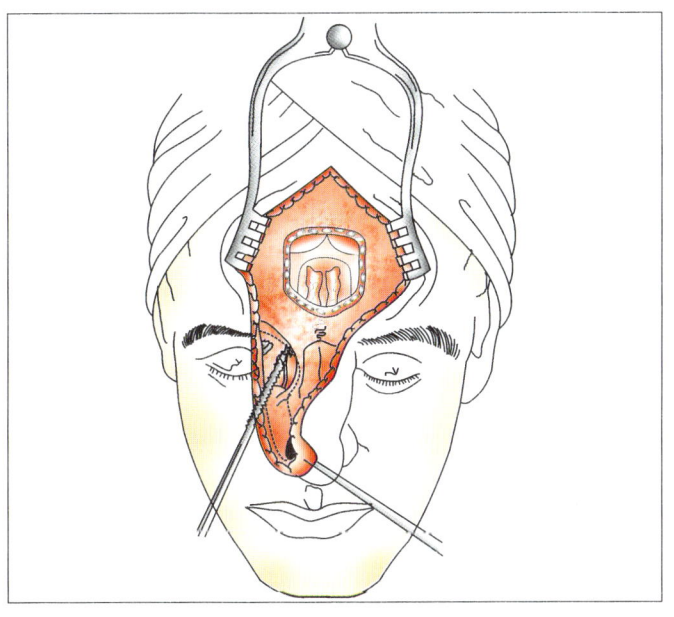

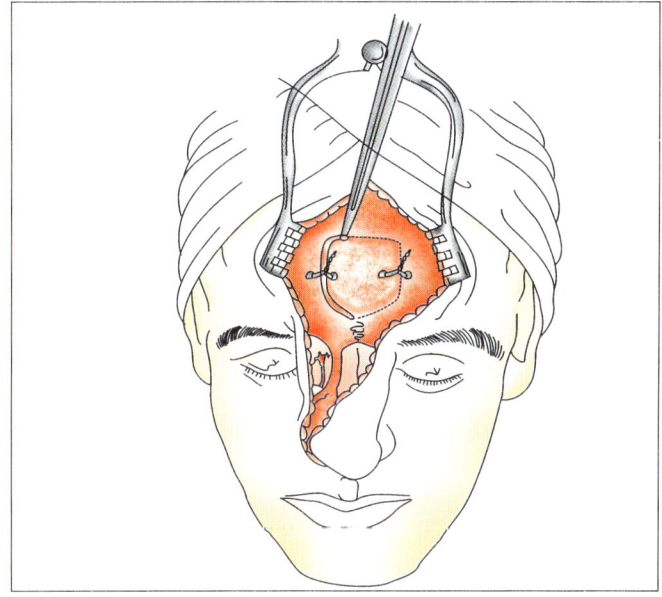

Fig. 7.74 Frontal osteotomy in conjunction with lateral rhinotomy for enblock resection of both ethmoid complex

Fig. 7.75 Window bone flap is replaced and refused with mini plates

The various types of skin incisions used in craniofacial resections

Cranial incisions

1. **The standard bicoronal frontal incision** The Bicoronal flap is placed approximately 2 cm posterior to the hairline. Extends from the tragus of one ear to that of the other, just within the hairline. It should be in true coronal plane. A short, forward directed, preauricular extension can be made on both sides to enhance scalp flap rotation.

2. **Small incision over the forehead** is preferred by Ketcham (1963). It is used to perform a but hole craniotomy, through which the floor of the anterior cranial fossa in the vicinity of the cribriform plate is transected. However, it affords much less exposure of the floor of the anterior cranial fossa.

3. **Extended lateral rhinotomy** incision on forehead to facilitate frontal window (Fig. 7.76).

Why coronal plane of incision is chosen for scalp?

1. It preserves the anterior branches of superficial temporal artery, superior orbital artery, vessels which in turn adds to the vascularity of the skin and enhances viability of the scalp flap.

2. It substantially increase the vascularized galea and pericranium available for reconstruction compared with incision along the anterior hairline, midforehead crease, or brow.

3. It facilitates a complete frontal craniotomy and affords excellent exposure (Fig. 7.77).

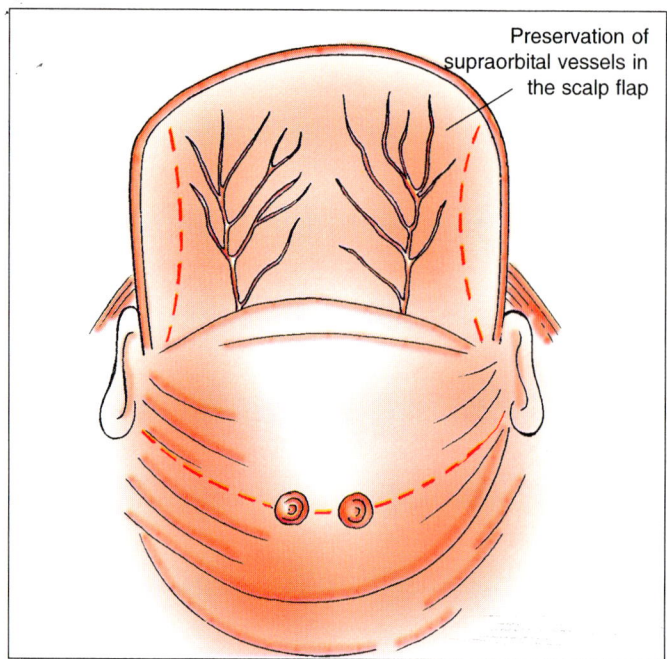

Preservation of supraorbital vessels in the scalp flap

Fig. 7.77 Showing the frontal craniotomy with two parasaggital burr holes (to aid protection of superior saggital sinus)

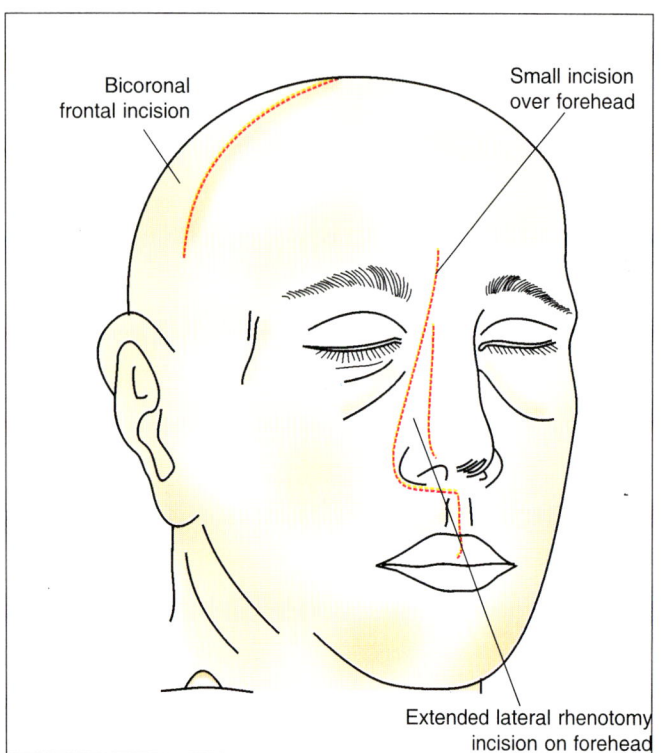

Bicoronal frontal incision

Small incision over forehead

Extended lateral rhenotomy incision on forehead

Fig 7.76 Showing various cranial incisions

Facial Incisions

1. The Weber-Dieffenbach (Fergusson) cheek incision with an ellipse to include in the resection, the margins of the upper and lower eyelid (which are sutured together) when the orbital contents of the orbit are to be removed. Removal of the lids is recommended when insertion of an orbital prosthesis is planned. If the globe is to be preserved, the upper horizontal incision is not performed and the edges of the lids are not resected.

The basic Weber-Ferguson incision is modified depending on the anatomical access required (Fig. 7.78).

- The upper lip is split in the midline if exposure of the lower half of the nasal cavity, hard palate, or maxilla is required. The cosmetic outcome after using this modified incision is considerably better because the scars situated at the borders adjoining the subunits of the nose are less conspicuous.

3. Contralateral lynch extension incision is at times utilized for additional exposure of the contralateral ethmoidal sinus when a bilateral total resection of the ethmoidal labyrinth is done. The incision is optional, depending on the extent of the disease and the exposure that may be necessary.

Three phases of craniofacial resection

1. Cranial resection
2. Facial resection
3. Reconstruction

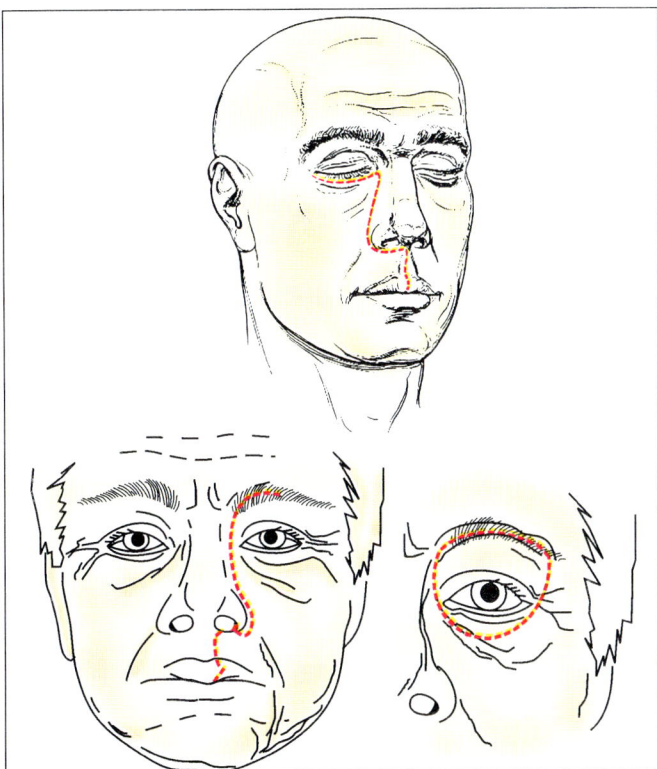

Fig. 7.78 Showing various modifications of Weber ferguson incision

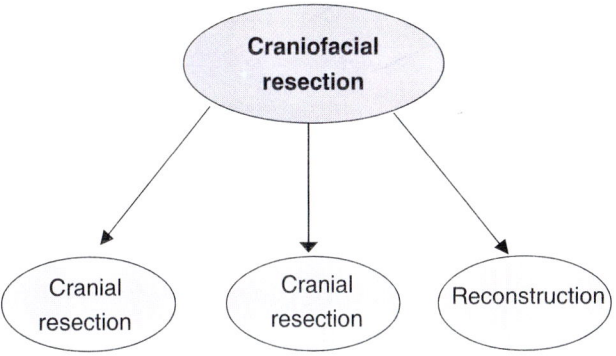

Where to begin?

There has been a lot of controversies regarding the first phase of the surgery i.e. whether it should be started with a cranial resection first or the facial resection. Various authors have described their own preferences depending on the type and the extent of the tumor.

The operation begins with the transfacial exposure in cases where.

- If a facial disassembly of the nasal bones is planned, the incision can be extended across the glabella up to the contralateral eyebrow.

- Alternatively, subciliary extension up to the lateral canthus can provide exposure for a total maxillectomy.

2. Lateral rhinotomy and various extensions (Fig. 7.79).

- The tumor is benign and most of it can be approached through the transfacial approach.

- Radiologically and clinically if the tumor appears to be extradural, resection can be tried through transfacial side before proceeding to craniotomy.

- Tumors involving the anterior wall of sphenoid only.

- Malignant tumors without dural invasion.

The operation begins with cranial resection first in cases where.

- Malignant tumors with cribriform plate involvement to ascertain the dural invasion i.e. superior and posterior extent.

- Dural invasion

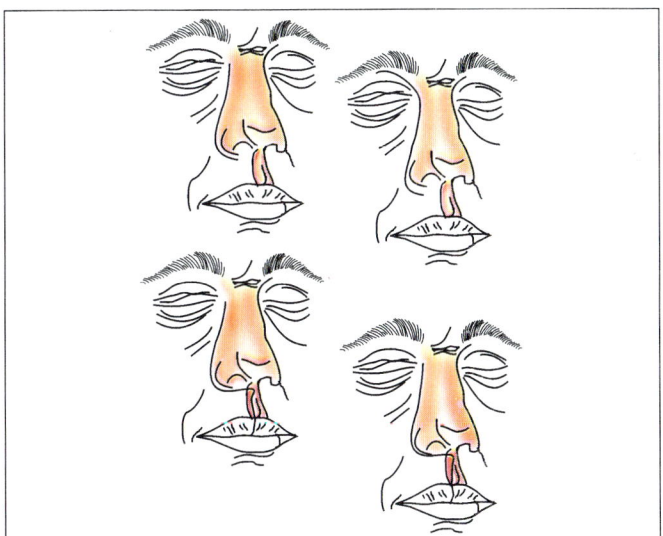

Fig. 7.79 showing various modifications of lateral rhinotomy

- Involvement of posterior wall of sphenoid.
- More posterior tumors involving planum sphenoidale, clivus etc.

Cranial phase of resection

Steps

1. Bicoronal incision is given (Fig. 7.80)
2. The scalp is incised down. The central portion of the anterior scalp flap (i.e. the portion between two superior temporal lines) is elevated in subperiosteal plane. Lateral to the two superior temporal lines, it is elevated in plane just above the deep temporal fascia. Therefore, at the temporal lines, the pericranium should be sharply incised to separate it from the origin of the deep temporal fascia.

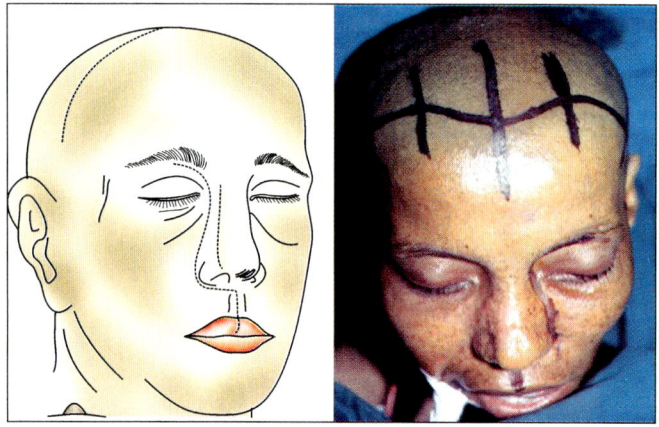

Fig. 7.80 Showing commencement of CFR, cranial and facial incisions

Note: This deep temporal fascia begins to split into superficial and deep layers beginning at approximately the level of the superior orbital rim. These facial layers diverge to envelop the lateral and medial surfaces of the zygomatic arch inferiorly, between the layers is the temporal pad of fad. The frontal branches of the facial nerve course just superficial to the zygoma along the superficial temporal fascia and are prone to injury if the dissection is done at the level. These injuries can be avoided by maintaining the plane of dissection at the level of the deep layer of the Deep Temporal Fascia.

3. Once the dissection reaches the level of the zygomatic arch, the arch is palpated and its superior surface is directly exposed by sharply incising the fat pad and periosteum.
4. Anterior flap elevation is advanced down the frontal area toward the supraorbital rims. Supraorbital vascular pedicle supplying the galea and pericrania are preserved. (Note: to avoid injury to this pedicle elevation of supraorbital periosteum is done in lateral to medial direction). If the pedicle is completely surrounded by bone, a 3 mm osteotome is used to fracture the inferior margin of the foramen, allowing it to be elevated along the pericranium and underlying periorbita (Fig. 7.82).
5. The posterior scalp flap is elevated in the loose areolar tissue plane between the galea and pericranium several centimeters posteriorly to expose the pericranium.

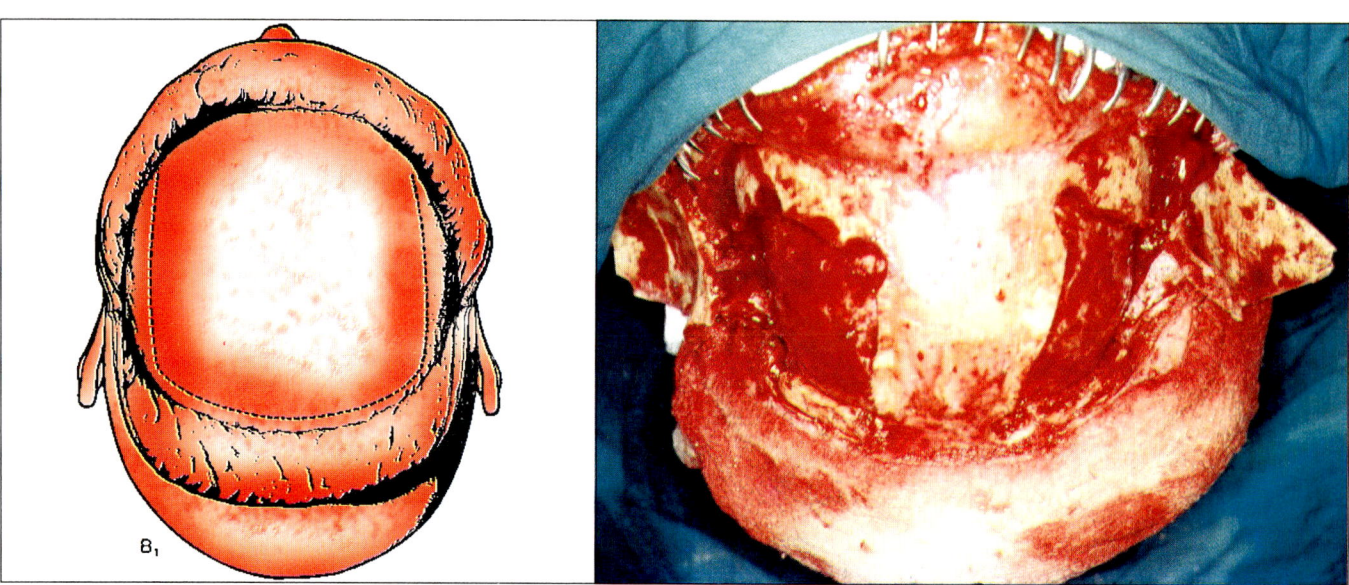

Fig 7.81 Showing elevation of anterior scalp flap

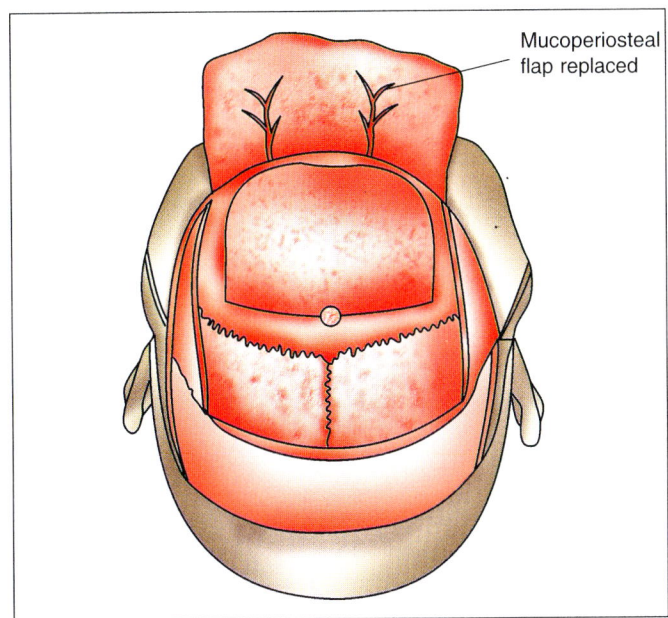

Fig. 7.82 Showing the elevation of scalp flap with preservation of vascular pedicle

Haemostatic Raney clips are applied to the cut edges of the scalp.

6. With the anterior scalp flap elevated to expose the glabellar region and the upper half of the nasal bones, the proposed craniotomy bone cuts are out marked with methylene blue on the anterior wall of the frontal sinus and the bone. Cosmetic saddle-nose deformity can be avoided by placing this bone cut so that the nasal bones are retained in situ and excluded from the bone plate.

Types of bone flap

a. Osteoplastic flap, it is preferred if patient has a large frontal sinus. In such cases thin posterior table of the frontal sinus is opened with burr to expose the dura and then removed.

b. Frontal bone flap preferred if the frontal sinus is small. It is performed with a guarded osteotome via burr holes created above the hairline. The lower frontal bone cut should be kept low to avoid brain retraction. The frontal lobes are elevated from the anterior cranial fossa by incising the dura and severing the olfactory nerves. This will result in a CSF leak that will require dural patch as well as permanent anosmia. The extent of resection is dictated by tumor involvement.

Technical variations of craniotomy include

a. Multiple frontal and parasagittal burr holes.

b. Single frontal burr hole and small osteotomy.

c. Anterior subcranial osteotomy.

d. Facial disassembly.

- The practice of using multiple burr holes has largely been abandoned bsecause of the associated cosmetic deformity. Here the frontal bone flap is developed using a guarded craniotome introduced via burr holes placed above the hairlines and in the temporal lines. Paramedian position of superior burr holes aids in protection of superior saggital sinus while the bone flap is being cut. Lower horizontal cuts should be kept low (with in 1cm of the superior orbital rims) to lessen the need of subsequent brain retraction (Fig. 7.83).

- **Single frontal burr hole and small osteotomy:** A single midline burr hole is made in the frontal bone approximately 5 cm above the glabella, and

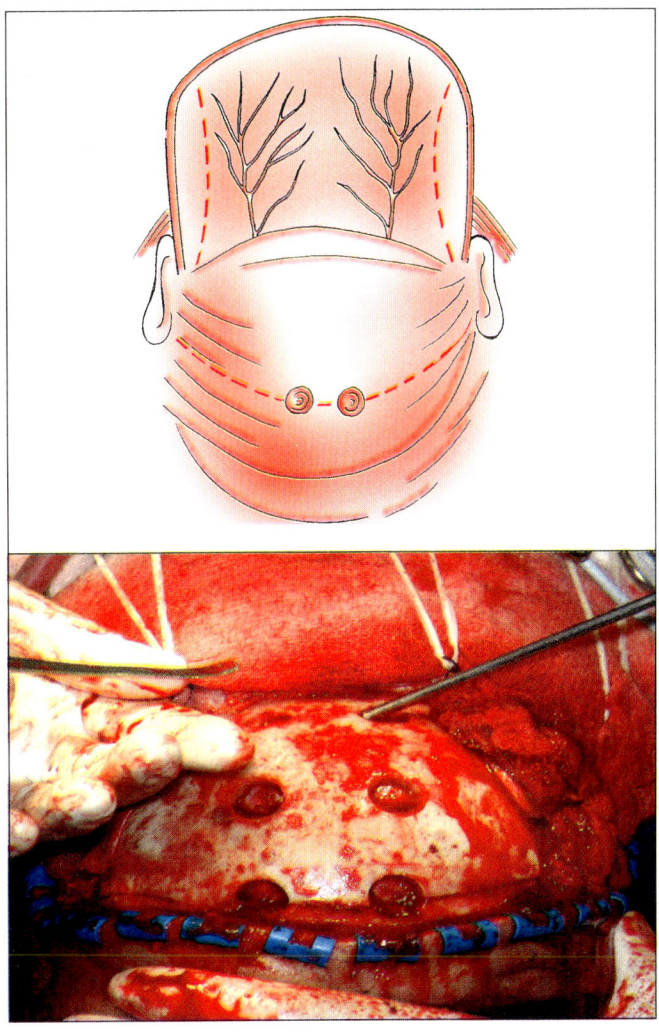

Fig. 7.83 showing frontal craniotomy with two parasaggital burr holes (to aid protection of superior saggital sinus)

the dura is separated from the under side of the bone. Arachnoid granulation bleeding is readily controlled using thrombin-soaked Gelfoam. The B1 bit on the Midas Rex drill is used to make bone cuts to approximately the level of the midorbits bilaterally without entering the frontal sinuses. The frontal sinus cuts are made using the 2-mm cutting burr through the anterior and posterior walls of the sinus. This procedural strategy has decreased the incidence of dural tears adjacent to the frontal sinus. A small frontal craniotomy is favored to increase the surface area of the frontal bones for the surgeon's hands to rest and consequently decrease the possibility of pressure inadvertently transmitted to the frontal lobes. Dissecting the saggital sinus and dura from the bone elevates the flap. The remainder of the posterior wall of the frontal sinus is removed using a rongeur and the mucosa is exenterated. A bone rongeur is use to remove the septal in the frontal sinus and all sharp spicules of bone are smoothed using a burr. It is important to curette the entire mucosa of the sinus and to cranialize the frontal sinus by excising its posterior wall. The nasofrontal duct openings are plugged with Gelfoam. A small frontal osteotomy in which a single frontal burr hole is made provides adequate access for exposure of the anterior skull base without the morbidity associated with multiple burr holes.

- The anterior subcranial approach has been reported to provide adequate exposure of the anterior skull base and the advantage of precluding frontal lobe retraction and lateral rhinotomy [13]. The size of the osteotomy can be varied depending on the exposure desired. Although effective in providing exposure for correction of craniofacial deformities and fractures, this approach does not allow retraction of the frontal lobe nor inspection or resection of the dura at the anterior skull bases, which are crucial steps for total enblock tumor excision in most cases requiring anterior CFR.

- The technique of facial disassembly allows the nasal bone complex to be removed en bloc to facilitate transfacial access to the nasal cavity. The bone complex is then replaced in its original position at the end of the procedure and fixated using miniplates.

7. Once the craniotomy is completed, the dura of the floor of the anterior cranial fossa is elevated, sharply

dividing its attachments to the crista galli. The dural sleeves along the olfactory nerves need to be individually divided and ligated. Immediate ligation of the dural sleeves ensures that contamination of the brain during subsequent phases of the operation is avoided. This segment of the dura along with the olfactory sleeves obviously needs to be resected in cases of esthesioneuroblastomas or other tumors that perforate the cribriform plate. Small dural defects can be repaired using a free graft of pericranium whereas larger defects require bovine pericardium or reconstituted cadaveric dura. Use of fibrin glue can be effective not only in supplementing repairs of dural tears and over the ligated olfactory dural sleeves but also as a sealant to prevent postoperative pneumocephalus (Fig. 7.84).

8. Once the dura is elevated, the exposed crista galli can

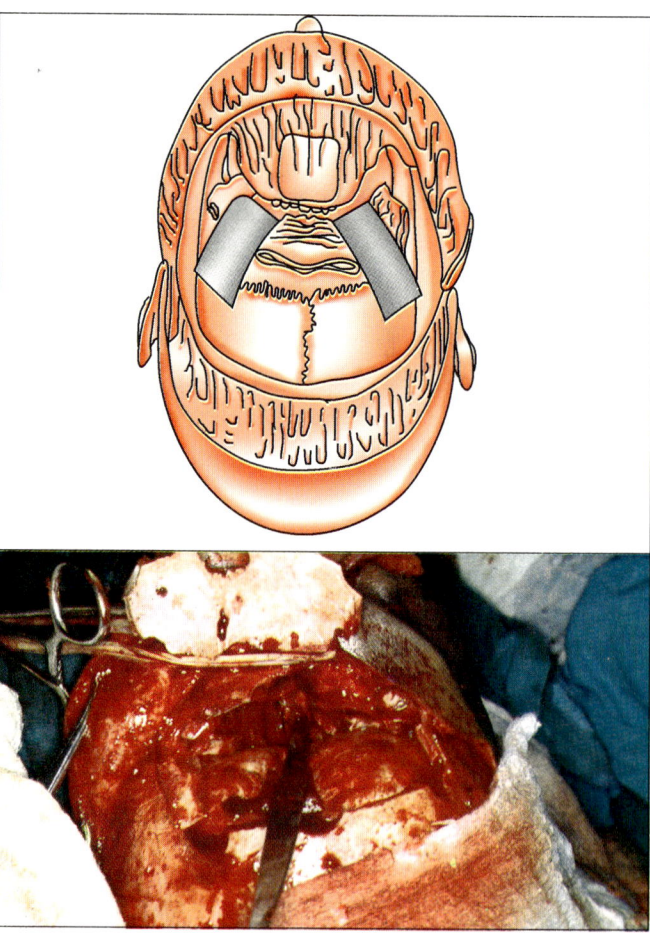

Fig. 7.84 shows intracranial exposure, showing dissection at the anterior skull base. Note that the frontal lobes have been retracted, dura has been excised leaving olfactory nerves and margin of the dura to be resected enbloc with the cribriform plate and the ethmoid labyrinth

be excised using a rongeur. The amount of dura and anterior cranial fossa floor resected depends upon the extent of the tumor. To enhance the exposure supraorbital bar can be included in resected specimen. (Fig. 7.85).

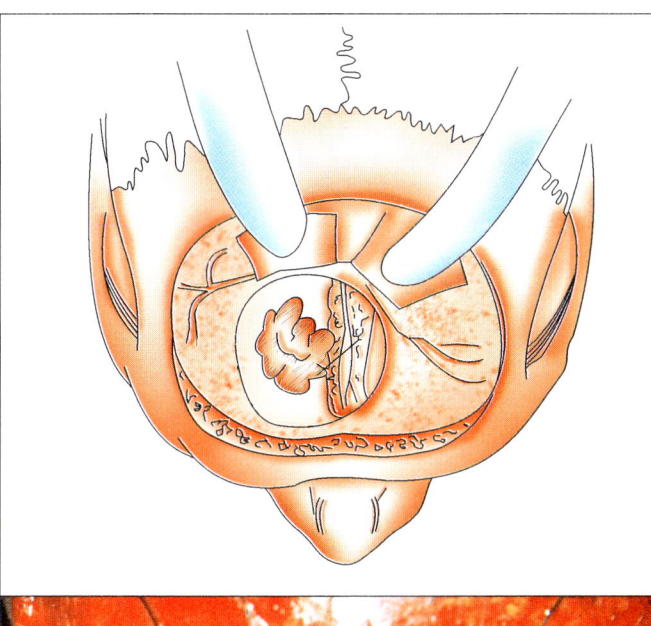

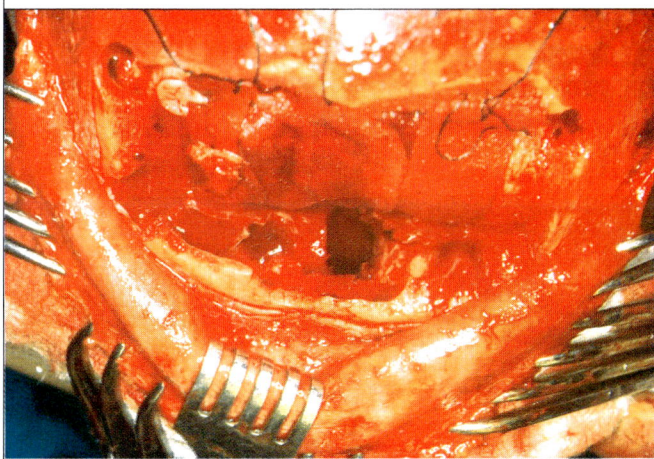

Fig. 7.85 Showing exposure of anterior cranial fossa floor with tumor

9. Dissection is then continued in a posterior direction to expose the posterior part of the cribriform plate and the planum sphenoidale. It must be reemphasized that retraction and handling of the brain should be minimized to avoid postoperative complications. Slackening of the brain by draining 30 to 60 ml of CSF via the intrathecal catheter is usually sufficient. A wide malleable retractor is used gently to protect the frontal lobes in the midline posteriorly to expose the planum sphenoidale and the cribriform plate. The

bone cuts in the floor of the anterior cranial fossa are completed using a fine burr on the high speed drill once the facial exposure is done.

10. Bone cuts are as follow:
    a. A sharp osteotome is used to mobilize the cribriform plate by transecting the floor of the anterior cranial fossa around it.
    b. Laterally, the osteotome is placed widely enough to encompass the medial walls of both orbital cavities, particularly on the side of maximal involvement.
    c. Posteriorly the osteotome enters the sphenoidal sinus.
    d. If the tumor involves the planum sphenoidale, the bony optic canal will need to be unroofed to protect the optic nerves.
    e. Anteriorly, the frontal sinus is entered and the posterior wall of the frontal sinus is included in the resection. The frontal sinus mucosa is curetted, and each sinus is drained into the nasal cavity.
    f. If the growth or tumor extends anteriorly the supraorbital bar can be removed with these osteotomies and replaced as a free graft if not involved.

11. In cases of tumors restricted to the midline of the anterior cranial fossa, a circumferential cut around the cribriform plate is adequate. More extensive tumors, such as those involving the lamina papyracea or the orbit, require the removal of appropriate amounts of the orbital roof to allow en bloc resection of the tumor.

    This concludes the first phase of the operation.

Facial phase of resection

The tumor can be approached from the inferior aspect via one of many transfacial approaches.

- Lateral rhinotomy (described earlier)
- Weber-ferguson (described earlier)
- Midfacial degloving
- Billers approach
- Le-fortes -I osteotomy

Although the sublabial approach avoids making facial scars, its exposure is generally adequate only for inferiorly located tumors. Facial incision may be avoided in cases of selected tumors of the superior nasal vault or ethmoid sinuses if adequate exposure and resection can be accomplished transcranially.

The transfacial exposure usually uses modifications of the lateral rhinotomy which may or may not transect the lip depending upon whether total maxillectomy will be performed. In most cases a complete en bloc ethmoidectomy will need to be performed necessitating a contralateral Lynch incision.

1. Depending upon the nature of the tumor incision is made. The skin incision is taken through the entire thickness of the soft tissue and musculature of the nasolabial region. A lateral cheek flap is developed to expose the facial surface of the maxilla as far as infraorbital foramen, leaving the nerve intact.

2. Fine periosteal elevators are used to dissect the nasolacrimal duct from its fossa, and the duct is divided flush with the rim of the orbit by using a scalpel. (Before the nasal pack is introduced, nasolacrimal drainage needs to be reestablished using silastic stents.) The attachment of the medial canthal ligament is sharply divided and tagged with a No. 4-0 Neurolon suture for subsequent reattachment to the nasal bone during closure. The orbital periosteum is incised medially and inferiorly and is separated from the medial and inferior orbital walls. The orbital contents are retracted laterally. Anterior and posterior ethmoidal arteries are identified and ligated.

3. **Nasal cavity** is entered by incising the soft tissue along the pyriform crest and osteotomy with outfracture of the nasal bone (rhinoplasty -type cuts are made to allow reflection and preservation of the nasal bones, thus minimizing postoperative deformity). A low lateral osteotomy is followed by superior one with a 2 mm chisel, 2 mm superior to the medial canthal ligament. The 2 mm chisel is also used to perform a perforating medial osteotomy with the aim of reflecting the nasal bone without detachment.

4. **Frontal bone is osteotomised** laterally and superiorly; complete vertical transection of the nasal septum anteriorly. The nasal septum is than transected inferiorly. This permits retraction of entire nose to expose the contralateral nasal cavity (Fig. 7.86).

5. It is vital to plan and make soft-tissue and bone cuts around the tumor so that total enbloc resection of the tumor is achieved. Tumors that are soft and friable may fracture during removal, but piecemeal resection should never be the aim of the procedure. Once the tumor has been surgically invaded into, blood obscures normal tissue planes and surrounding margins. If preoperative imaging studies or intraoperative observations confirm the presence of tumor with in

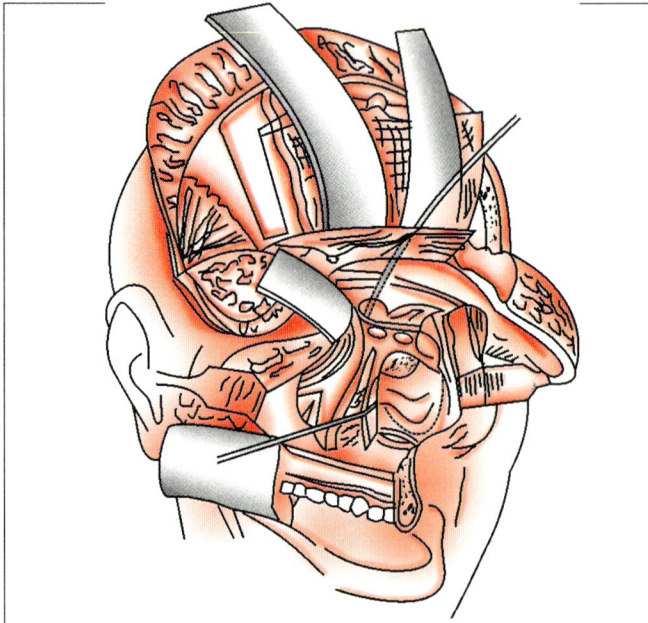

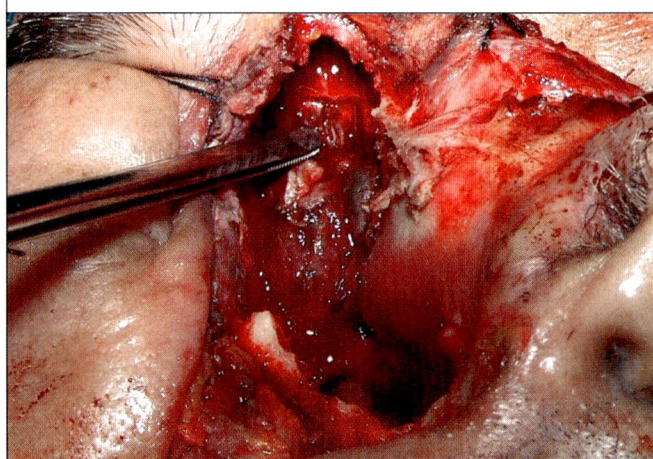

Fig. 7.86 Extended lateral rhinotomy incision has been performed, frontal bone is osteotomized laterally and superiorly. Vertical transaction of nasal septum anteriorly.

the soft tissues of the orbit, then orbital exentration may be facilitated by extending the skin incision laterally to include a portion of eyelids. Depending on the nature and extent of the tumor, ostetomies may also be made to include part or all of the maxilla.

6. **Creation of defect in anterior maxilla:** The antrum is entered by perforating the anterior wall. The opening is enlarged using Hajek's forceps. This manoeuvre allows visualization of the posterior wall of the antrum when forming the bone cuts (Fig. 7.87).

7. **Bone cuts** on the ipsilateral side are done through the medial wall of antrum inferiorly and through the roof

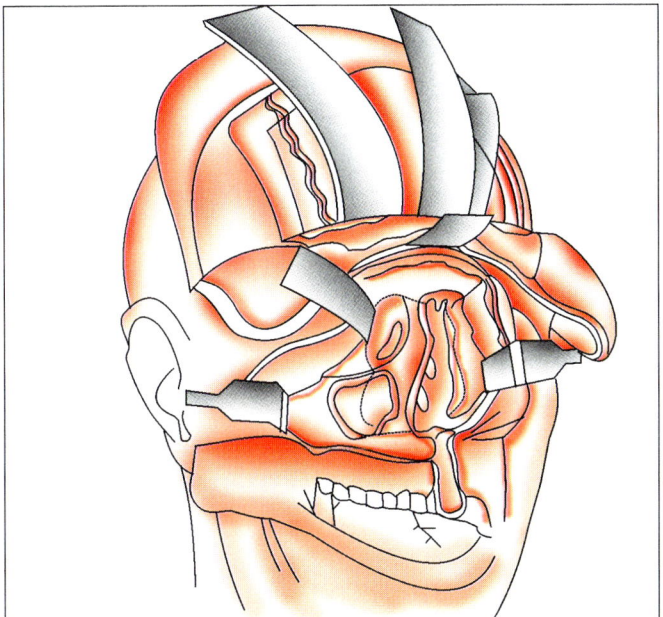

Fig. 7.87

of antrum, extending back to the level of posterior antral wall. The lateral wall of nose is mobilized by dividing between superior and inferior turbinates. The contralateral bone cuts are than made via intranasal or intracranial approach. Resection may include the entire medial orbital wall, or it may include the entire medial antral wall as well (Fig. 7.88).

8. Following this attention is returned to anterior fossa and cuts are made through fovea on each side and through the posterior part of the cribriform plate. Cutting through the anterior ethmoid cells allows the whole segment to be removed in block.

9. Final mobilization of specimen done by downward pressure on the cribriform plate as the specimen is delivered into the facial wound (Fig. 7.90).

10. The residual mucosal attachment are cut with scissors.

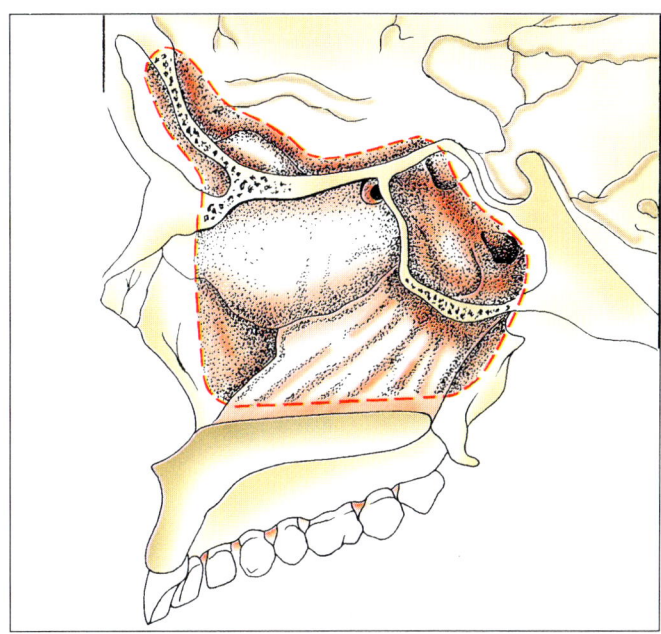

Fig. 7.89 Area of sinus tissue usually removed in craniofacial resection

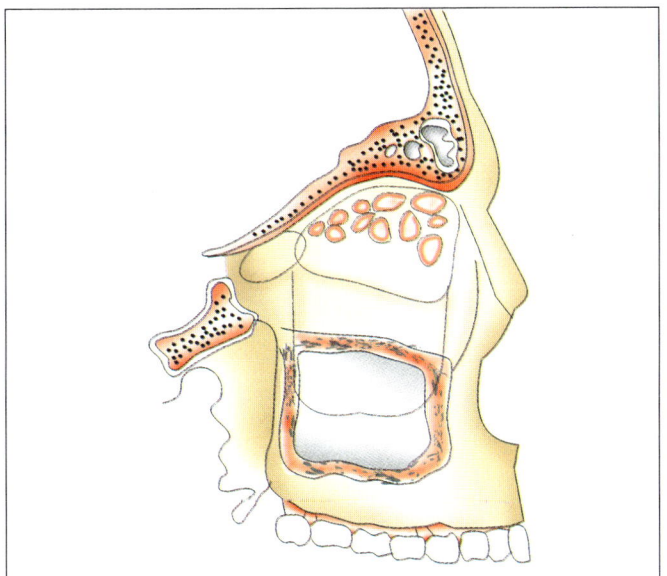

Fig. 7.88

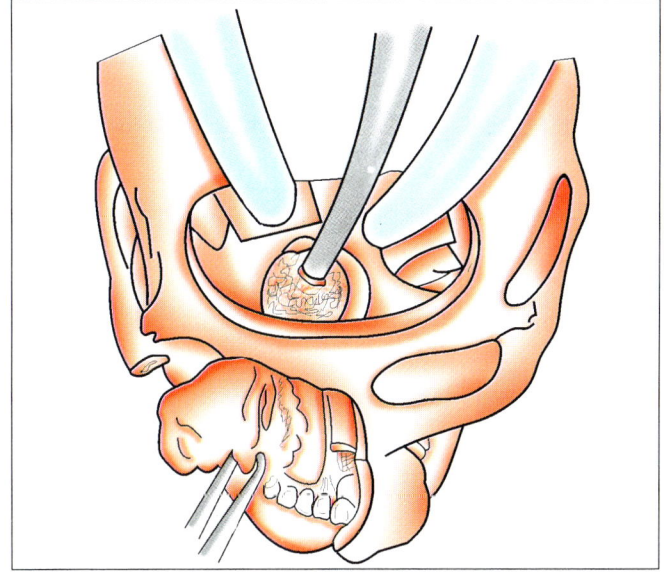

Fig. 7.90 The cut is made with the drill through the fovea on each side and through the posterior part of the cribriform plate

11. The specimen is then removed completely resulting in the large defect present in the roof of the nose continuing with the anterior cranial base (Fig. 7.91a, b & c).

12. All the exposed paranasal sinus mucosa is removed by curettage.

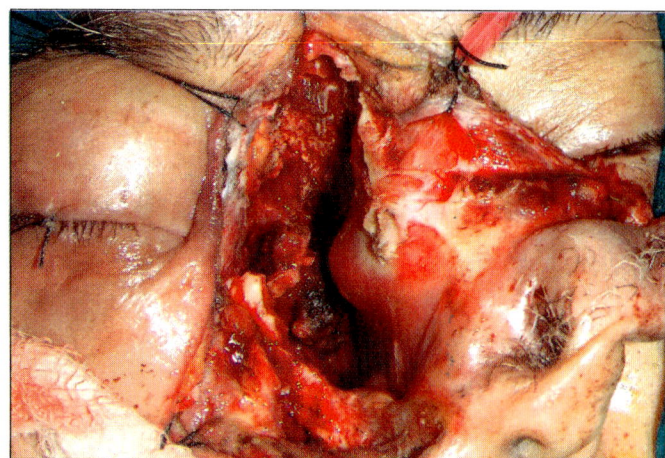

Fig. 7.91c Defect after the tumor removal

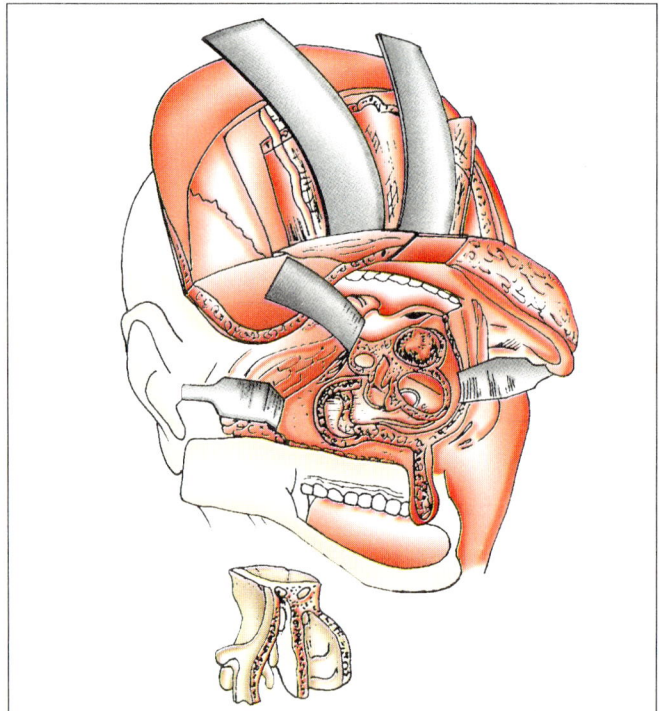

Fig. 7.91a The specimen removed in a enblock fashion resulting in large defect in the roof of the nose containing with anterior cranial base

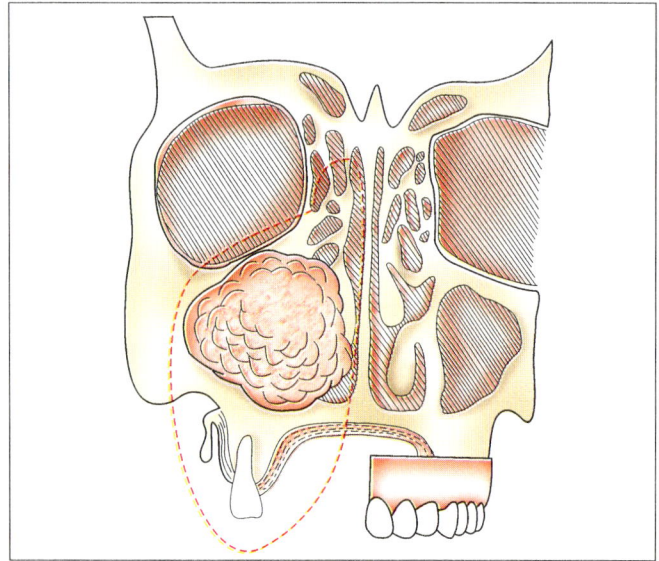

Fig. 7.91b Showing the extent of the resection in coronal section

13. Skull base defect is then closed using galeal flap (after dural repair) (Fig. 7.92a & b). The galeal flap is turned into form the floor of the anterior cranial fossa. This galeal flap is necessary for the prevention of osteomyelitis, because the free frontal bone flap would otherwise be exposed to the nasal cavity. If a craniotomy is placed just above the eyebrow (*e.g.*, to be able to resect the frontal sinuses, with the glabella and frontal process that forms the suture line with the lamina papyracea), then the galeal flap can be based at the anterior (inferior) edge of the scalp flap. The galeal flap is then turned inferiorly to cover the dura where the cribriform plate is resected. A portion of the frontal bone inferiorly has to be removed with the resection of the frontal sinus. This affords space for the turned-in galeal flap, thus preventing impingement or pressure on the flap. Although the dura may be intact in most of the cases, a portion may require resection and patching with fascia.

14. The frontal bone flap is replaced and secured with tie wires placed through drill holes. Wire sutures are avoided if postoperative radiotherapy is anticipated, because "local electron scatter and osteoradionecrosis do not subsequently develop."

15. A split-thickness skin graft is placed to cover the inner bare area of the cheek flap as well as other large bare areas. However, a skin graft should not be buried. It is better that the other bare areas be covered by regrowth of mucosa to facilitate a moist surface. The septal columella and dorsum of the septum have to be preserved for support of the nasal tip, alar nasi and nasal bridge. The remaining portion of the septum can be resected.

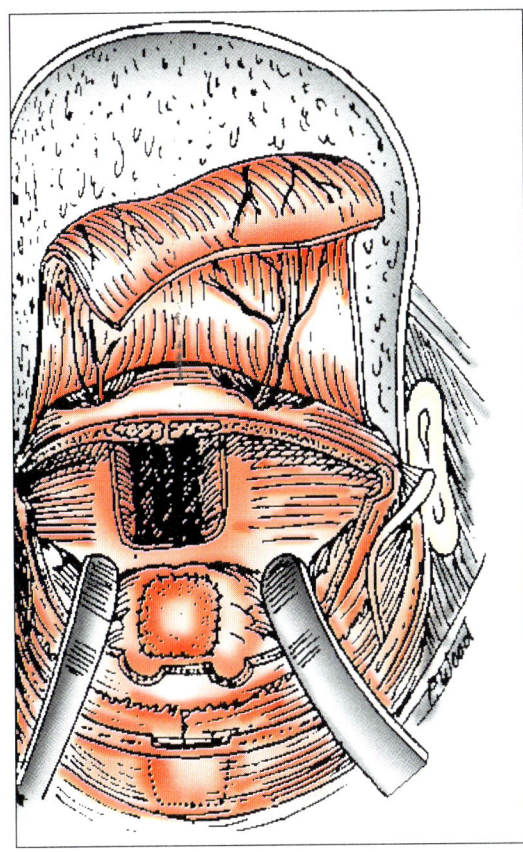

Fig. 7.92a

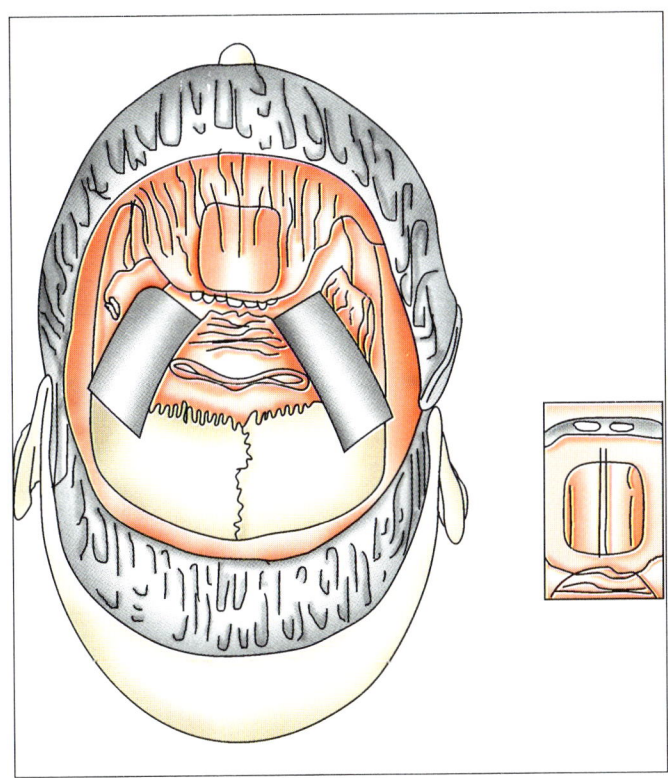

Fig. 7.92b

16. If there is any significant bone defect of the cranium over the frontal lobe, a free-septal cartilage graft or bone graft can be placed between the dura and the cranium. A nasal septal flap can also be placed over the cranial base defect.

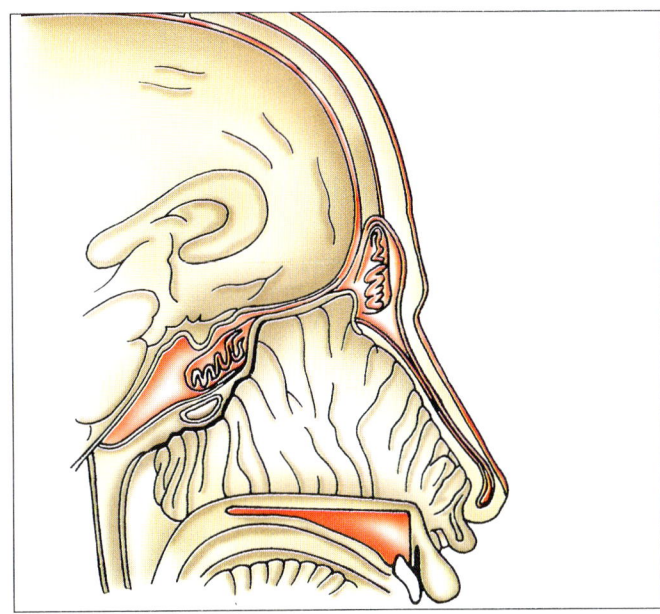

Fig. 7.93 showing nasal packing

17. The entire nasal cavity is then packed snugly with a Xeroform roller gauze packing to provide support to the galeal pericranial flap superiorly and the medial orbital periosteum laterally.

18. The nasofrontal ducts are obliterated and the sinus is obliterated or cranialized. The facial incisions are closed with attention to the medial canthal tendon and lacrimal apparatus.

19. Skin closure is done in layers.

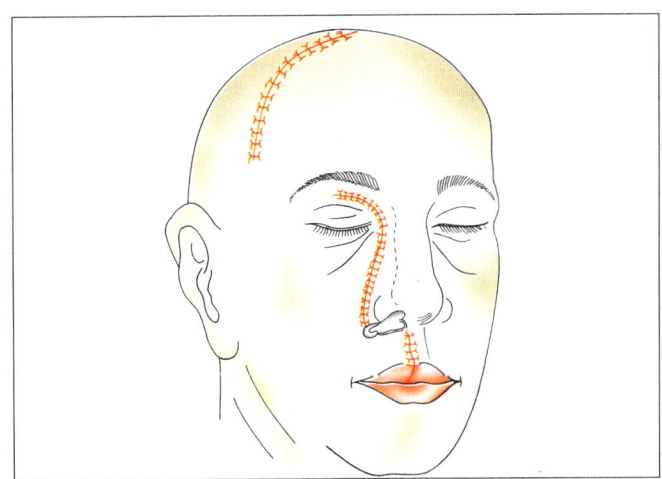

Fig. 7.94 Facial and scalp incisions sutured in layers

20. Towards the end of the 1st postoperative week (maintain patient on intravenous antibiotics). The nasal pack is removed in stages over a period of 2 to 3 days via the nostril.

Reconstruction procedures

The concept of combining facial and anterior cranial surgery has been known for many years, but newer surgical approaches and expanded applications of these approaches have resulted in a greater surgical challenge from the standpoint of reconstruction following surgical ablation of neoplasms involving the floor of the anterior cranial fossa.

Why reconstruction is important?

- Defects resulting form craniofacial resection frequently result in exposure of dura and vital structures such as the brain and various cranial nerves. Soft tissue is required to cover these vital structures
- Prevent the development of cerebrospinal fluid leaks by providing watertight seals.
- Reconstruction must provide sufficient structural support to prevent brain herniation.
- Failure to achieve a watertight seal may result in CSF fistula, meningitis, intracranial abscess or a wound infection that compromises the graft.

Flap selection, design, and insetting are the primary components in preventing postoperative complications.

Technical considerations and tissue flap selection

1. Dural repair.
2. Reconstruction of skull base defects.
3. Reconstruction of medial canthus.
4. Reconstruction of nasolacrimal drainage.
5. Palatal obturators and others methods of reconstruction of maxillectomy defects.

Consideration of size of defects

The complexity of reconstruction is related to the size of the violation of normal boundaries between a sterile intracranial cavity and a bacteria-laden extracranial environment.

Small defects, closure of the dura with a graft may suffice if primary closure is not possible.

Larger skull base tumor resections, the key is to provide a barrier for the intracranial compartment to protect the dural closure.

The reconstructive needs, functional and esthetic, must be balanced against donor-site morbidity.

1. Dural repair

Types of dural repair

a. Primary

b. Graft

c. Flap

- **Primary** closure of dura is always preferred.
- **Grafts:** If primary closure is not possible, cadaveric dura, autologous facial grafts or pericranial flaps can be used.

Torn dura must be repaired and resected dura must be replaced.

A rim of dura should be preserved posteriorly to facilitate dural patching with fascia late. A second layer of fascia late may be placed across the roof to the nose and secured to bone laterally, acting as a hammock to support the brain. A split thickness skin graft is placed on the nasal surface of this free graft. The skin graft is secured to the fascia in the upper nasal passage for 10 days, utilizing nasal packs saturated with a liquid suspension of tetracycline or terramycin. To enhance the structural support of the frontal lobes, iliac crest bone or nasal cartilage can be fashioned to span the gap across the resected cribriform plate and fovea ethmoidalis. The graft is places superior to the bone defect, overlapping the bone margins of the resection. The implant is placed between the dural patch graft above and the free fascia late graft below.

Soft tissue coverage of the anterior skull base and repair of the dural defects may be accomplished in one step by developing a galeal flap, which provides support for the frontal lobes and sufficient vascularity to nourish a split thickness skin graft. The flap is developed by dissecting galeas and subcutaneous tissues through a brow incision. The soft tissue flap is based on the supraorbital artery and vein and is rotated as an anteriorly based flap downward and backward and sutured to the remaining dura laterally and posteriorly. The nasal surface of the galeal flap is covered with a split thickness skin graft.

2. Reconstruction of skull base defects

Types of reconstruction

- Local or regional flaps.
- Pedicled flaps or free flaps (free tissue transfer).

LOCAL TISSUE FLAPS

Pedicled galeal pericranial flap

The pedicled galeal pericranial flap is considerably more robust than a pericranial flap and is the flap of choice when reconstructing the skull base defect. It is important to harvest a sufficient length of the flap posteriorly so that it can extend to the skull base defect without undue tension. To provide additional length to the graft, the skin incision is made well posterior on the scalp and through the pericranium.

During reconstruction of the skull base, the galeal pericranial flap is separated from the anterior scalp flap, remaining superficial to the galeal. Sufficient length of the flap is separated to obtain adequate tissue for repair, without compromising its blood supply from the supraorbital and - trochlear vessels. The galeal-pericranial flap is dissected using a No. 15 blade and wrapped in a bacitracin, soaked gauze throughout the procedure. A 1-cm cuff of galea should be preserved on the anterior flap for subsequent scalp closure. The incision should be fashioned to provide approximately 8 cm of pericranial-galeal graft to cover the skull base deficit. The remaining 10 cm of pericranial graft can be folded over to create third layer of closure. On occasion, the scalp incision may be limited to one side if only unilateral exposure is desired as, for example, in cases of orbital tumors that do not approach or cross the midline

Pericranial flaps

The most commonly used flap for reconstruction of anterior skull base defects is the pericranial flap. The vascular supply is usually derived from the supraorbital and supratrochlear arteries. During the transbasal approach for craniofacial resection, a vascularized pericranial flap can be harvested from the bicoronal incision. The flap is suspended to the adjacent skull base with sutures passed through drill holes and in some instances is fastened to the skull base with titanium screws directly. Alternatively, it may be sutured to the dural margin beyond the region of dural repair. If the orbital roofs are intact, the pericranial flap may be sufficient in achieving adequate support without formal bone reconstruction. This has become a standard technique in repairing simple midline anterior skull base defects after tumor ablation. Alternatively, an extended pericranial flap can be used for defects extending beyond the clivus into the nasopharynx and cervical spine.

Temporalis muscle flaps

Medial transposition of the temporalis muscle is very effective for reconstruction of anterolateral skull base defects. This muscle can be transferred with calvarial bone for orbital rim reconstruction.

- Its use was first described for reconstruction of orbitomaxillary defects.
- Unsightly and potentially dangerous defects of the orbit and periorbital regions.
- Limited by its narrow arc of rotation, the temporalis muscle can cover ipsilateral defects of the orbitofrontal region, maxilla, temporal bone, and infratemporal fossa.
- The temporalis muscle flap is most useful for blanking out the orbit after exenteration when eyelid skin has been preserved.

Disadvantages

- Transfer of the entire muscle can result in a significant cosmetic depression in the donor-site area.
- With larger medially situated defects that communicate with the nasopharynx, temporalis muscle flaps are less reliable and free flaps are usually indicated.

Access to the temporalis muscle

- Through a coronal incision above the auricle.
- The muscle with its deep periosteum and superficial fascia is elevated from above downward.
- The facial attachment to the zygomatic arch is divided transversely to make possible free forward rotation of the muscle. To preserve its blood supply from the internal maxillary artery, the muscle must remain attached to the coronoid process.
- The muscle is rotated into the orbit through a fenestration in the lateral orbital wall. The window should be large enough to avoid attrangulation of the muscle. In mobilizing the muscle forward, care must be taken not to injure branches of the facial nerve.
- The fascia of the temporalis muscle may be sutured to the fibrous tissue in the region of the medial canthal ligament to prevent retraction of the muscle.

Nasal septal flap

A nasal septal flap can also be placed over the cranial base defect in case of significant bone defects below the frontal lobe.

Regional flaps

The loss of the eyelids, orbital contents and the maxilla

following large craniofacial resections results in a formidable rehabilitation task. Traditional methods of reconstructing large orbital maxillary defects include the use of the forehead flap, nape of the neck flap, and medially based deltopectoral flap. Except for the forehead flap, all these skin flaps should be delayed because of the relatively long distance between the surgical defect and the flap donor site. The disadvantages of these regional skin flaps include insufficient bulk to fill in the orbital defect and skin, which may tend to be less pliable than adjacent facial skin.

Pedicled myocutaneous flaps

More contemporary methods of rehabilitating patients with orbital maxillary defect include the use of regional musculocutaneous flaps pedicled on their dominant blood supply. The need to reconstruct more extensive anterior skull base defects led to the development of pedicled musculocutaneous (muscle and overlying skin) flaps. These may be derived from the pectoralis major, trapezius, latissimus dorsi, or sternocleidomastoid muscles. Musculocutaneous flaps offer more coverage for larger skull base defects and may provide greater protection against bacterial invasion when compared with skin flaps. Both the pectoralis major and posterior trapezius myocutaneous flaps have been advocated for the reconstruction following temporal bone resection. Because of its proximity, the trapezius myocutaneous flap is favored for reconstructing laterally situated defects of the posterior skull base.

The most distal aspect of the pedicled myocutaneous flap is often the most tenuous area of blood circulation. Tension on the vascular pedicle from excessive reach can result in ischemia. A small area of marginal necrosis can lead to introduction of pathogens and subsequent ascending meningitis. Authors of some reports have suggested that pedicled myocutaneous flaps are associated with high complication rates and do not always provide a watertight seal of the nasopharynx.

The two most versatile flaps are the pectoralis major and the trapezius musculocutaneous flaps. Both may be mobilized to reach the orbital area without delay. The latissimus dorsi musculocutaneous flap has been used to reconstruct the orbital region as an island pedicle flap tunneled beneath the skin of the neck form the axilla. In the case of the pectoralis major musculocutaneous flap, necrosis of the distal portion of the flap may occur when the cutaneous territory is extended beyond the sixth rib. This extension is often necessary to gain sufficient length to reach the level of the eyebrow superiorly and thus delay of the distal portion of the flap is prudent.

Free tissue transfer (Free flaps)

The major advancement in skull base reconstruction is free tissue transfer, which is regarded by most authors as the best method to cover large defects of the skull base. Free flaps have revolutionized skull base reconstruction by providing large quantities of flexible, well-vascularized tissue to cover more medial and extensive defects, especially when multiple cavities (nasal, oral, and pharyngeal) are violated. By providing additional vascularized tissue, these grafts are ideal for extensive resections that involve the removal of dura, bone, muscle, and skin.

The large size and conformal ability facilitates obliteration of dead space and isolation of the intracranial cavity from the nasopharynx. They are also optimal for reconstruction of the skull base in patients who have undergone previous surgery or radiation therapy. The wide selection of free flaps includes latissimus dorsi, rectus abdominus, greater omentum, radial forearm, scapula, parascapula, and tensor fascia lata. The use of free flaps for reconstruction should be reserved for situations in which local and regional flaps are not suitable and when vascularized tissue is required. Many authors have reported that free flaps are associated with fewer complications and are superior to local and pedicled flaps in creating a watertight seal.

3. Reconstruction of craniectomy defects

If extirpation of the tumor requires craniectomy, reconstruction- related options include no osseous support, alloplastic material, split calvarial graft, or free flap reconstruction. Small craniectomy defects may be left open, without bone reconstruction, if the patient is able and willing to take measures to protect the underlying brain from injury. Alloplastic material such as acrylic plates, titanium plates, or synthetic mesh and methylmethacrylate cement may interfere with healing and delay initiation of radiotherapy. The approach-related risks and benefits need to be carefully considered to avoid compromising the quality of treatment.

4. Reconstruction of medial canthus

Reconstruction of the surgical defect entails repositioning the divided medial canthus to its normal position, providing watertight support across the anterior skull base, reestablishing nasolacrimal drainage, and accurate re-approximation of the facial incisions. It is important to match the position of the divided medial canthal ligament accurately to the contralateral side to avoid telecanthus. The previously tagged end of the medial canthal ligament is sutured via an appropriately positioned drill hole in the nasal bone.

If functioning of eye has been preserved, the floor of the orbit must be reconstructed using a split calvarial graft or rib graft to avoid postoperative diplopia.

5. Reconstruction of nasolacrimal drainage

Needs to be reestablished to avoid postoperative epiphora. A silastic stent is used to cannulate the puncta of the nasolacrimal duct, and the stent is kept in place by knotting its two ends within the nasal cavity.

6. Reconstruction of maxillectomy defects

The traditional approach has been to surface the cavity with a split thickness skin graft and rehabilitate the patient with a palatal obturator. The advent of microvascular surgery allows these defects to be reconstructed using vascularized flaps that provide lining, soft-tissue bulk, and osseous support. A bulky intraoral component of the flap can interfere with dental prosthetic rehabilitation, but patients who retain healthy dentition after resection are able to function without being inconvenienced by the necessity for care of the prosthesis. In such patients the external appearance can be greatly improved by a facial prosthesis. The services of a skillful maxillofacial prosthetist are invaluable in rehabilitating patients with facial deformity following extensive CFS.

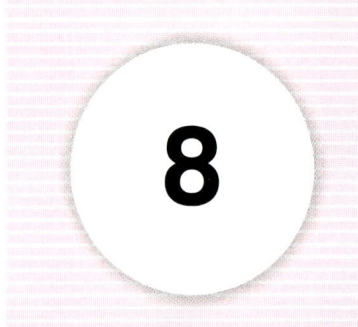

8

Approaches to Lateral Skull Base

APPROACHES TO INFRATEMPORAL AND PTERYGOPALATINE FOSSA

1. Patient selection

Patients in whom an ITF approach or dissection are contraindicated include:

- Those with lymphoreticular tumors, which are best treated with radiation and/or chemotherapy.

- Pulmonary, cardiac, renal, or other significant comorbidity.

- Patients with disseminated disease or distant metastasis.

- Patient must not have neoplastic involvement of intracranial course of any cranial nerve except facial or trigeminal nerve. Sphenoid sinus or cavernous sinus as clear margins of normal tissue cannot be safely removed beyond these structures. Posterior oropharynx as the tumour will have extent into posterior mediastinum which is non-resectable.

- An ITF approach is a complex procedure involving significant time, effort, and cost; therefore, under most circumstances, consider the procedure only as part of a curative therapeutic plan.

- Patient should be willing to accept: Possibility of facial distortion. Need for palatal prosthesis. Permanent unilateral hearing loss in certain surgeries (like Type C Fisch). Prolonged hospitalization. Neurological complications that may arise especially in intra cranial extension.

  Example: stroke, meningitis.

2. Patient evaluation

Assessment of Local extent and distant metastasis is made by:

Physical examination

- *Neurological examination*

  1. Ophthalmoscopy

  2. Indirect Laryngoscopy and rigid telescopy of Larynx.

  3. Otomicroscopy

  4. Diagnostic nasal endoscopy

- *CT and MRI*

- *Angiography :* MR angiography (MRA) and CT angiography (CTA) are noninvasive tests that demonstrate the arterial anatomy of the ITF and brain. Angiography is preferred over MRA and CTA when preoperative embolization of the tumor is indicated (*e.g.,* juvenile nasopharyngeal angiofibromas [JNA], paragangliomas).

  But collateral blood supply is better evaluated using single-photon emission computed tomography (SPECT) with balloon occlusion, transcranial Doppler, or angiography and balloon occlusion with xenon-enhanced computed tomography (ABOX-CT) scan.

3. Preoperative embolisation

Prior to this, angiography has to be done which tells about vascular supply of lesion, angioarchitecture and potential anastomotic connections. Gelfoam is commonly used however it is short lived. Its life being 7-21 days. On table injection of embolus may be done into external carotid artery above the superior thyroid branch.

4. Biopsy

Whenever possible. FNAC, truecut, frozen section.

5. Staging

Staging done after CT neck, CT scan of the chest and abdomen and a bone scan. A lumbar spinal tap for cerebrospinal fluid (CSF) cytology and a spinal MRI to rule out "drop metastasis".

Preoperative details

1. Preexistent lower cranial neuropathies (*e.g.*, CNS IX-XII) are common in patients with tumors at the parapharyngeal space, tumors that extend to the jugular foramen, or both. These patients present with hypernasal or slurred speech, nasal regurgitation, dysphagia, aspiration, and dysphonia (CNS X and XII). Lower cranial neuropathies presenting with aspiration have life-threatening consequences patients with a proximal vagal paralysis may benefit from a medialization laryngoplasty and an arytenoid adduction procedure with speech and language and swallowing therapy.

   - A tracheostomy to facilitate tracheal toilet.

   - A gastrostomy tube to facilitate postoperative feeding and to decrease the risk of post prandial aspiration.

   - Velopharyngeal insufficiency (VPI) may be corrected by a palatal lift prosthesis, a pharyngeal flap or a palatoplasty.

   - Myringotomy, amplification, or both in case of conductive or sensorineural hearing loss.

   - Preoperatively evaluate corneal sensation and protective mechanisms.

   - Facial weakness or paralysis, facial spasms, and epiphora. A gold weight, tarsorrhaphy.

   - Trismus due to pain resolves with the induction of general anesthesia. Mechanical trismus may require a nasotracheal intubation performed while awake or, if the trismus is expected to persist even after tumor removal, a tracheostomy is performed while the patient is under local anesthesia.

2. Arrange for adequate blood replacement.

3. Wide-spectrum perioperative antibiotic prophylaxis with good penetration of the blood-brain barrier.

4. Somatosensory evoked potential (SSEP) monitoring of the median nerve proximity to nerves. Facial nerve monitoring is routinely used for transparotid or transtemporal approaches.

Choice of anesthetic agent and technique depends on various factors

1. The extent of intracranial dissection.

2. The potential for brain or vascular injury.

3. Systemic hemodynamics.

4. The need for monitoring of cortical and brainstem functions (*e.g.*, brainstem-evoked response, SSEP, EEG)..

5. The need for CN monitoring (i.e., CNS VII, X-XII).

On table preoperative preparation

- Secure the endotracheal tube with a circumdental or circummandibular wire ligature (*e.g.*, #26 stainless steel wire). Insert a spinal drain when intradural dissection is anticipated.

- Measures to diminish the intracranial pressure, such as hyperventilation, osmotic diuresis or corticosteroids.

- Pass and secure a nasogastric tube and Foley catheter.

- Antiembolic sequential-compression stockings are recommended to prevent deep venous thromboses.

- Position the head of the patient on a horseshoe-shaped head holder. Use "egg-crate" padding to avoid ischemic ulcers of the scalp or back during a prolonged surgery. When intracranial neurovascular dissection is anticipated, secure the head with a 3-pin head fixation system. When the need for proximal control of the ICA is anticipated, position the head in slight extension to facilitate access to the neck.

- Place tarsorrhaphy sutures for protection of the eyes.

- Shave the scalp, following the planned incision line (*e.g.*, bicoronal)

- Infiltrate the incision line with a solution of lidocaine and epinephrine (1:100,000-1:400,000).

Approaches to infratemporal and pterygopalatine fossa

1. Infratemporal fossa approaches

   - Infratemporal fossa approach of FISCH
   - Transparotid approach
     • Conservative total parotidectomy
     • Lateral conservative parotidectomy
     • Radial lateral parotidectomy
   - Extended rhytidectomy approach
   - Lateral transtemporal - sphenoid approach
   - Lateral facial approach
   - Subtemporal - preauricular infratemporal approach
   - Superior approach
   - Infratemporal fossa approach to sphenoid sinus

2. Transfacial approaches

   - Facial translocation approach
   - Extended anterolateral approach
   - Modified Barbosa approach
   - Transantral approaches
     • Lateral rhinotomy
     • Extended lateral rhinotomy
     • Weber fangusson
     • Mid facial degloving
     • Mid facial split approach

3. Tanscervical approach

   - Infuse approach
   - Biller's approach

4. Transpalatal approach

   - Wilson's transpalatal approach
   - Combined sublabial and transpalatal approach of Sardana's
   - Mishra and Bhatia's modification of transpalatal approach

5. Trans-endoscopic approach

Infra temporal fossa approach of lateral skull base

1. Fisch's approach

Infratemporal approaches to the lateral compartment have three distinct variations described by Fisch. All three of these approaches involve mastoidectomy, dissection and transposition of the facial nerve, and obliteration of the eustachian tube, middle ear, and external auditory canal (EAC). The type A approach provides access from the sigmoid sinus to the condylar fossa and is designed to reach the petrous apex and infralabyrinthine regions (Fig. 8.1).

The type B approach extends from the sigmoid sinus to the petrous tip with exposure of the horizontal petrous ICA and foramen ovale to provide access to the clivus (Fig. 8.2).

Finally, the type C variant extends the field of dissection to include the parasellar region to reach the cavernous sinus and foramen rotundum and lacerum. Removal of the pterygoid plates during the type C approach allows exposure of the nasopharynx (Fig. 8.3).

These techniques essentially extend the limit of dissection of the basic transtemporal approaches anteriorly by affording control of the petrous ICA. Conductive hearing loss is a result (Fig. 8.4a, b).

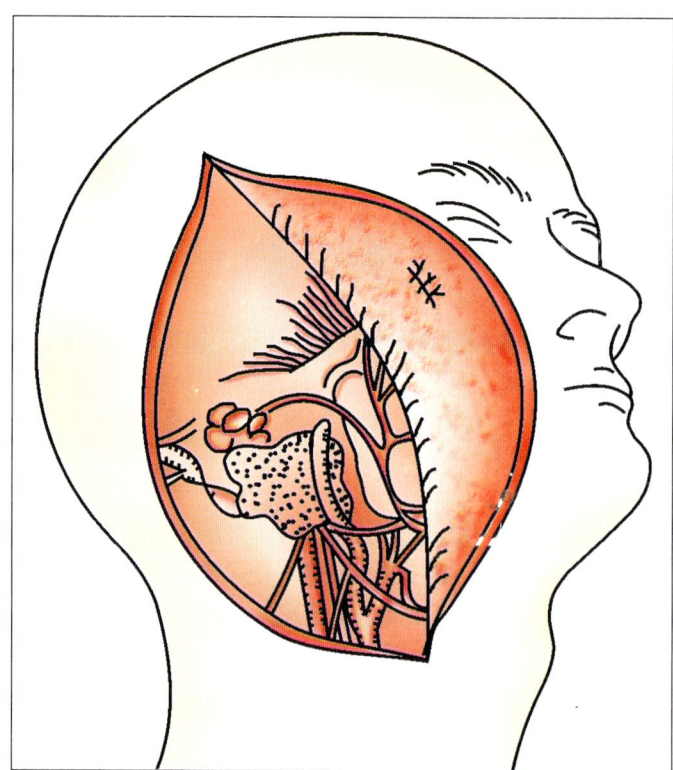

Fig. 8.1 Tumor exposure achieved by Type A approach

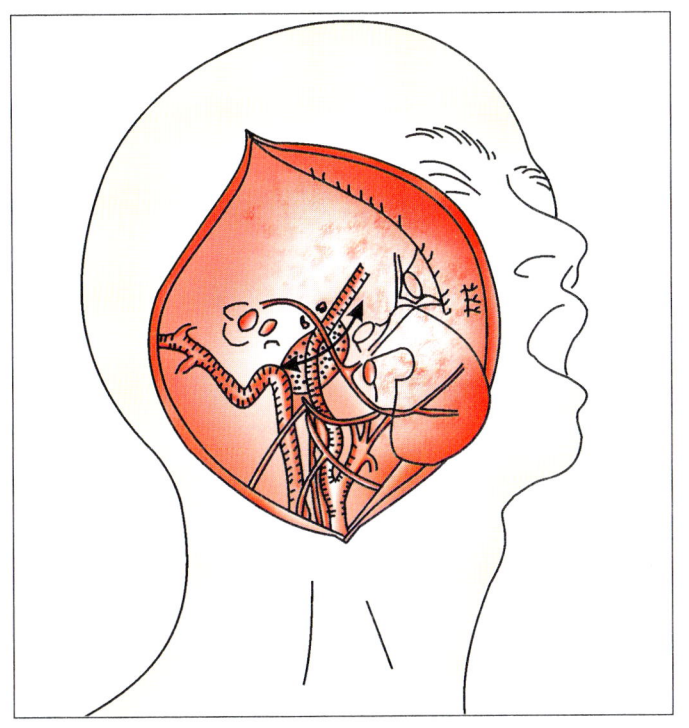

Fig. 8.2 Tumor exposure achieved by Type B approach

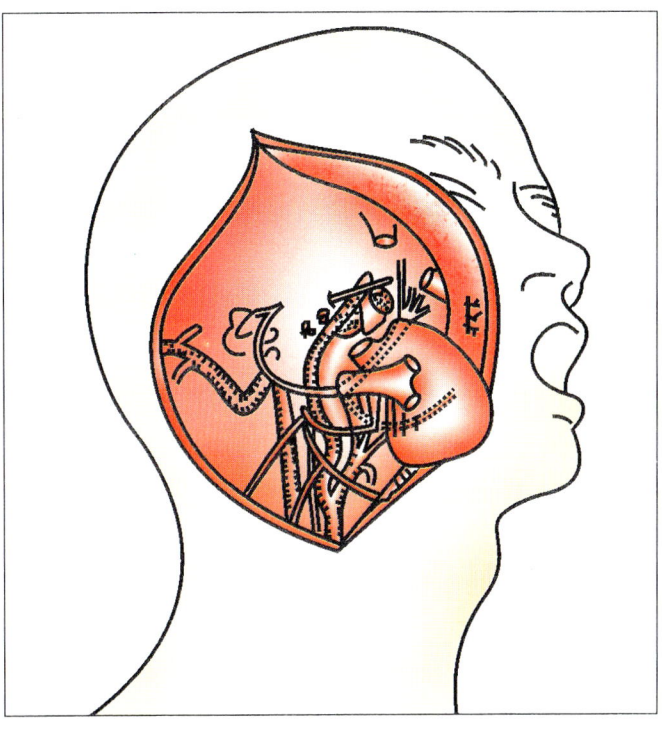

Fig. 8.3 Tumor exposure achieved by Type C approach

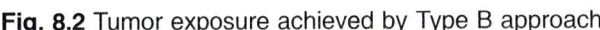

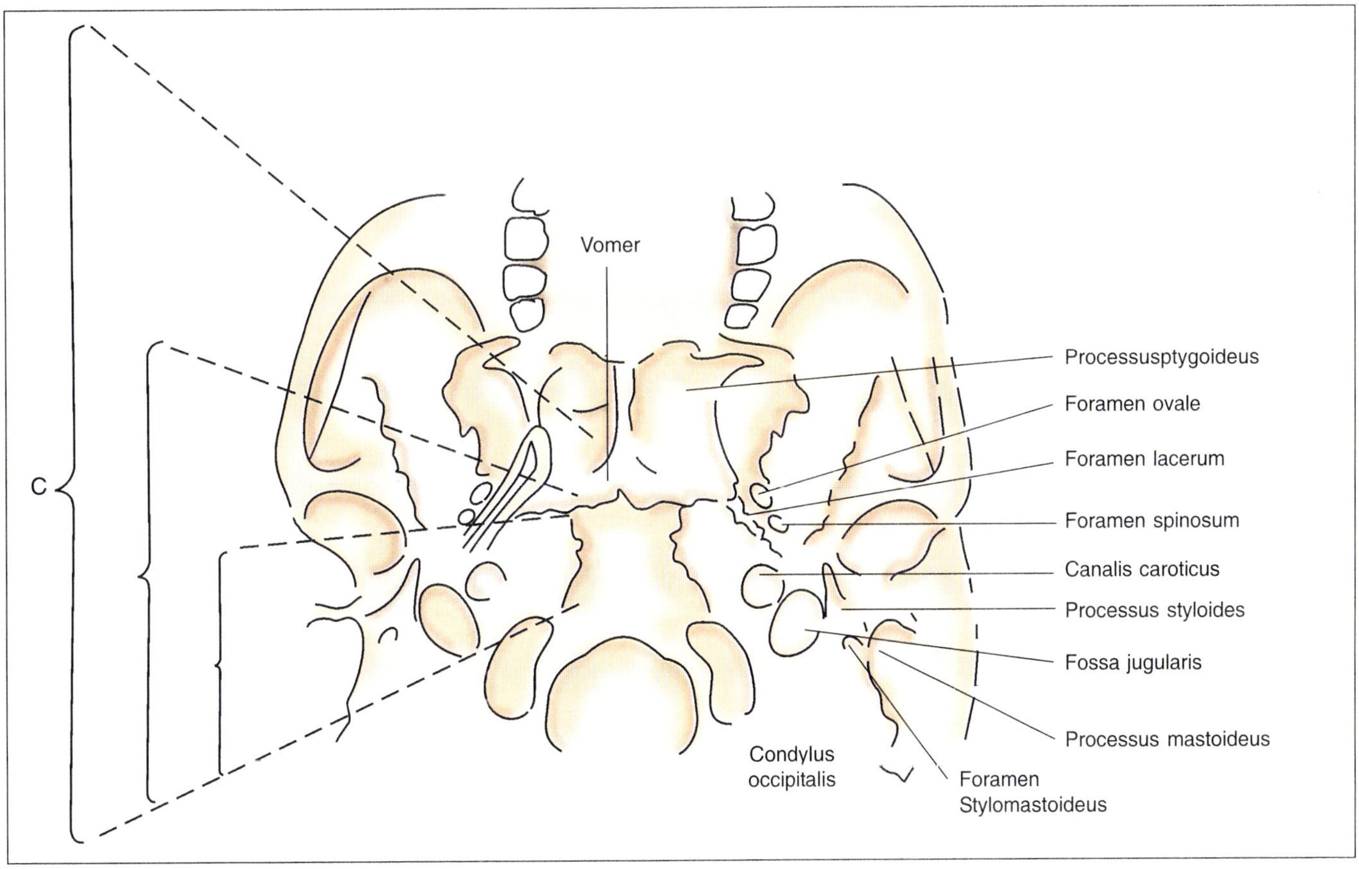

Vomer

Processusptygoideus

Foramen ovale

Foramen lacerum

Foramen spinosum

Canalis caroticus

Processus styloides

Fossa jugularis

Processus mastoideus

Condylus occipitalis

Foramen Stylomastoideus

C

Fig. 8.4a Schematic diagram showing the limits of FISCH type A, B, C

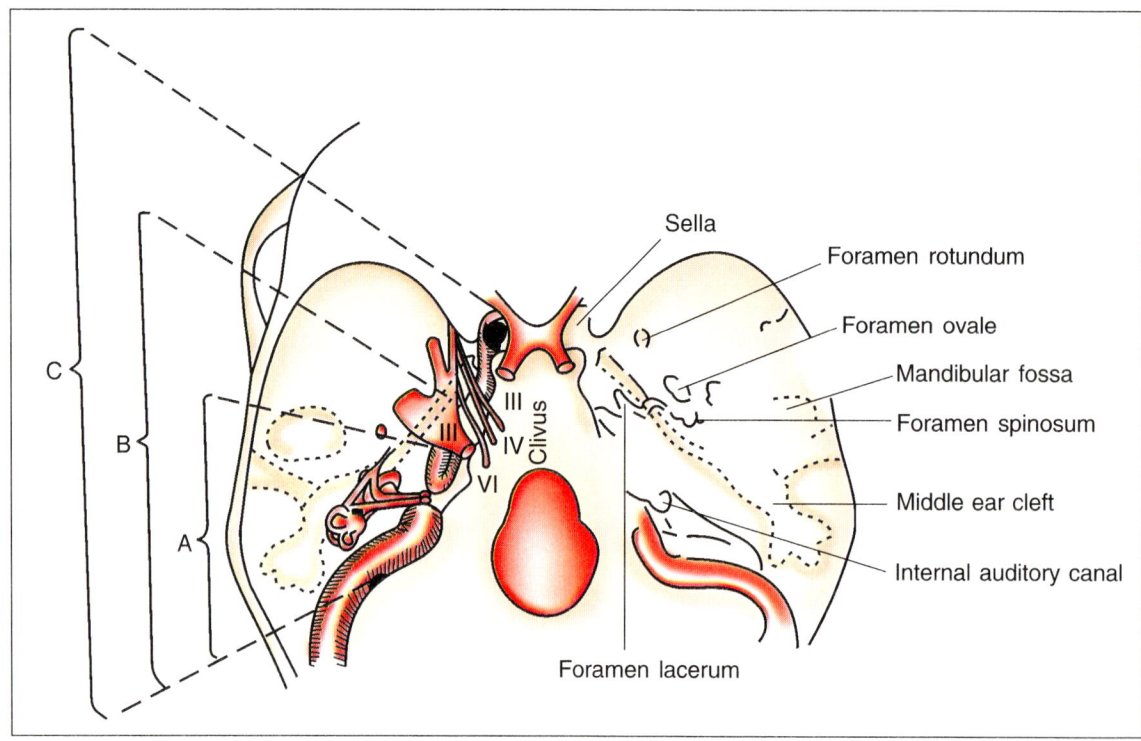

Fig. 8.4b Schematic diagram showing the limits of FISCH type A, B, C

Type A approach

Surgical technique

The skin incision involves undermining of anterior skin edge. A periosteal flap based on posterior aspect of the membranous canal wall is elevated as shown in figure (Fig.8.5 a & b).

Blind sac closure of the external auditory Canal

- The external auditory canal is transected at the bone-cartilage junction.

- The lateral canal skin is freed from the underlying cartilage, everted, and sutured using 4-0 Vicryl.

- The periosteal flap seals the inner surface of this suture line.

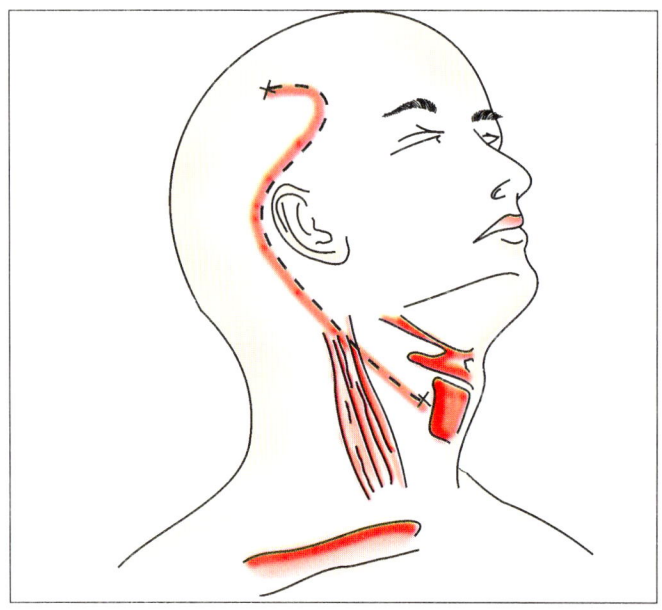

Fig. 8.5a Showing the marking for skin incision

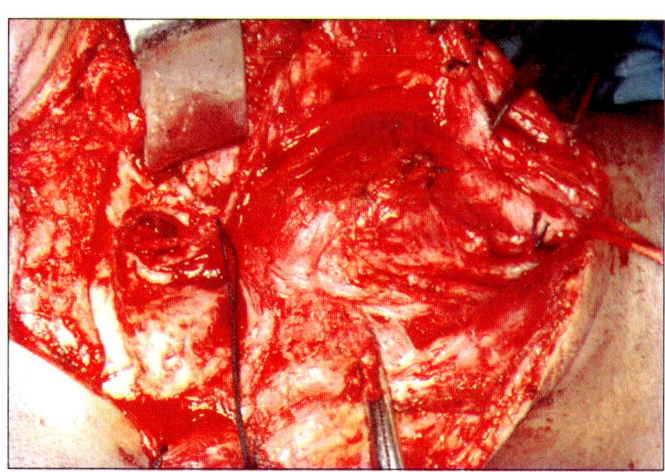

Fig. 8.5b

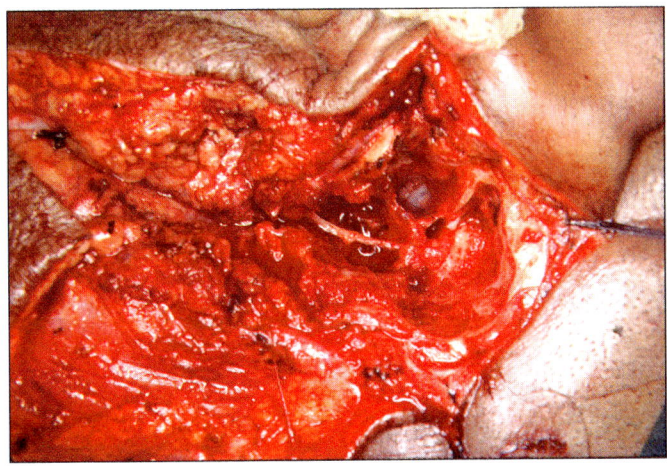

Fig. 8.6

Peripheral facial nerve

The facial nerve trunk is identified distal to the stylomastoid foramen along the axis formed by the bisection of a line drawn between the pointer of the tragal cartilage and the mastoid tip. The peripheral banches as far as the point of second division are exposed by lateral dissection of the superficial lobe of the parotid gland.

Dissection in the neck

Cranial nerves IX to XII, the carotid arteries and branches and the internal jugular vein are identified.

The tumor feeding arteries, namely, the ascending pharyngeal, occipital, and external carotid, are ligated. Heavy silk ligatures, to be tied at a later stage, are left loosely around the internal jugular vein.

Subtotal petrosectomy

The concept of subtotal petrosectomy embraces not only an extended radical mastoidectomy but exenteration of the complete petrous air cell system and all its contained mucosa. The surgical details are as follows:

1. Removal of the remaining skin of the bony external auditory canal, the tympanic membrane, the malleus, incus and stapes arch.

2. Detachment of the sternocleidomastoid muscle from the mastoid tip and removal of the mastoid tip.

3. Skeletonization of the middle cranial fossa dura.

4. Removal of all bone from the lateral sinus and from the posterior fossa dura in front of and behind the sinus.

Skeletonization of the fallopian canal from the geniculate ganglion to the stylomastoid foramen, using a diamond bur, suction irrigation, and the all purpose microraspatorium.

5. The protympanum is exenterated, removing at this time the lateral part of the tympanic bone. Care is taken to leave enough bone in the supratubal recess (anterior attic) to allow formation of a new fallopian canal. The internal carotid artery is identified medial to the eustachian tube, which is followed to its bony isthmus with the diamond bur and then obliterated with bone wax (Fig. 8.7a).

Permanent anterior transposition of the facial nerve

1. Creation of new fallopian canal in the anterior attic wall.

2. Vertical incision in the parotid tissue anterior: to the temporomandibular joint.

3. Repositioning of the nerve in the new canal and parotid groove. The edges of the parotid groove are sutured together to retain the nerve in position (Fig. 8.7b).

4. Use of an aluminium strip, attached to the self-retaining retractor, to protect the facial nerve in the new bony canal.

Permanent obliteration of Eustachian tube

The lateral wall of the bony eustachian tube is drilled away until the isthmus is revealed. The lumen of the eustachian tube is then packed with bone wax and a free fascia-muscle graft. Fibrin glue is used to secure the seal.

Double ligation of the sigmoid sinus

Double ligation of the sigmoid sinus is performed over the upper half of the sinus. Removal of all bone covering the sinus avoids any danger of laceration by a bone fragment when the ligatures are tied. The standard aneurysm needle is used to pass the ligature medial to the sinus.

Insertion of an infratemporal retractor and further exposure of the internal carotid artery

The infratemporal fossa retractor is inserted in such a way that the long anterior blade lies against the lower part of the posterior margin of the mandibular ramus. The short posterior blade goes under the corresponding part of the posterior margin of the wound. The styloid process and the attached portion of the tympanic bone covering the carotid foramen are removed with rongeurs. This permits further anterior retraction of the soft tissues of the retromandibular

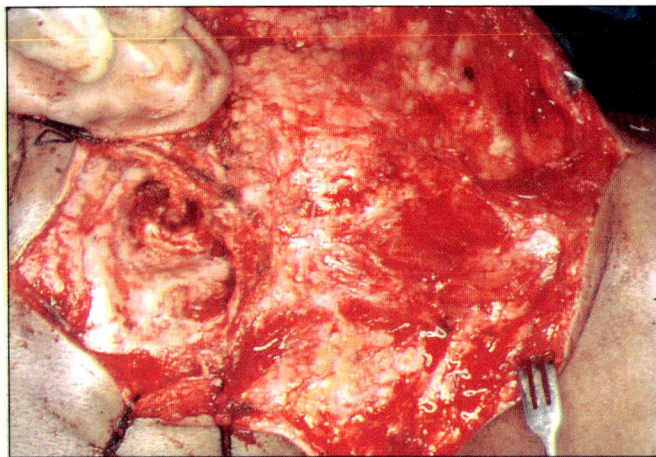
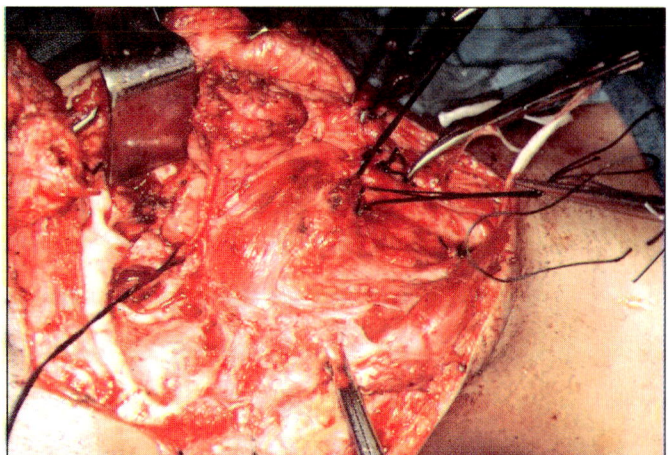

Fig. 8.7 A) Complete Radical Mastoidectomy with skeletonization of facial nerve and sigmoid sinus **B)** anterior transposition of facial nerve and double ligation of sigmoid sinus

fossa, exposing the internal carotid artery and the anterior pole of the tumor. The artery, which has been identified medial to the bony eustachian tube, is followed centripetally until the tumor is reached. Residual tympanic bone, lateral to the artery, is removed with a diamond bur.

Mobilization of tumor poles

The anterior pole is freed from the internal carotid artery. In most cases a plane of cleavage will be found at the level of the carotid foramen between the adventitia of the artery and the periosteum of the carotid canal. If the adventitia has been infiltrated, a small layer of tumor is left in situ for later separate removal. This maneuver allows coagulation of the caroticotympanic arteries when the anterior pole of the tumor is separated from the internal carotid artery.

The superior pole is freed from the otic capsule. Cochlear function can be lost at this time if there is a significant fistula into the basal turn of the cochlea. Tumor invasion into the internal auditory canal can lead to operative damage to cranial nerves VII and VIII if the surgeon has not been made aware of this condition by high resolution computed tomography.

The posterior pole is approached after opening the sigmoid sinus below the double ligature. Although the tumor frequently invades the lateral wall of the sinus, the medial wall is never involved. This provides the necessary plane of cleavage for separation of the tumor along the posterior fossa dura, as the posterior pole of the tumor is rolled forward.

The inferior pole is approached after ligation and transaction of the internal jugular vein below the contained intravenous extension of the tumor. The vein is elevated as far as the intradural extension of the tumor within the jugular bulb. Cranial nerves X to XII can be dissected free up to this point. Nerve IX has to be sectioned to begin development of a plane of cleavage between the internal carotid artery and the medial aspect of the tumor (Fig. 8.8a & b).

The medial surface of tumor

Cranial nerves IX, X, and XI are intimately connected with the medial surface of the tumor. When infiltrated by tumor, these nerves have to be sacrificed to ensure completeness of tumor removal. Nerve XII can be separated from the tumor intact if its function is normal preoperatively. The inferior petrosal sinus, with its several openings, is reached as the tumor is elevated out of the jugular foramen. Bleeding occurring from the sinus at this stage is stopped by packing with Oxycel or bone wax. The extradural portion of the tumor is now mobile and is separated by sharp dissection from any intradural extension (Fig.8.9a & b).

The intracranial intradural extesion

When bleeding from the previous stage of surgery (particularly from the posterior fossa dura) is under complete control, any intracranial intradural extension up to 2 cm can be removed. Dural vessels supply the intracranial intradural tumor to a larger extent than the vertebral artery. Wide dural cautery and excision considerably reduce tumor blood flow and facilitate removal of the intracranial tumor extension by favoring its extrusion by cerebrospinal fluid pressure through the dural defect that has been created. Any extension larger than 2 cm. is left in

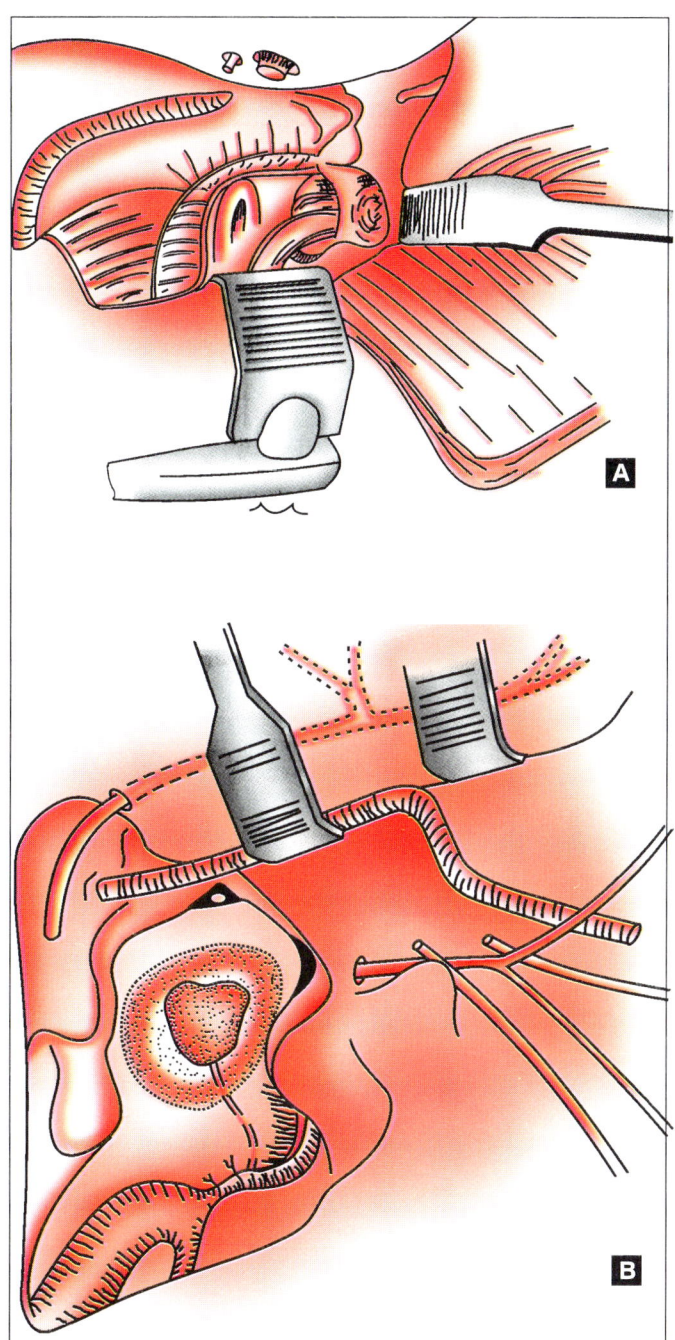

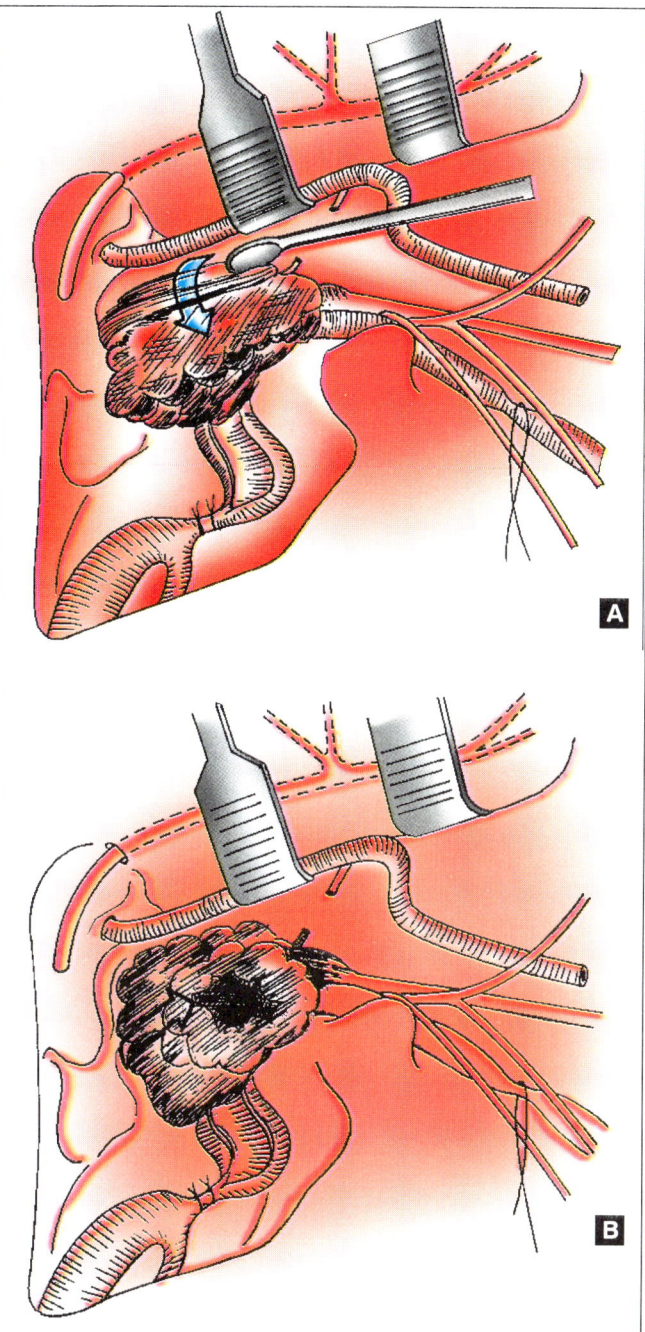

Fig. 8.8 A) Mobilization and separation of anterior pole of the tumor pole **B)** mobilization of the superior pole of tumor along the remaining labyrinthine bony capsule

Fig. 8.9 A) Mobilization of tumor pole following the opening of the lateral sinus below the double ligature .The medial wall of lateral sinus is seen to be free of tumor. **B)** Mobilization of the inferior pole of the tumor. The internal jugular vien has been ligated. Cranial nerves IX to XI have been transected because of tumor invasion.

situ for later neurosurgical removal because of its possible extensive communication with large venous vessels situated at the pontomedullary junction.

Wound closure

Wound closure is carried out with meticulous hemostasis. Lyophilized dura or temporalis fascia is used with fibrin glue to seal the dural defect. Obliteration of the cavity is effected with abdominal fat and pedicled temporalis muscle, which is sutured to the margins of the operative defect Negative suction catheters are used with a two layer closure.

Type C

For access to infra temporal fossa, pterygopalatine fossa, parasellar region and nasopharynx.

Indications

- Large Juvenile nasopharyngeal angiofibroma extending into infra temporal fossa, orbit, parasellar region and cavernous sinus.

- Nasopharyngeal carcinomas.

- Craniopharyngiomas

- Pituitory adenoma.

- Postauricular incision extending from frontal region to the neck.

- External auditory canal is transected with formation of periosteal flap. Facial nerve branches exposed in parotid region.

- Frontal branch of facial nerve identified. Zygomatic arch sectioned as anterior as possible and may include a part of lateral orbital wall.

- Temporalis muscle, zygomatic arch with masseter and frontal branch of facial nerve are retracted inferiorly.

- External auditory canal is closed like a blind sac and then covered by periosteal flap serving as a second layer of closure.

- Mandibular condyle is retracted inferiorly with a special infra temporal fossa retractor.

- Extended radical mastoidectomy is done to expose internal carotid artery from the middle ear to the foramen Lacerum.

- Middle meningeal artery and mandibular nerve are sectioned at their respective foramina that are foramen spinosum and foramen ovale respectively.

- This exposes the structures situated in infra temporal fossa which are Eustachian tube, levator and tensor palatine muscles and medial and lateral pterygoid muscles.

- Soft tissues of infra temporal fossa and lateral parapharyngeal space including Eustachian tube are removed in one block. This gives exposure to nasopharynx. In the nasopharynx, resection of tumour is carried out up to pharyngeal wall of opposite side.

- Temporalis muscle is used to fill the operative cavity.

- Zygomatic arch is rewired in place. Middle ear cavity is filled with fat from abdominal wall. Wound closed in 2 layers with two negative suction drains.

Advantages

- Provides complete visualization of internal carotid artery, and cranial nerves during tumour manipulation so that there is safety in tumour manipulation to these of vital structures.

- Intra cranial extension can be safely managed.

- Dura of middle cranial fossa can be followed medially upto optic chiasm.

- Internal carotid artery is exposed up to foramen lacerum.

- Cavernous sinus can be approached if required.

- A very short working distance.

- Ideal illumination, magnification and binocular vision owing to use of operating microscope.

Disadvantages

- Permanent conductive hearing loss.

- Facial and tongue anaesthesia due to sectioning of maxillary and mandibular nerve. However in cancer patients this may provide pain relief.

- CSF leak and meningitis are however prevented by blind sac closure of external auditory canal and obliteration of middle ear cavity and Eustachian tube orifice.

- Slight temporal depression due to transposition of temporalis muscle to fill the surgical defect. However, it remains well hidden with in the temporal hairline.

Type D

For access to infra temporal fossa, floor of middle fossa, petrous apex, lateral clivus, pterygopalatine fossa and orbit.

Indications

- Juvenile angiofibroma extending into pterygopalatine fossa, infratemporal fossa or orbit and not encroaching upon the internal carotid artery.

- Cholesterol granuloma

- Hemangioma

- Trigeminal nerve schwannoma

- Chondrosarcoma

- Adenoid cystic carcinoma

- Incision: Extended preauricular incision which ascends up on to scalp and curves forward up to hairline above the orbit (Fig. 8.10).

Steps

- A pre-auricular incision as described above is given with a plane of dissection anterior to the middle ear, petrous horizontal carotid artery and eustachian tube.

- In a fashion similar to the Type C approach, the main trunk and frontal branch of the facial nerve are identified and dissected.

- The zygomatic arch is transected, pedicled on the masseter muscle and temporarily displaced inferiorly and anteriorly.

- The temporomandibular joint is left intact.

- The temporalis muscle is detached from the squama of the temporal bone and retracted inferiorly and anteriorly. The bony base of the middle cranial fossa is removed using a high-speed drill (Fig. 8.11).

- In contrast to the Type C approach no subtotal petrosectomy is done and hence the middle ear and

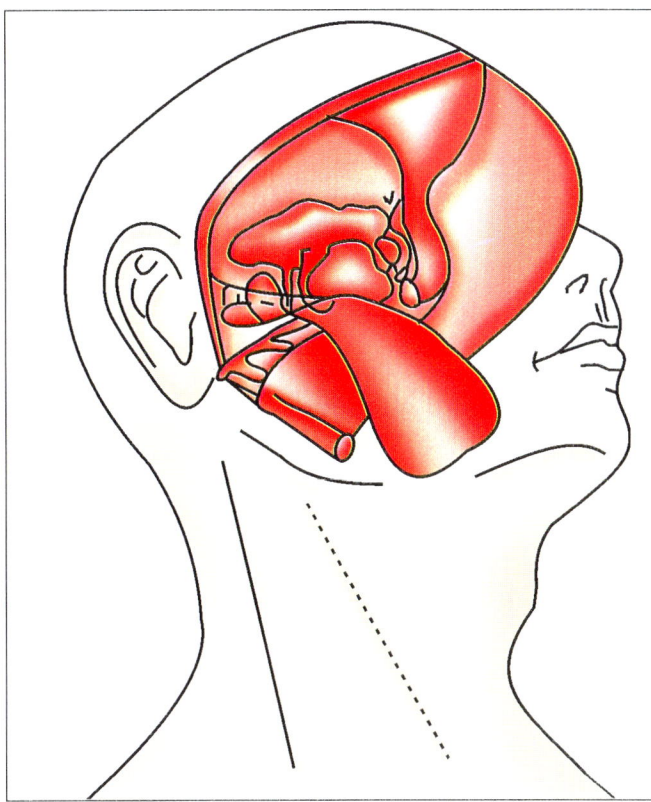

Fig. 8.11 The temporalis muscle is detached from the squama of the temporal bone and retracted inferiorly and anteriorly. The bony base of the middle cranial fossa is removed using a high-speed drill

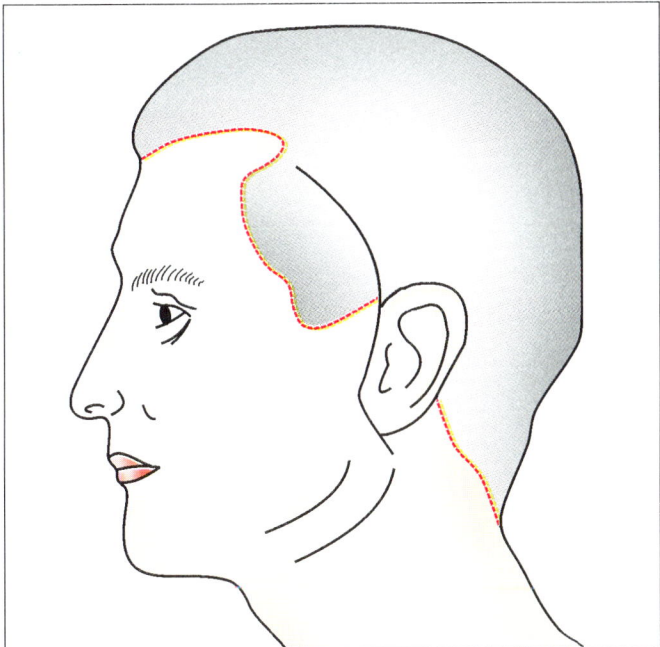

Fig. 8.10 Showing extended preauricular incisions in type D approach

the eustachian tube are left intact. The horizontal internal carotid artery is not necessarily directly identified or dissected in this approach.

- The middle meningeal artery is sacrificed at the foramen spinosum. The third branch of the trigeminal nerve (V3) is transected at the foramen ovale after careful electrocauterization. The second branch of the trigeminal nerve (V2) is also sacrificed in approximately 75% of the time at the foramen rotundum. This allows the superior and posterior margins of the tumor to be dissected and detached from the bony skull base.

- Type D approach gives access to the lateral orbital wall, the infratemporal and pterygopalatine fossa.

Type D1: (Posterior variant of Type D)

Apart from above steps glenoid fossa is removed to expose tumour in vicinity of maxillary nerve. And bone is removed from roof of infratemporal fossa.

Type D2 (Anterior variant of Type D)

Hemicoronal incision for lesions involving pterygopalatine fossa and/or orbit only.

All steps are same as D1 except osteotomy is made at lateral orbital rim instead of anterior root of zygoma. So entire lateral orbital complex in continuity with zygomatic arch is reflected inferiorly to provide good exposure to orbit. Temporomandibular joint is kept intact.

Advantages

- No conductive hearing loss.

- Normal facial contour maintained.

- Less time consuming as radical mastoidectomy and ICA control are not necessary.

- Can be converted to Type C if necessary.

- Direct access into the fossae.

New combined infratemporal and trans maxillary approach

Starts with and infratemporal fossa (Type D) which allows dissociation of the posterior and superior margins of the tumor from the bony skull base combined with a transmaxillary approach which would subsequently deliver the tumor through a large maxillotomy 'this is done in two stages.

2. Transparotid approach: Conservative lateral approach

Indications

- Extracranial meningiomas.
- Deep lobe tumors of parotid gland.
- Recurrent plemorphic adenoma of parotid.
- Pterygoid or infratemporal masses.

Steps

- Superficial parotidectomy is performed through an extended parotidectomy incision.

- Branches of facial nerve are traced and freed from temporalis fascia, zygomatic arch and masseter.

- After separations of temporalis fascia, zygomatic arch is divided anteriorly as zygomaticomalar suture and posteriorly at its root.

- Zygomatic arch along with masseter is retracted inferiorly to expose ascending ramus of mandible.

- After ramus is made bare by elevating the poriosteum, it is sectioned in a trifurcate manner. Coronoid segment along with temporalis muscles is retracted superiorly and lower segments are retracted inferiorly and now infratemporal fossa can be entered.

- Encapsulated masses are delivered with ease by inserting a finger in the nasapharynx and by pushing lateral nasopharyngeal wall outwards. For more extensive masses, the medial and lateral pterygoid muscles may be divided to provide better exposure.

- Once tumour is out, mandible and zygomatic arch are rewired and wound closed with drainage (Fig. 8.12a, b, c & d).

Disadvantage

- Restricted exposure and technique is limited to encapsulated benign lesions.

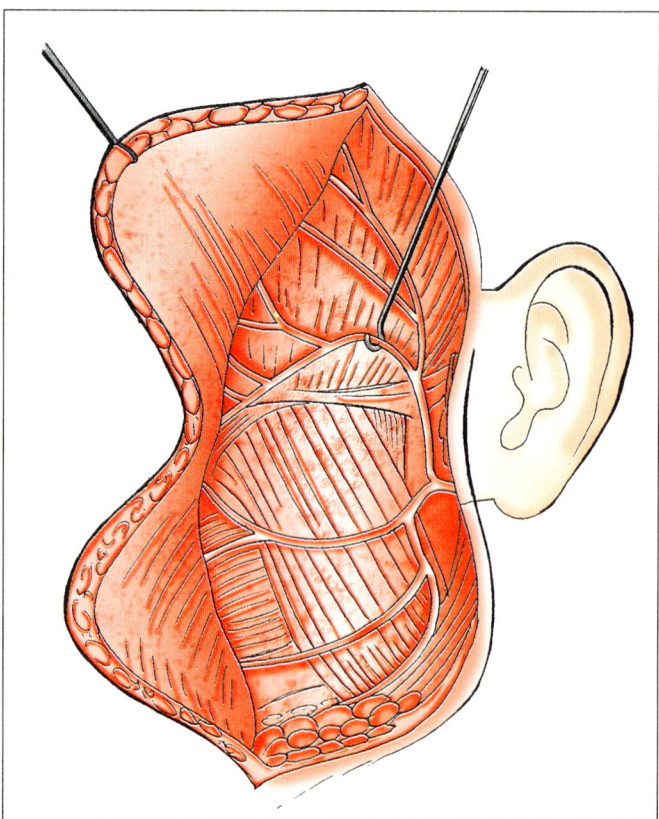

Fig. 8.12a Branches of the facial nerve are dissected as far distally as possible

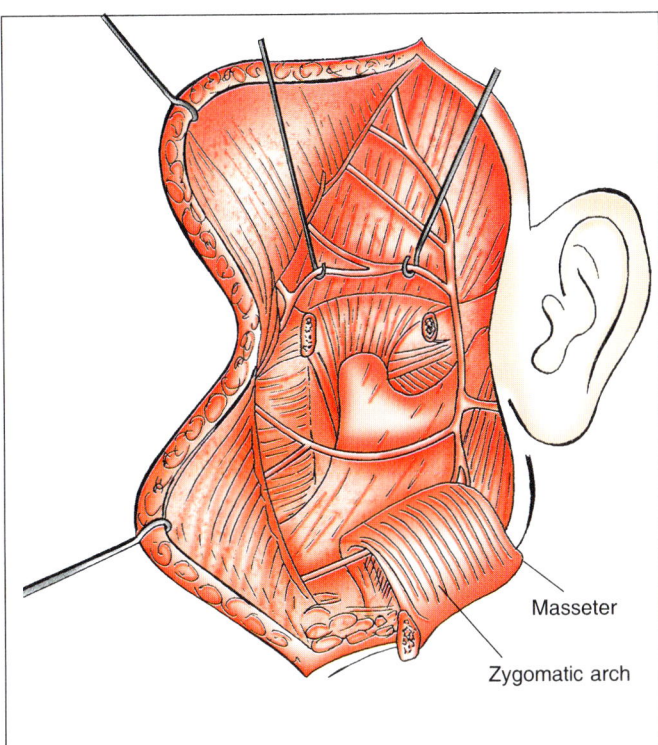

Fig. 8.12b Detachment and downward displacement are dissected of the zygomatic arch and massive muscle

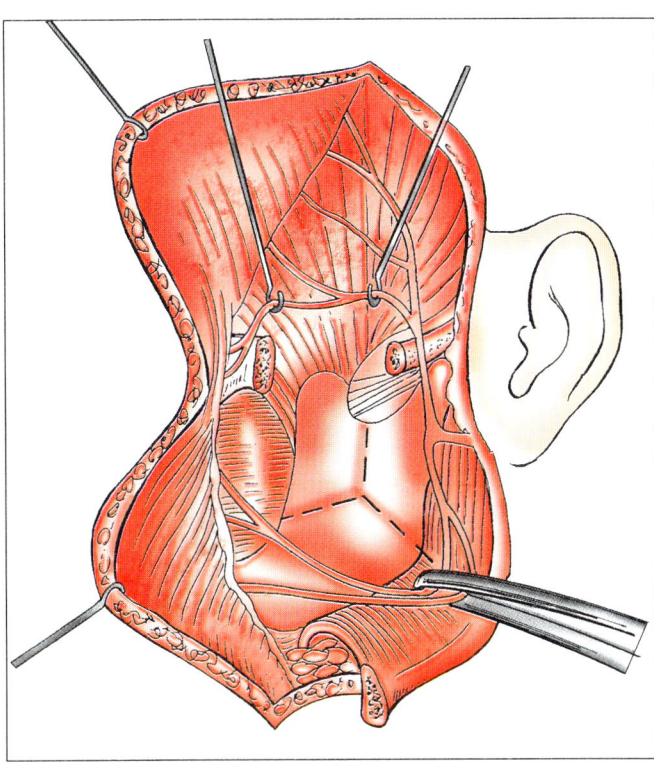

Fig. 8.12c The ascending ramus is sectioned in a trifuecate manner

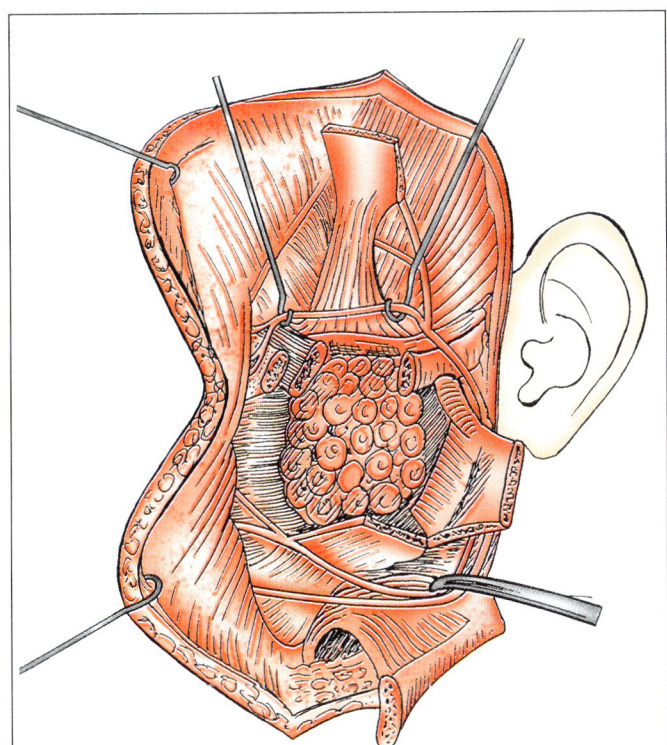

Fig. 8.12d Retraction of the bony fragment exposes the infratemporal fossa with tumor

Complications

- Facial neuropraxia
- Damage to inferior dental nerve and lingual nerve
- Trismus

3. Infratemporal extension of lateral parotid approach

Indications

Extensions of infratemporal fossa tumors into facial muscles or skin or posteriorly into temporal bone.

Incision

Incision is similar to an extended parotidectomy incision except that it carries a posterior limb 2-3 cm superiorly behind the lobule in postauricular crease. Thus it becomes a 'Y' shaped incision.

Steps

- Access is achieved into mastoid, middle cranial fossa and superior aspect of infratemporal fossa by retracting the auricle superiorly.

- Steps of this technique are almost similar to earlier approach except that through the posterior limb mastoid and transverse sinus can be exposed and transverse sinus may be controlled by packing its lumen with surgical cotton if Jugular bulb is to be resected.

- After mobilization of posterior surface of parotid gland if mass is felt deep to digastric muscle, just a biopsy may be taken by staircase mandibulotomy at mandibular angle. Because at this site mass could be cranial nerve IX, X, XI, XII Schwannoma or mesenchymal tumour or aneurysm.

Advantages

- Exposure to mastoids, middle cranial fossa and infratemporal fossa at the same time.

4 . Extended Rhytidectomy approach without facial nerve dissection

(Facial biflap procedure)

Indications

- Tumors involving more inferior portions of infra temporal fossa, pterygoid space, nasopharynx, parapharyngeal space and posterior maxilla.

- Infratemporal fossa is approached by first elevating a skin flap based anteriorly then elevating, the mimetic muscles, facial nerve and parotid gland as a unit based posteriorly, exposing the facial skeleton.

Steps

- Double modified Blair incision as shown below in the diagram (Fig. 8.13)

- Cephalic extension of incision is necessary only when intra cranial extension is suspected.

- Facial skin flap elevated from underlying muscles based anteriorly (Fig. 8.14)

- Anterior limit is a line drawn from lateral canthus to corner of mouth. Vermillion is included in facial skin flap.

- Facial muscles are elevated from the facial skeleton and are based posteriorly (Fig. 8.15).

- Elevations is done in following order.

  - Orbicularis oris - lateral 1/3rd with underlying labial mucosa.

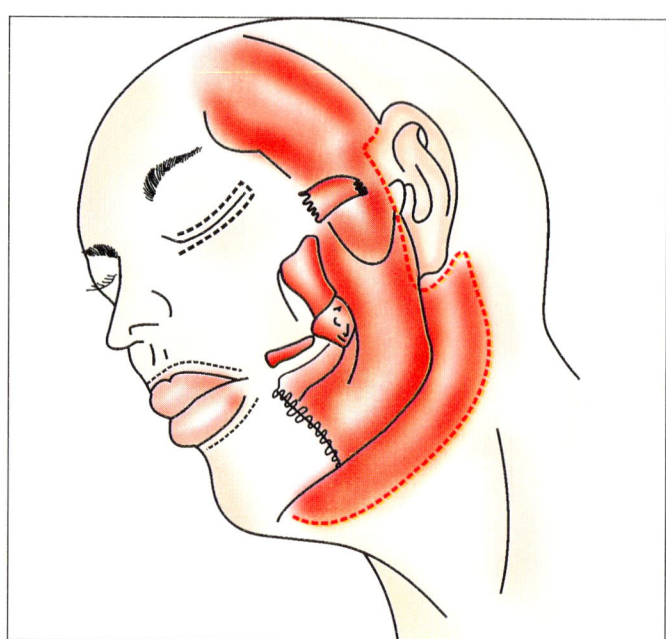

Fig. 8.13 Doubel modified Blair incision

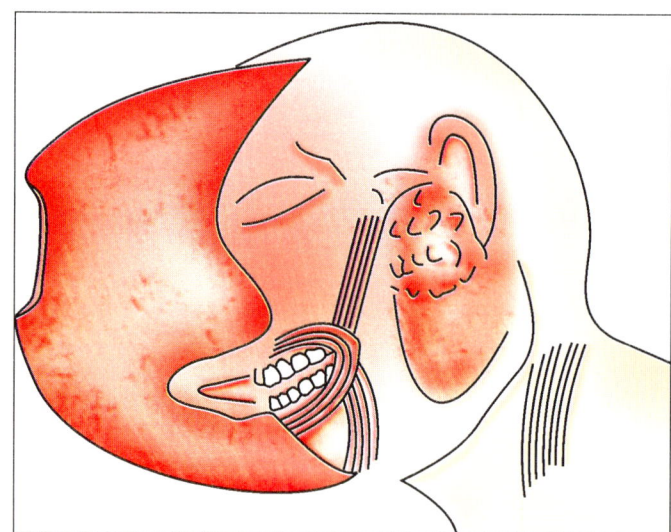

Fig. 8.14 Facial skin flap elevation

- Buccal mucosa detached from vestibular attachments.

- Zygomaticus minor and major, labii superioris reflected posteriorly off the maxilla.

- Nasalis muscle is transected on a vertical plane at lateral edge of pyriform aperture.

- Facial muscles, parotid gland and buccal and labial mucosa are reflected laterally, along with facial nerve and its branches.

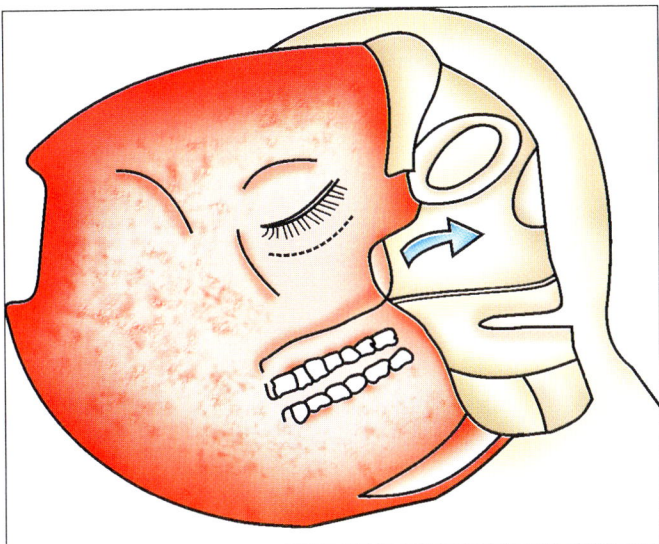

Fig. 8.15 Facial muscle elevation, based posteriorly

- Masseter elevated from mandible.
- Mandibulotomy and transaction of zygomatic arch to expose the infratemporal fossa (Fig. 8.16).
- Tumour is resected.
- Facial muscles replaced in original position.
- Facial skin flap is replaced and closed in 2 layers.

Advantages

- Avoids facial nerve injury
- Quicker
- Good exposure
- Good cosmetic result

5. Lateral transtemporal sphenoid approach to skull base (Holliday in 1986)

Indications

- Temporal / Infratemporal fossa lesions.
- Parasellar lesions.
- Clival and nasopharyngeal lesions.
- Pterygopalatine fossa lesions.
- Petrous apex lesions.
- Posterosuperior maxillary sinus lesion.

This approach reach infratemporal fossa from a superior direction by displacing zygomatic arch inferiorly and reflecting temporalis muscle.

Incision

- Curvilinear incision begun superiorly along temporal hairline posterior to lateral aspect of superior orbital rim. It is continued downwards and posteriorly 1 finger breadth above and parallel to zygomatic arch and curved inferiorly at preauricular crease up to the lobule (Fig. 8.17).

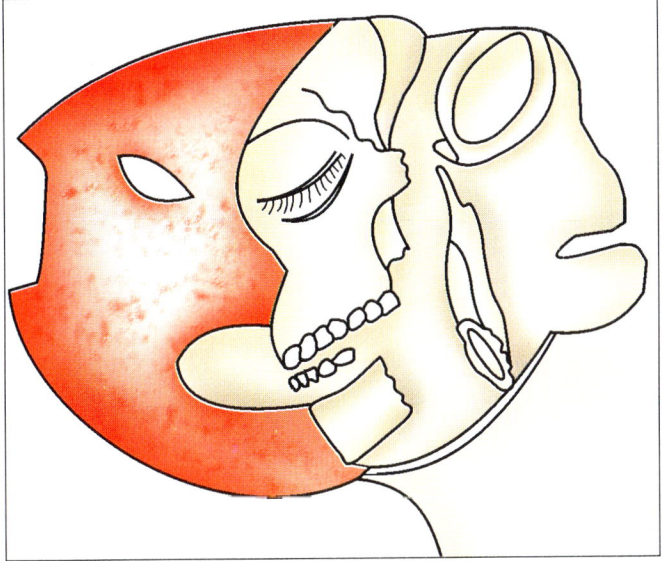

Fig. 8.16 Mandibulotomy and transaction of zygomatic arch to expose ITF

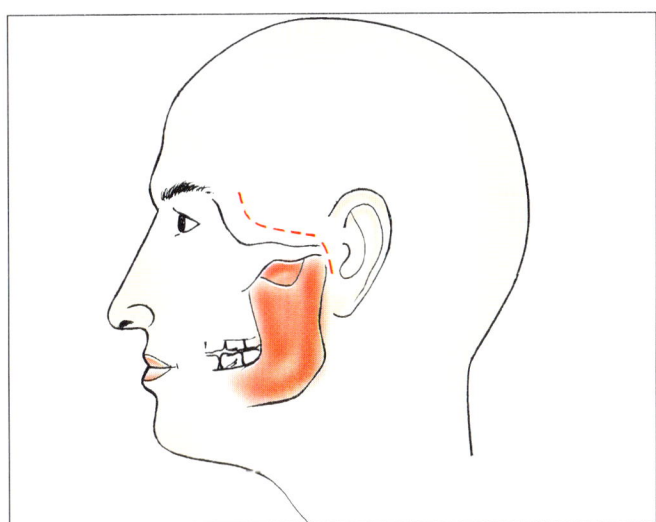

Fig. 8.17 Shows Subtemporal craniotomy incision

- Subcutaneous flaps raised superiorly and inferiorly to expose temporalis fascia.

Steps

- Temporalis fascia incised parallel to zygomatic arch and 3 cm above it up to 1 cm posterior to posterior aspect of lateral orbital rim. This avoids injury to frontozygomatic branch of facial nerve.

- Fascia is reflected off the zygomatic arch using electrocautery over superior aspect of the arch.

- Periosteum is elevated and arch exposed.

- Temporalis muscle transected and reflected upwards (Fig. 8.18).

- Arch is transected at its anterior and posterior attachments with drill or saw and reflected inferiorly with masseter. Greater wing of sphenoid is thinned out using high-speed drill under operating microscope (Fig. 8.19).

- For exposing superior orbital fissure and orbital areas bone over periorbita and lesser wing of sphenoid may be thinned.

- TM joint and capsule is elevated and retracted inferiorly and this provides exposure of carotid artery, Eustachian tube or petrous apex.

- Squamotympanic fissure can be identified and it forms an important landmark to middle meningeal artery and Eustachian tube.

- Just medial to the most medial extent of this fissure is present spine of sphenoid.

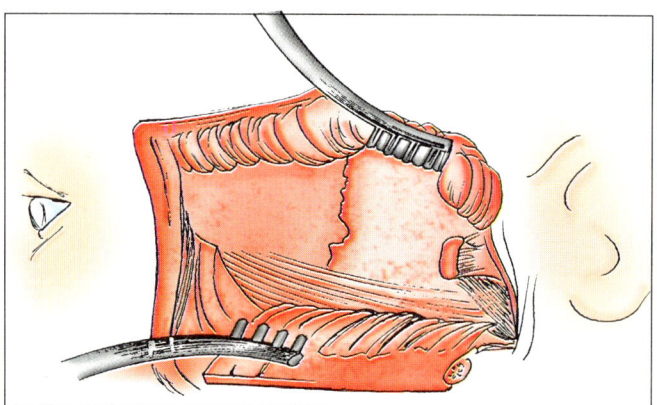

Fig. 8.18 Showing retraction of temporalis muscle to expose greater wing of sphenoid in lateral transtemporal sphenoid approach

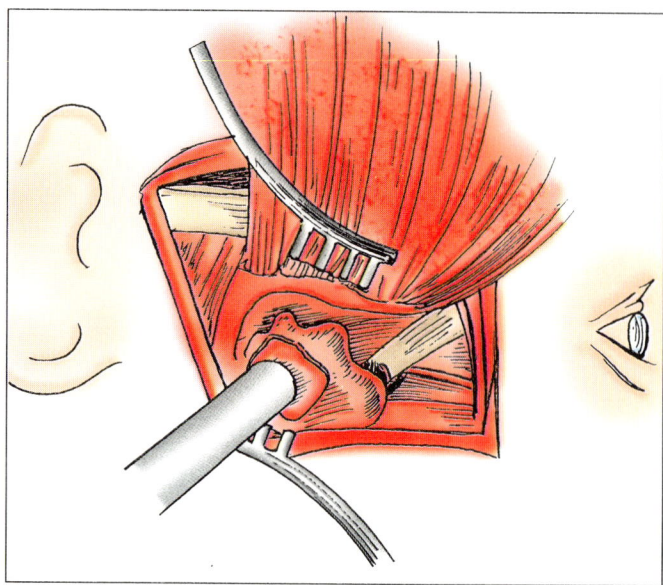

Fig. 8.19 Showing subtemporal craniotomy to expose the orbital apex in lateral transtemporal sphenoid approach

- Once this spine is drilled, middle meningeal artery can be identified on its anterior aspect and bonycartilagenous junction of Eustachian tube can be found on its medial aspect.

- Tympanic bone just posterior to this fissure is drilled to expose internal carotid artery (Intratemporal part).

- Further microsurgical drilling dissection of ICA exposes superior compartment of petrous apex.

- Further drilling between Foramen ovale, Foramen Rotundum and Superior orbital fissure will expose dural reflection of cavernous sinus.

- Middle meningeal artery and mandibular nerve may be divided and further bone removed medially to expose ICA, Eustachian tube and foramen lacerum.

- Once the tumour is removed zygomatic arch is rewired and TM joint repositioned and wound closed under suction drain.

6. Lateral facial approach (Fig. 8.20 & 8.21)

Steps

- Incision extends from preauricular region upwards along temporal hairline up to level of lateral edge of superior orbital rim.

- Temporalis muscle and zygomatic arch are exposed.

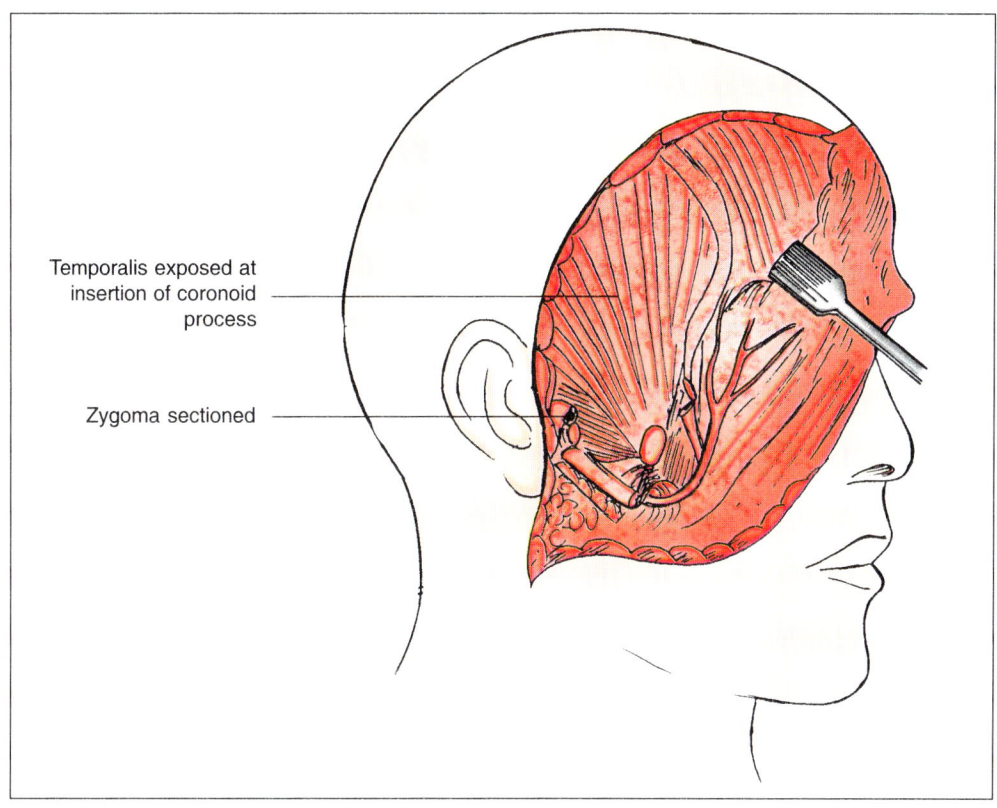

Fig. 8.20 Lateral facial approach using temporal and preauricular incision, temporalis muscle and zygomatic arch are exposed. Zygoma is sectioned to allow access to temporalis insertion at coronoid

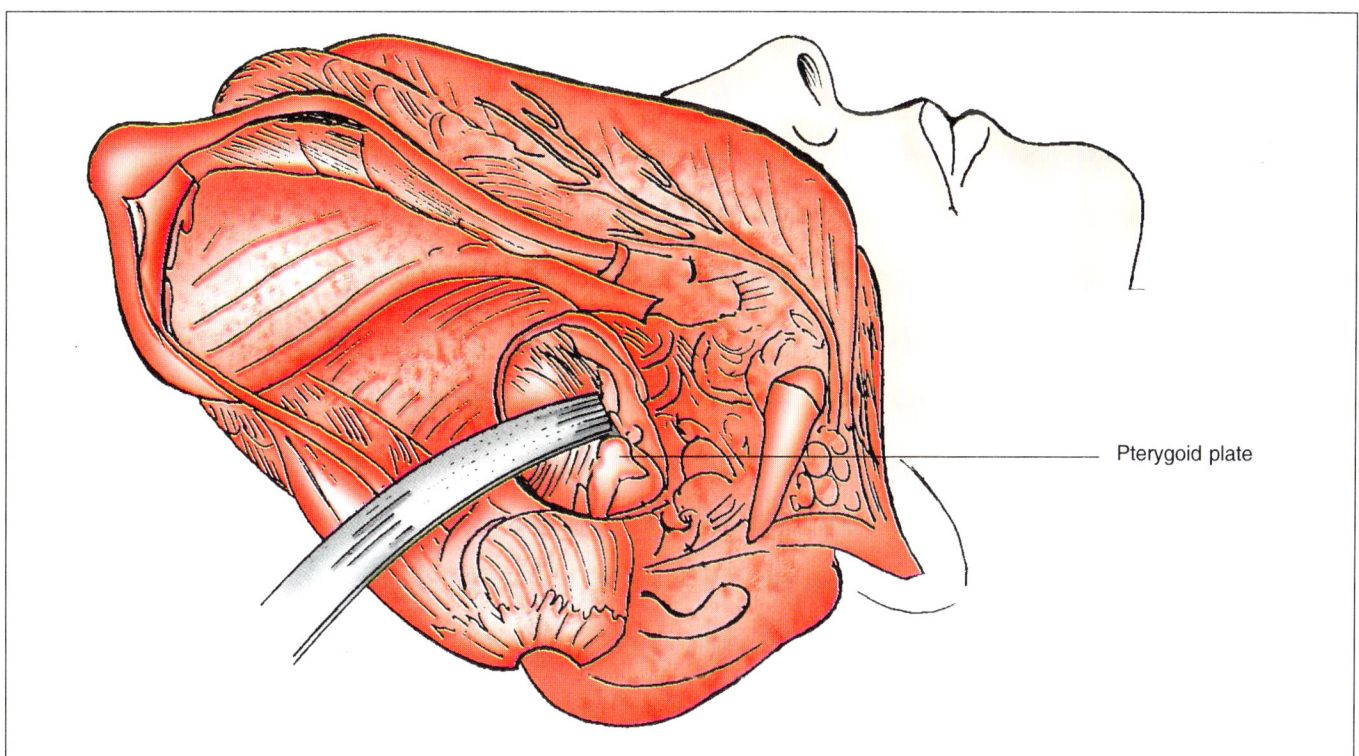

Fig. 8.21a Lateral facial approach to cranial base Temporalis muscle retracted, greater wing of sphenoid partially removed retraction of temporal to be dura done, exposing branches of trigeminal nerve, pterygoid plate at skull base

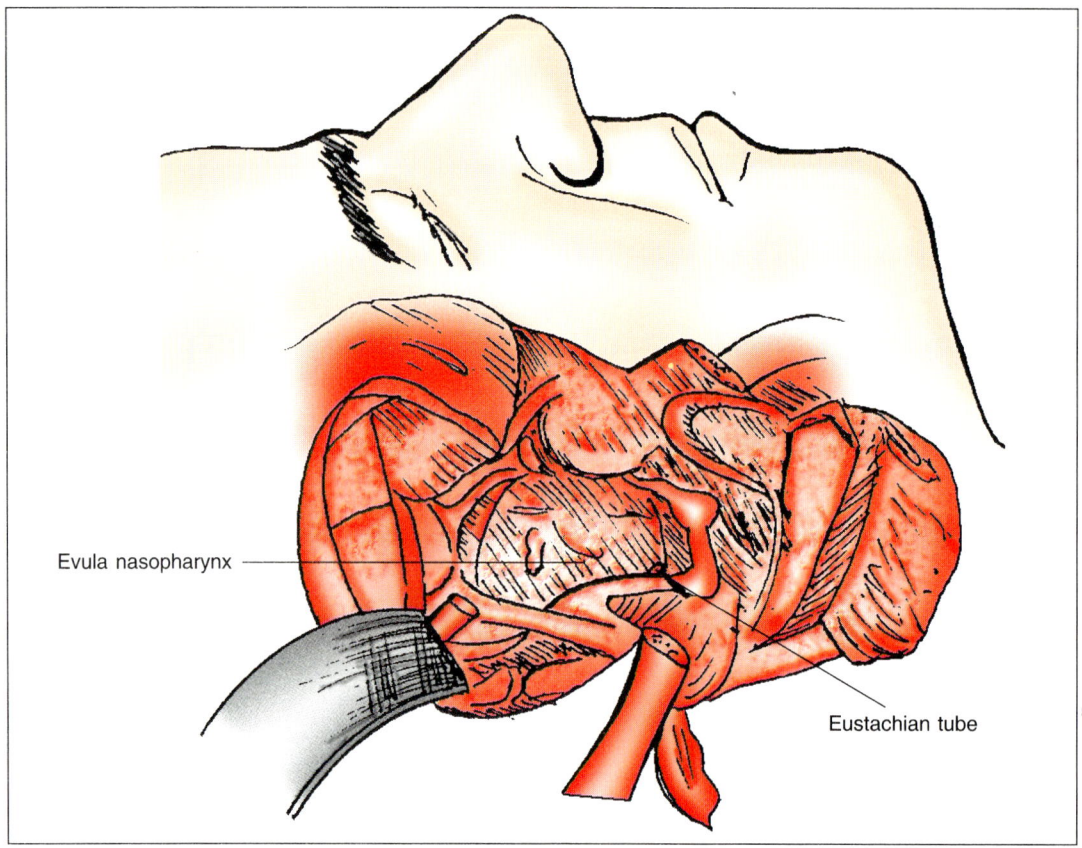

Fig. 8.21b Division of maxillary nerve, resection of pterygoid plate to expose nasopharynx

- Zygomatic arch is sectioned at anterior and posterior roots to allow excess to coronoid and attachment of temporalis muscle.

- Frontal branch of facial nerve is preserved with skin flap.

- Temporalis muscle is retracted to expose greater wing of sphenoid.

- Subtemporal craniectomy is done by removing greater wing of sphenoid partially.

- Temporal lobe dura is retracted to expose trigeminal nerve branches.

- Pterygoid plate is seen at its attachment to base of sphenoid.

- Maxillary nerve and pterygoid plate are resected to expose nasopharynx.

- Tumour from superior parts of infratemporal fossa, nasopharynx can be resected out.

- Sphenoid bone is secured with microplates, temporalis muscle is replaced back.

- Zygomatic arch is replaced and secured.

- Wound closed in layers.

Advantages

- Avoids facial nerve rerouting.

- Avoids sensorineural hearing loss unlike translabyrinthine and transcochlear approaches.

- Avoids disability of permanent conductive hearing loss unlike intratemporal fossa approach.

- Avoids mastoid, middle ear, facial nerve and otic capsule dissection therefore saves time.

- Sterile approach.

- Minimal functional or cosmetic deformity.

- Option of temporalis myocutaneous flap usage.

Disadvantage

Can not be used for lesions posterior to carotid canal that are intrasellar and for CP angle, parapharyngeal space lesions.

Expected complications

- Facial numbness - in patients where V3 was sectioned.
- Trismus
- Frontalis palsy
- Loss of Eustachian tube function
- Diplopia

7. Subtemporal - Preauricular infra temporal fossa approach (Shekhar in 1987)

Exposure: Sphenoid, clivus, petrous medial half, infra temporal fossa, nasopharynx retro/parapharyngeal area, paranasal sinuses (Fig. 8.22 a, b & c).

Indications

- Meningiomas
- Chordomas
- Nasopharyngeal carcinoma

Incision

Started in frontal scalp curved in front and below the external auditory canal and extended anteriorly on neck along skin crease. Cervicofascial flap elevated and is anteriorly based.

Steps

- Temporalis fascia and muscle elevated.
- Zygomatic arch divided anteriorly and posteriorly and resected out.
- Mandibular condyle and capsule of TM joint are dislocated anteriorly.
- Neck dissection is done to expose and trace ICA, cranial nerves X, XI, XII and IJV. Styloid process with its muscles and ligaments is resected.
- A frontotemporal bone flap is fashioned and removed along with root of zygomatic arch and glenoid fossa.
- Maxillary nerve, mandibular nerves are exposed at thin foramina after greater wing of sphenoid is drilled.

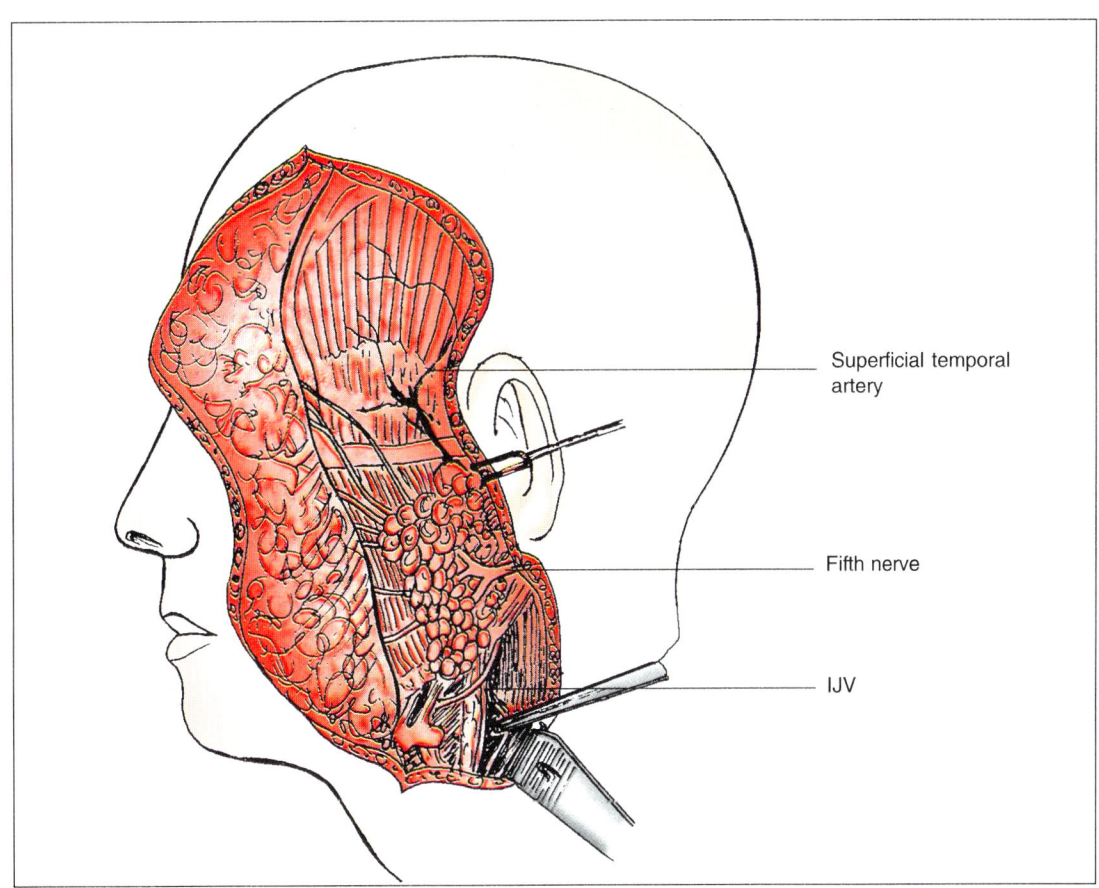

Superficial temporal artery

Fifth nerve

IJV

Fig. 8.22a Preauricular and infratemporal approach to the cranial base. Initial exposure showing branches of facial nerve, frontal branch being included in skin flap

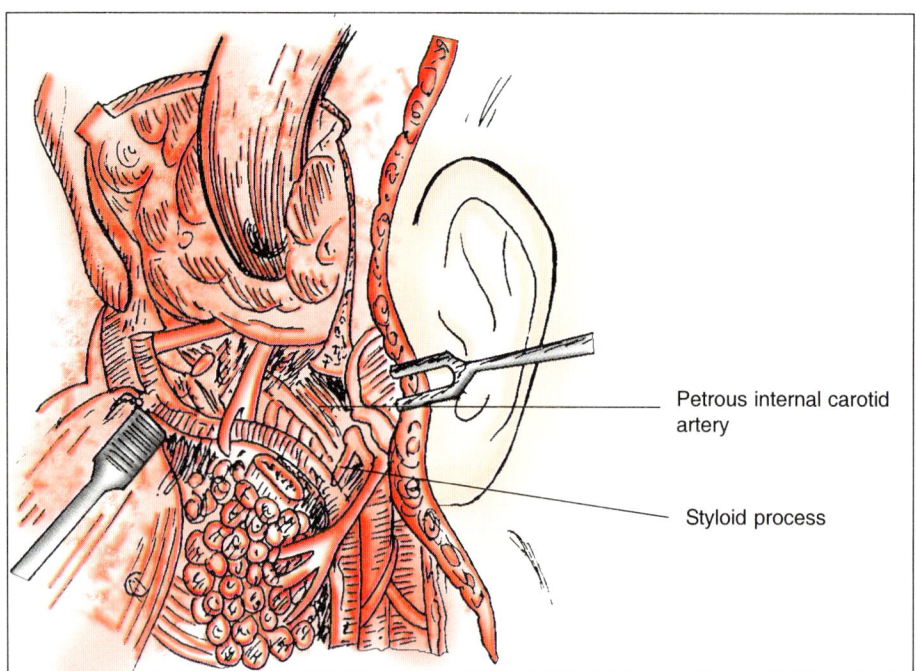

Petrous internal carotid
artery

Styloid process

Fig. 8.22b Zygomatic arch removed temporarily, temporalis muscle retracted inferiorly. Subtemporal cranioctomy being performed. Styloid process devided and carotid artery traced distally and separated from tumor

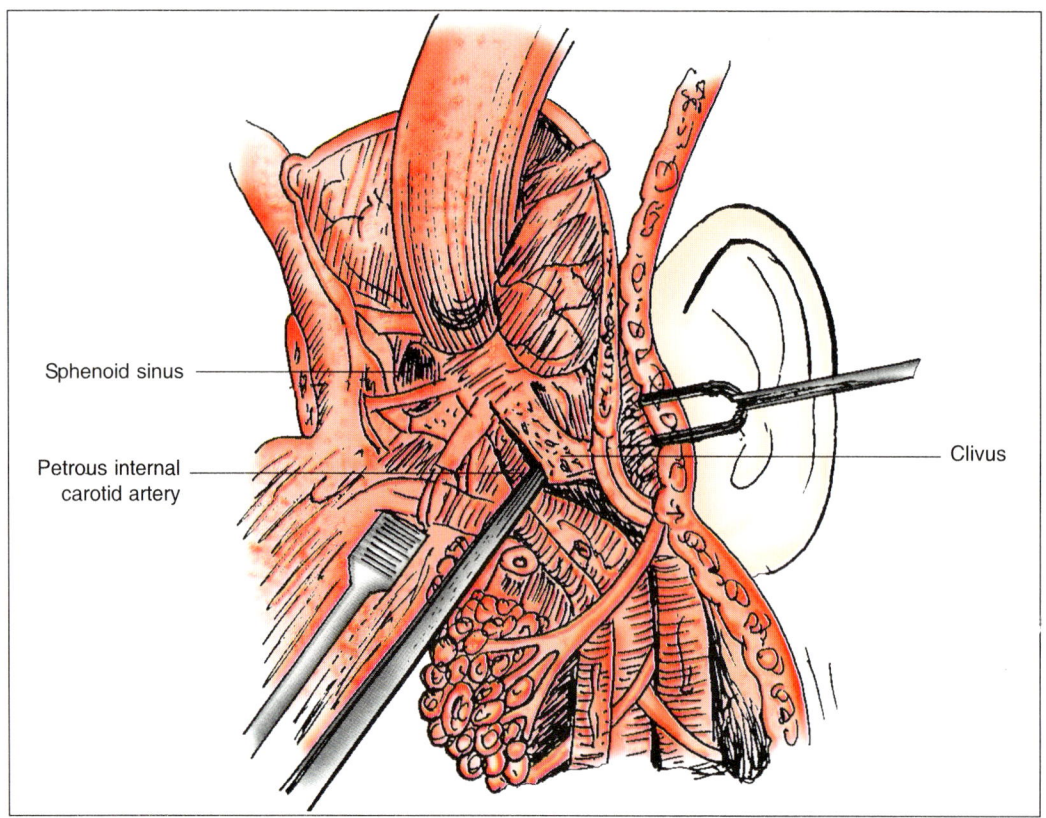

Sphenoid sinus

Petrous internal
carotid artery

Clivus

Fig. 8.22c Showing exposure of clivus, sphenoid and adjacent meneal and vascular structures

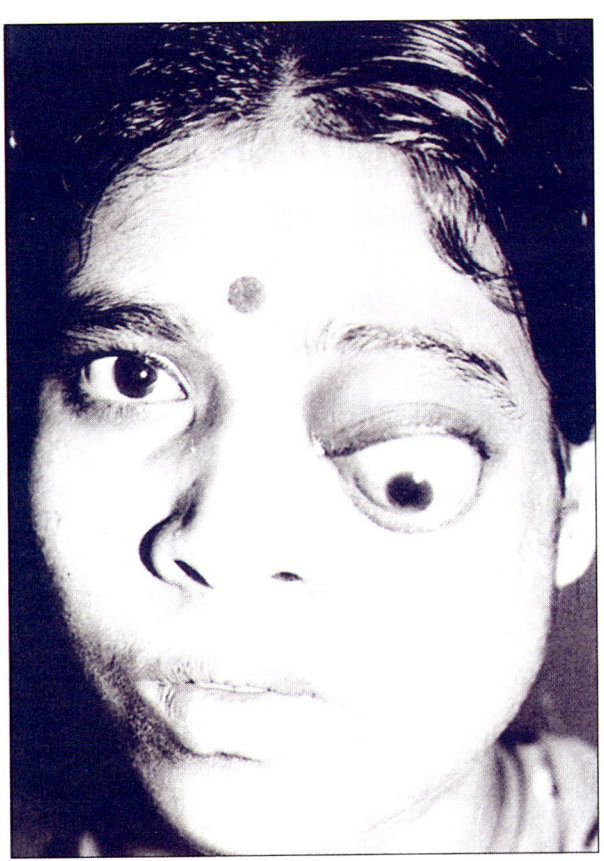

Fig. 8.23 Showing the proptosis and facial swelling in osteogenic sarcoma of sphenoid bone (Courtesy JLO)

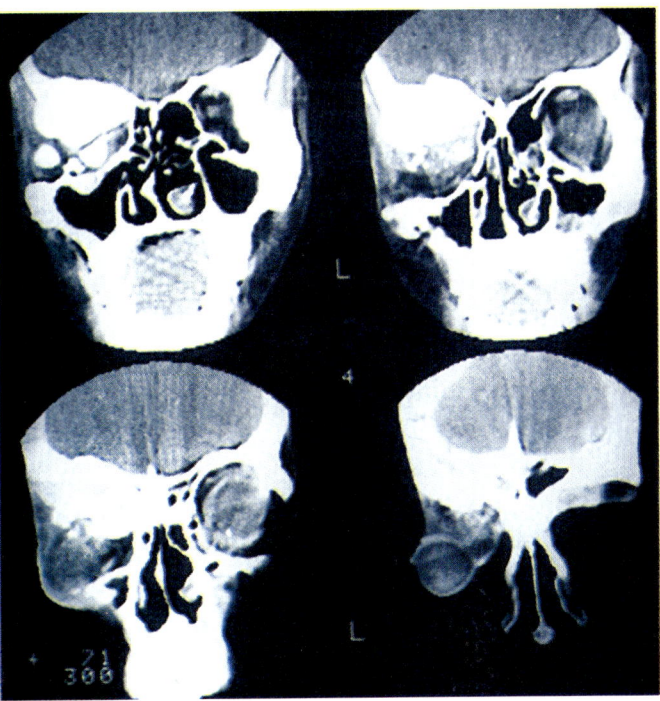

Fig. 8.24 CT scan showing bony mass arising from sphenoid wing involving left orbital root and left frontal bone (Courtesy JLO)

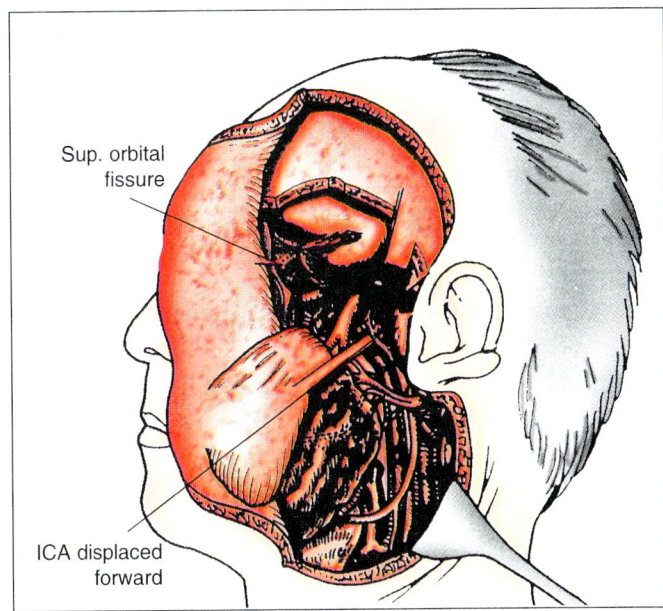

Fig. 8.25

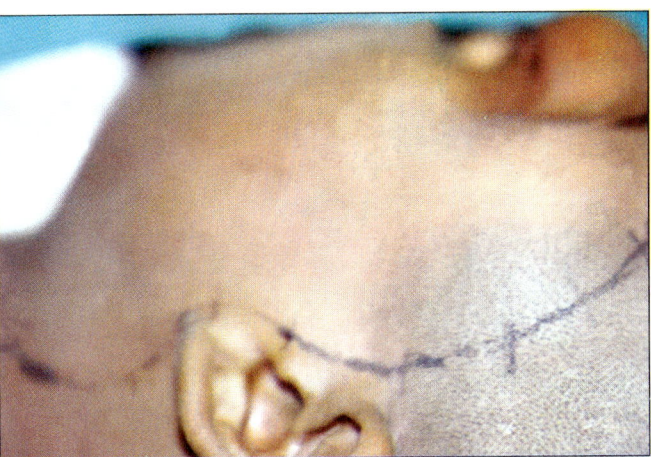

Fig. 8.26 Showing skin incision for subtemporal preauricular infra temporal fossa approach

- Medially, bony Eustachian tube and its muscles are exposed and excised. Vertical and then horizontal segments of petrous ICA are traced upto cavernous sinus.

- Bone of petrous apex and clivus region may be drilled to exposure dura from petrous apex area upto foramen magnum.

- Reconstruction of Dural breach by autologous fascia/ temporalis fascia/fascia lata. Reconstruction of

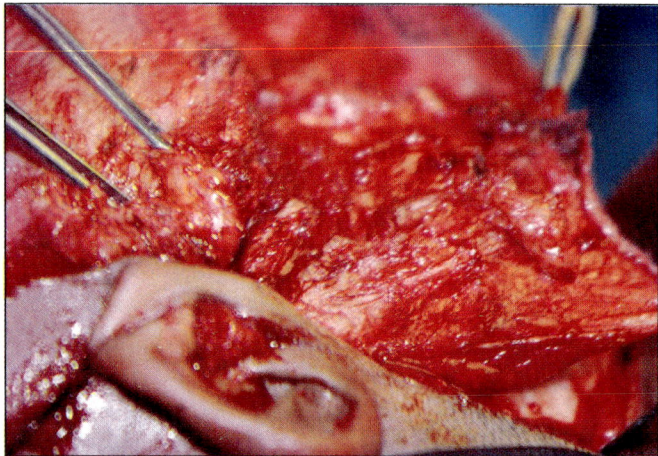

Fig. 8.27

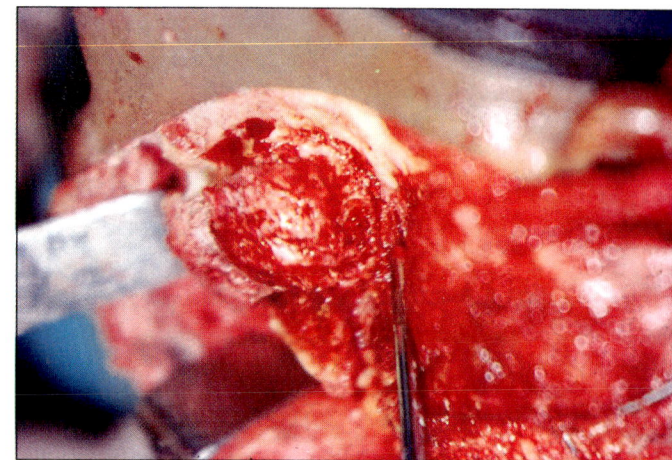

Fig. 8.28

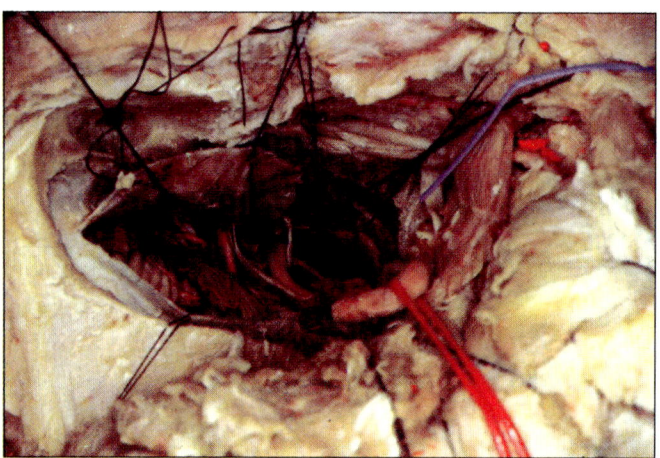

Fig. 8.29

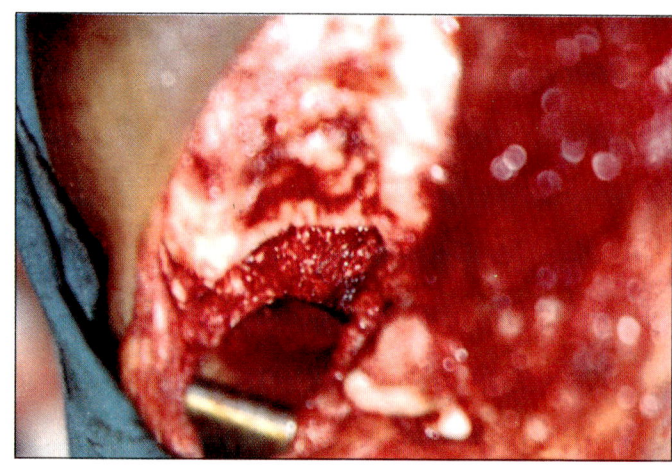

Fig. 8.30

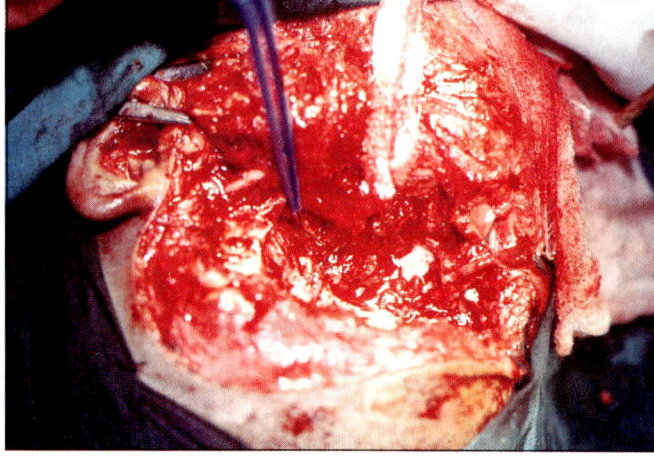

Fig. 8.31

surgical defect by temporalis muscle transposition or rectus abdominus flap.

Advantages

- Preservations of hearing.
- Minimal brain retraction.

Disadvantages

- Exposure to intra petrous carotid artery is difficult without entering the ear.
- Although petrous apex lesions such as cholesterol granuloma may be reached with this approach, dependent drainage via mastoid is not obtained (as the process is prearticular).

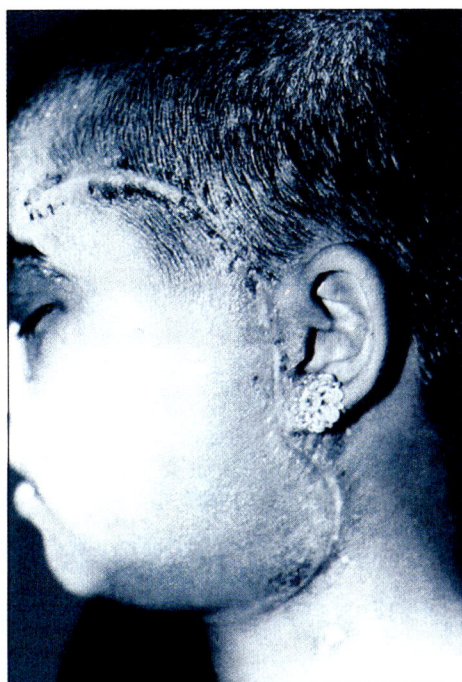

Fig. 8.32 Post operative picture after subtemporal transparotid transzygomatic incision

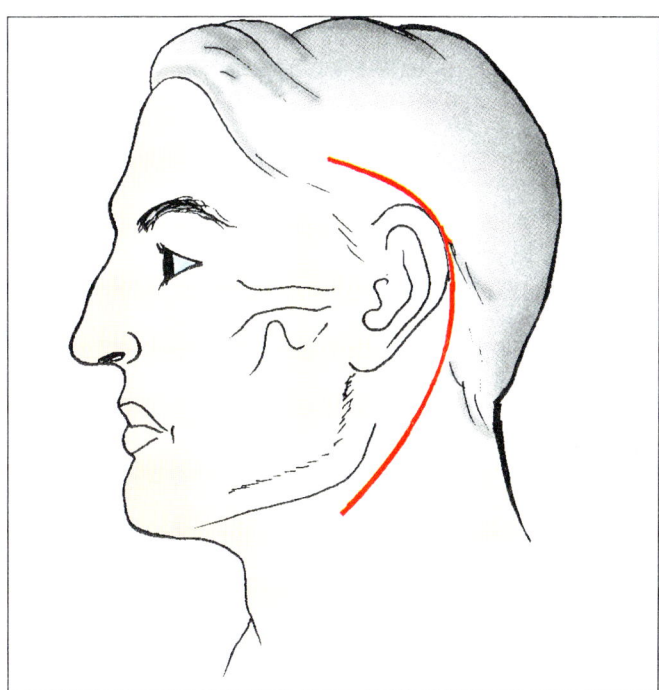

Fig. 8.33 The incision for the superior approach to the infratemporal fossa

8. Superior approach

Indications

- As exposure is limited and provides access to upper lateral part of infratemporal fossa, it is suitable for:
    - Osteoblastomas of skull base
    - Low-grade malignancies
    - Biopsy from the tumour

Incision

Postauricular incision is extended along temporal hairline above the ear upto just lateral to lateral orbital rim.

Steps

- Incision is deepened up to bone pinna reflected downwards and forwards after division of external auditory meatus.
- Temporalis muscle is detached from side of skull by periosteal elevator and retracted downwards and forwards. Temporalis fascia is separated from the upper border of zygomatic arch. Arch is fractured at its anterior and posterior roots. By retracting the arch and temporalis muscle exposure can be enhanced. Further exposure of skull base can be achieved by drilling the infratemporal crest till dura is exposed.

Advantage

- In case of a small sized low-grade malignancy this approach may be favoured as the facial nerve is out of risk of injury.

9. Infratemporal fossa approach to sphenoid sinus

This approach may be necessary for extensive sphenoid sinus neoplasms that have invaded the cavernous sinus, pterygomaxillary space, ITF and nasopharynx. This is actually a combined middle cranial fossa ITF approach. If skull base extension has not occurred then the craniotomy portion of the procedure can be avoided.

The skin incision extends from the vertex of the scalp into the neck and flaps are elevated from the angle of the mandible to the lateral orbital rim to the calvarial vertex.

The temporalis muscle is then elevated into the ITF to where it inserts on the coronoid process. Zygomatic osteotomies are made on the zygomatic arch, lateral orbital wall, and malar eminence. The soft tissues are then completely dissected from the medial end of the glenoid fossa to the foramen spinosum, foramen ovale, and base of the lateral pterygoid plate.

The craniotomy is made and elevated along the dura. The craniotomy usually fractures across the eustachian tube which is the key maneuver in finding the internal carotid artery.

The carotid is further defined with the a cutting burr. V3 is next identified as it crosses the carotid. Dissection will then lead to the cavernous sinus and parasellar region.

Tumor dissection then proceeds.

II. Transfacial approaches

- Barbosa approach and modified Barbosa approach.
- Lateral rhinotomy and external lateral rhinotomy.
- Weber fergusson approach.
- Midfacial degloving.
- Midfacial split approach.
- Facial tranlocation approach.
- Extended anterolateral approach.

II. TRANSNASAL TRANSANTRAL APPROACH

This approach was designed to remove benign well circumscribed mass, angiofibroma being a classical example. However, extensive angiofibromas can also be removed by modified Weber Fergusson or midfacial degloving approach.

Advantages of transantral approaches

- Removal of antral extension.
- Posterior antral wall can be assessed for any destruction.
- If posterior antral wall is eroded, pterygopalatine fossa can be opened and extension tackled.
- Sublabial incision can be extended as far as necessary to remove cheek extensions.
- If still not sure of complete removal then modified Weber Fergusson approach can be used as a radical measure.

A. Lateral rhinotomy approach (described under approaches to anterior skull base)

Extensions of lateral rhinotomy

- Extended superiorly under the medial eyebrow (like that of Lynch - Howarth approach).
- Inferiorly around the alar margin, through the medial

philtrum and upper lip, further extended as lip cutting and continued in gingivobuccal sulcus.

- Superior and inferior extents may be combined.

SURGICAL APPROACHES SPECIFIC TO PTERYGOPALATINE FOSSA

A. Caldwell-Luc Approach

Caldwell and Luc developed the concept of combining canine puncture and stripping of the diseased sinus mucosa with known technique of creating inferior metal antrostomy to allow long lasting drainage into nose.

Indications

- Ligation of internal maxillary artery to control epistaxis.
- Section of vidian nerve in vasomotor rhinitis.
- Resection of sphenopalatine ganglion for facial pain.
- For resection of maxillary nerve for tic douloureaux.

1. Ligation of internal maxillary artery (Seiffert's Operation)

Steps

Local infiltration with 2% xylocaine with adrenaline given over incision size.

Incision

- From lateral incisor tooth to the area of first molar tooth in the gingivobuccal sulcus.
- Anterior cheek flap is elevated off the face of maxilla. Infraorbital nerve identified and preserved as it emerges from its foramen.
- Sinus is entered through canine fossa. Posterior wall of maxillary antrum visualised. Mucosa of posterior wall is scraped with a curette.
- Posterior bony antral wall is removed about 15 x 15 mm piece.
- Underlying periosteum is incised.
- Fatty tissue inside the pterygopalatine fossa is directed out to expose the maxillary artery which is seen to be pulsating.

- A clip is applied to main trunk and then descending palatine and sphenopalatine branches are individually clipped.

Pitfalls during surgery

- Avoid injury to maxillary nerve and sphenopalatine ganglions, as it can lead to cheek and palatal anaesthesia, dryness of eyes and nasal mucosa.

- If special clip-applying instrument is not available. A deschamps forceps is to be used for ligation.

- If artery tears and bleeds, another ligation should be attempted at a more lateral position.

- Opening of posterior wall of maxillary antrum should be temponaded for 6-8 minutes to obtain less blood on operation field.

- With an atypical origin of ophthalmic artery from middle meningeal artery (seen in 0.1%) ligation of maxillary artery may incite a reflex spasm of ophthalmic artery which can cause blindness.

Contraindications

- Small underdeveloped antrum.

- Severally sclerosed antrum due to infection or prior surgery.

2. Vidian Neurectomy (Golding Wood's Operation)

It is done in patients with uncontrolled vasomotor nasal symptoms. As the symptoms are similar to allergic rhinitis, Allergic rhinitis is ruled out first.

Steps

- Similar steps as for maxillary artery ligation upto exposure of pterygopalatine fossa.

- Maxillary artery is identified, clipped and divided for exposure. Large veins are also dealt with similarly.

- Search is made for crest of bone on posteromedial wall of fossa. This crest is bone lies in direct line with medial wall of antrum and is medial and inferior to infraorbital nerve. Just medial and inferior to the crest lies vidian nerve existing from pterygoid canal.

- Nerve is sectioned and Bone wax is used to control bleeding from foramen.

- Mucoperiosteum of posterior wall of antrum is replaced and wound closed.

Complications

- Bleeding from small vessels controlled by electrocoagulation.

- Bleeding from pterygoid canal.

- Dryness of Ipsilateral eye treated with methylcellulose eye drops.

- Inadvertent vidian neurectomy may occur.

- Chronic sinusitis may occur but not a major problem if intranasal antrotomy is adequate.

V. Temporal bone resection

Surgical considerations in general

In general, surgery or radiation therapy, alone or in combination, are the treatment options for squamous carcinoma of temporal bone. Tumors confined to the EAC are considered localized in the absence of middle ear cleft invasion or facial nerve involvement.

The steps in the decision-making process involve the following

1. Histopathologic confirmation of malignancy.

2. Radiologic determination of disease extent and metastatic spread.

3. A realistic appraisal of whether surgery is aimed at palliation or cure.

4. The need to include the parotid, TMJ, infratemporal fossa, neck exploration, carotid artery and dural or cerebral resection or reconstruction as part of the planned resection.

5. The necessity or type of reconstruction options.

6. A radiation oncology consultation in anticipation for postoperative radiation.

7. A neurosurgery consultation if skull base surgical resection needed.

8. An internal medicine, cardiology, or anesthesiology consultation.

A number of surgical approaches are feasible that largely depend on the extent of the tumor. Complete surgical resection with a clear microscopic margin is the preferred initial primary treatment goal in a patient with a resectable cancer.

For small tumors, radiation therapy is an alternative. When resection is contemplated, a team comprising a head and neck surgeon, neurosurgeon, neurootologist, and plastic surgeon may be required.

In general, four types of resection are performed.

1. Excisional biopsy (including sleeve resection)
2. Lateral temporal bone resection
3. Subtotal temporal bone resection
4. Total temporal bone resection

Lateral temporal bone resection and subtotal temporal bone resection, the two most commonly performed procedures (Fig. 8.34 a & b).

Management of the primary site

Hirsch and Chang have described the operative procedures in detail and the indications based on the location and stage of the tumor (Hirsch, 1997).

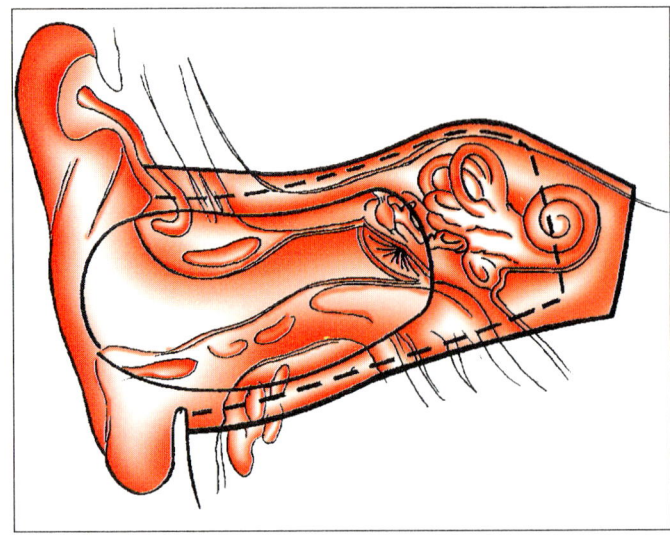

Fig. 8.34a Coronal section showing schematic representation of extent of resection (a) Lateral (b) Subtotal (c) Total

Forman ovale

Forman spinosum

Superior petrosal sinus

Inferior petrosal sinus

Sigmoid petrosal sinus

Zygomatic arch

Sulcus for middle menengeal artery

Lateral temporal bone resector

Sub total temporal bone resector

Total temporal bone resector

Mastoid tip

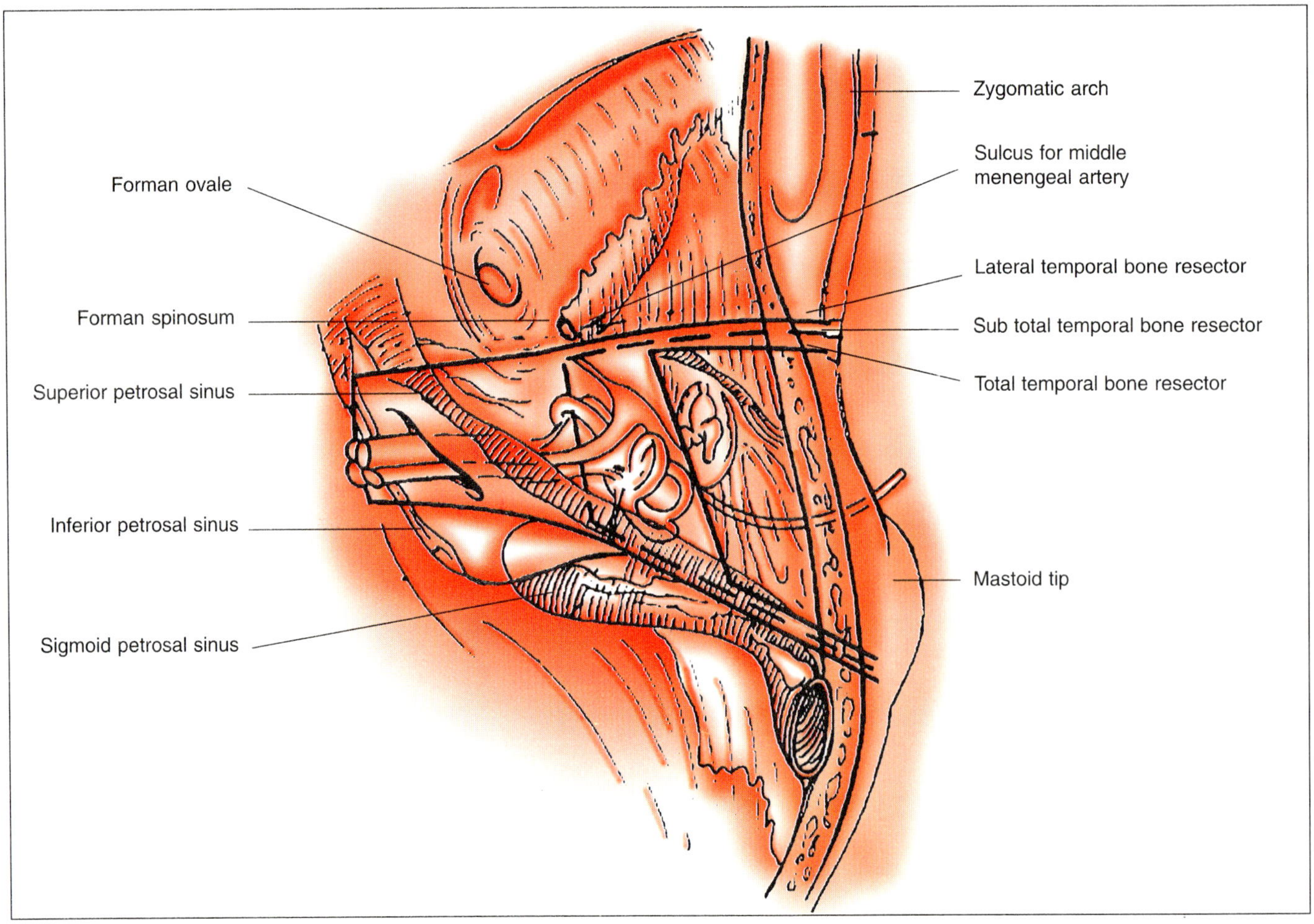

Fig. 8.34b Axial schematic representation showing extent of (a) Lateral (b) Subtotal (c) Total temporal bone resections

1. Excisional biopsy

Rarely, when a tumor is small and does not invade bone or cartilage, it can be excised with an adequate margin of normal skin. This is usually basal cell in type. A so-called sleeve excision can be done.

2. The LTBR includes resection of the EAC, tympanic membrane, malleus, and incus.

The boundaries are the middle ear cavity and stapes medially, the mastoid cavity posteriorly, the epitympanum and zygomatic root superiorly, the temporomandibular joint (TMJ) capsule anteriorly, and the medial tympanic ring or infratemporal fossa (ITF) inferiorly. The lateral margin depends on the extent of spread. The otic capsule and facial nerve are preserved. The LTBR is appropriate for T1 and T2 tumors.

The LTBR begins with a long, postauricular incision extending from the temporal fossa into the neck. If the pinna is to be preserved, a second incision is made within the concha lateral to the lesion. If the pinna is to be resected, a preauricular incision is incorporated to the postauricular incision allowing the pinna and surrounding skin to be included in the specimen. A cortical mastoidectomy is performed and the facial nerve identified. Bone removal is extended into the zygomatic root and to the digastric ridge. An extended facial recess is made, and the incudostapedial joint is separated. The facial recess is continued inferiorly and anteriorly lateral to the facial nerve, but medial to the annulus, until the specimen is attached only at the anterior canal bony wall at the level of the temporomandibular capsule. An osteotome is used to separate the bony specimen. The parotidectomy is performed in bloc.

Medina (1990) described several modifications of the lateral temporal bone dissection (LTBR) based on the location of disease.

A Modified LTBR removes the EAC and leaves the uninvolved tympanic membrane intact. This type of resection is appropriate for tumors originating in the concha without involvement of the EAC.

3. A subtotal temporal bone resection (STBR)

STBR is performed when invasion medial to the tympanic membrane or into the mastoid (T3 disease) is evident. In this case, the medial margin may be obtained in a piecemeal fashion, usually with a drill.

The specimen includes the LTBR with additional dissection of the otic capsule and the medial bony wall of the middle ear and mastoid. The margins of resection are the sigmoid sinus and posterior fossa dura posteriorly, middle fossa dura superiorly, internal carotid artery anteriorly, jugular bulb inferiorly, and petrous apex medially. Based on the extent of tumor spread, dissection may include the condyle of the mandible, the facial nerve, dura, sigmoid sinus, and contents of the infratemporal fossa. The carotid artery is skeletonized and becomes the medial margin.

Tumor involvement of the jugular bulb requires ligation of the internal jugular vein and proximal control of the sigmoid sinus. The facial nerve is traditionally sacrificed, with the proximal margin taken in the labyrinthine or internal auditory canal segment. However, the surgeon may elect to preserve the nerve if no indication of nerve involvement exists.

The medial extent of dissection at the level of the otic capsule depends on the depth of involvement and is done piecemeal. Tumor extension into the protympanum, eustachian tube, or carotid artery is addressed with an infratemporal fossa dissection. The temporalis muscle is reflected and the zygomatic arch removed. The mandibular condyle is resected. The dissection proceeds based on the extent of disease but may include identification of the pterygoid plate, the mandibular nerve (V3), and the horizontal carotid artery and may include a temporal craniotomy.

4. A total temporal bone resection

A total temporal bone resection can be used to address T4 disease. However, this procedure is associated with significant morbidity and may not significantly improve survival in these cases of advanced disease.

The total TBR includes the STBR with the additional resection of the petrous apex. The internal carotid artery may be isolated, mobilized, and preserved or resected. The sigmoid sinus, jugular vein, carotid artery, dura and CNS are removed as indicated by the extent of the tumor.

Management of the parotid and temporomandibular joint

The intraparotid lymph nodes are a first echelon drainage site for cancers of the EAC and middle ear. An adequate anterior margin for the temporal bone resection routinely involves resection of the parotid gland, temporomandibular joint, and condyle. Resection of these soft tissues will also address minimal soft tissue extension beyond the temporal bone.

Ideally, this is performed enbloc with the temporal bone. A superficial parotidectomy is performed with preservation of the facial nerve for T1 and T2 tumors. When the facial nerve is resected for more advanced lesions, a total parotidectomy may be performed.

SURGICAL TECHNIQUE IN DETAIL

Lateral Temporal Bone Resection

The first step of the procedure is to outline the lesion emanating from the EAC with an adequate margin of skin and conchal cartilage. Incisions are extended superiorly and inferiorly (Fig. 8.35) to permit adequate exposure for mastoidectomy, condylar resection, and parotidectomy, when these latter two adjunctive procedures are required. The superior extension into the scalp is required if the zygomatic root is invaded or limited middle fossa exposure is necessary. The remnant of the pinna is left attached to the skin flap.

In rare instances, there may be CT or MRI evidence of invasion of the mandibular condyle. In other instances, condylar resection may be required to achieve an adequate margin in the mesotympanum or even the anterior canal wall. In such cases, an incision in the fascia over the condyle is made to resect it. The temporalis fascia is elevated over a broad plane to avoid injury to the temporal branch of the facial nerve The fascia over the joint capsule is incised and the capsule itself transected, exposing the condylar head and overlying meniscus. A subperiosteal dissection encircles the neck of the mandible, and the Condyle is surgically isolated.

The next step in the procedure, which many times will precede the condylectomy, is to do a complete mastoidectomy. The basic landmarks in the standard mastoidectomy are exposed, but the completeness of air cell removal is not necessarily as thorough as in surgery for cholesteatoma. The exception to this is the anterior part. Careful skeletonization of the fallopian canal is done such that the facial recess can be exposed with maximum exposure of the middle ear, especially the mesotympanic side of the tympanic membrane. An atticotomy is done, the incudostapedial joint severed, and the incus removed. If the zygomatic root is invaded, extension of the atticotomy is required to expose this portion of the disease. If the disease falls short of the tympanic membrane, the incus and malleus are preserved and the atticotomy is done meticulously, drilling the bone to a fine shell over the ossicles and carefully removing the thinned bony plate with a stapes curette.

If tumor is found to invade the TMJ, then, as previously mentioned, a mandibular condylectomy is done that includes the condyle, meniscus, glenoid fossa, capsular ligaments, and insertion of the lateral pterygoid muscles. Although controversial, it is probably wise to do a parotidectomy with facial nerve sparing in most cases of carcinoma of the EAC. The easy passage of tumor through the fissures of Santorini in the cartilaginous external canal to the parotid make the gland particularly vulnerable to tumor spread, and thus parotid resection is an important aspect of safe tumor clearance.

The final stage of tumor resection is at hand. In the usual type of tumor without zygomatic extension, a fissure is cut with the bur from the anterior attic into the glenoid fossa. A similar fissure is made from the inferior extremity of the

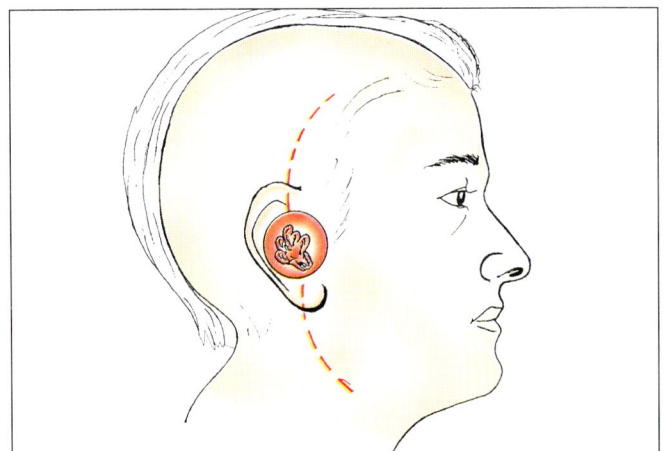
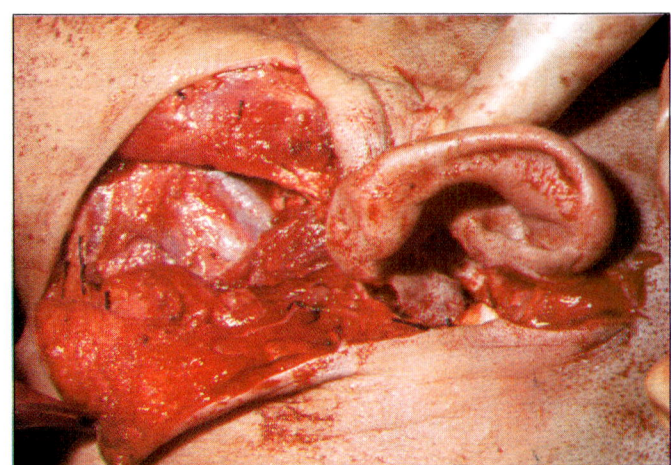

Fig. 8.35a & b Showing incision for lateral temporal bone resection

Pinna along
with scalp flap

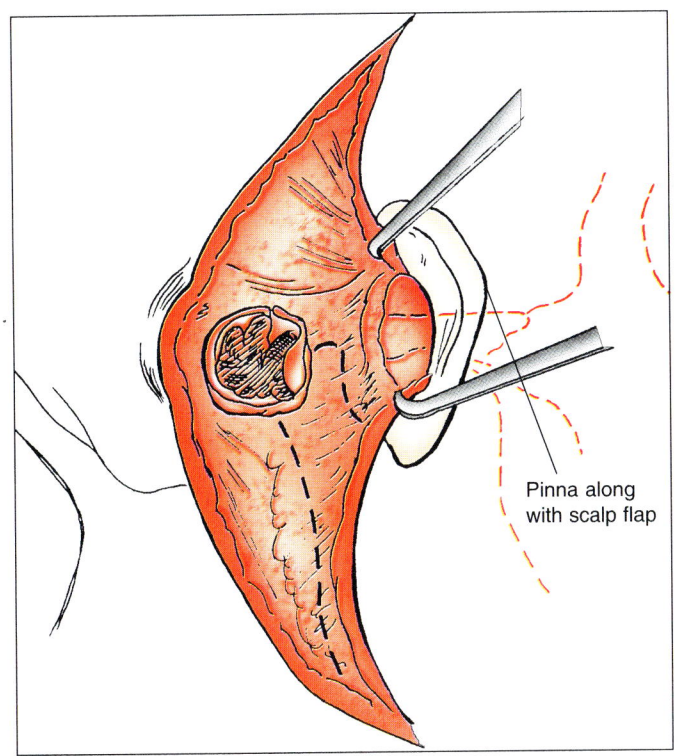

Fig. 8.36 The tumor is encompassed by a soft tissue cuff down to the mastoid cortex

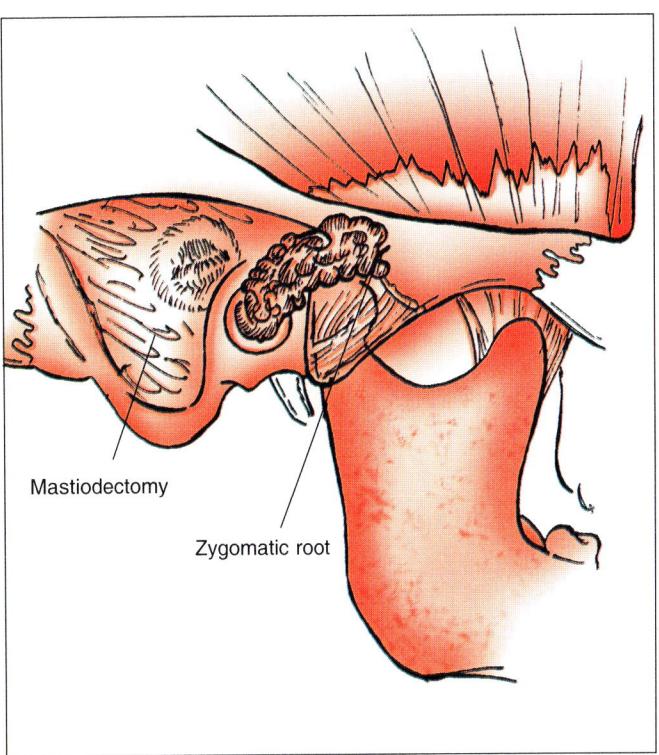

Mastiodectomy
Zygomatic root

Fig. 8.37 Mastoidectomy completed. Tumor shows invasion to zygomatic root

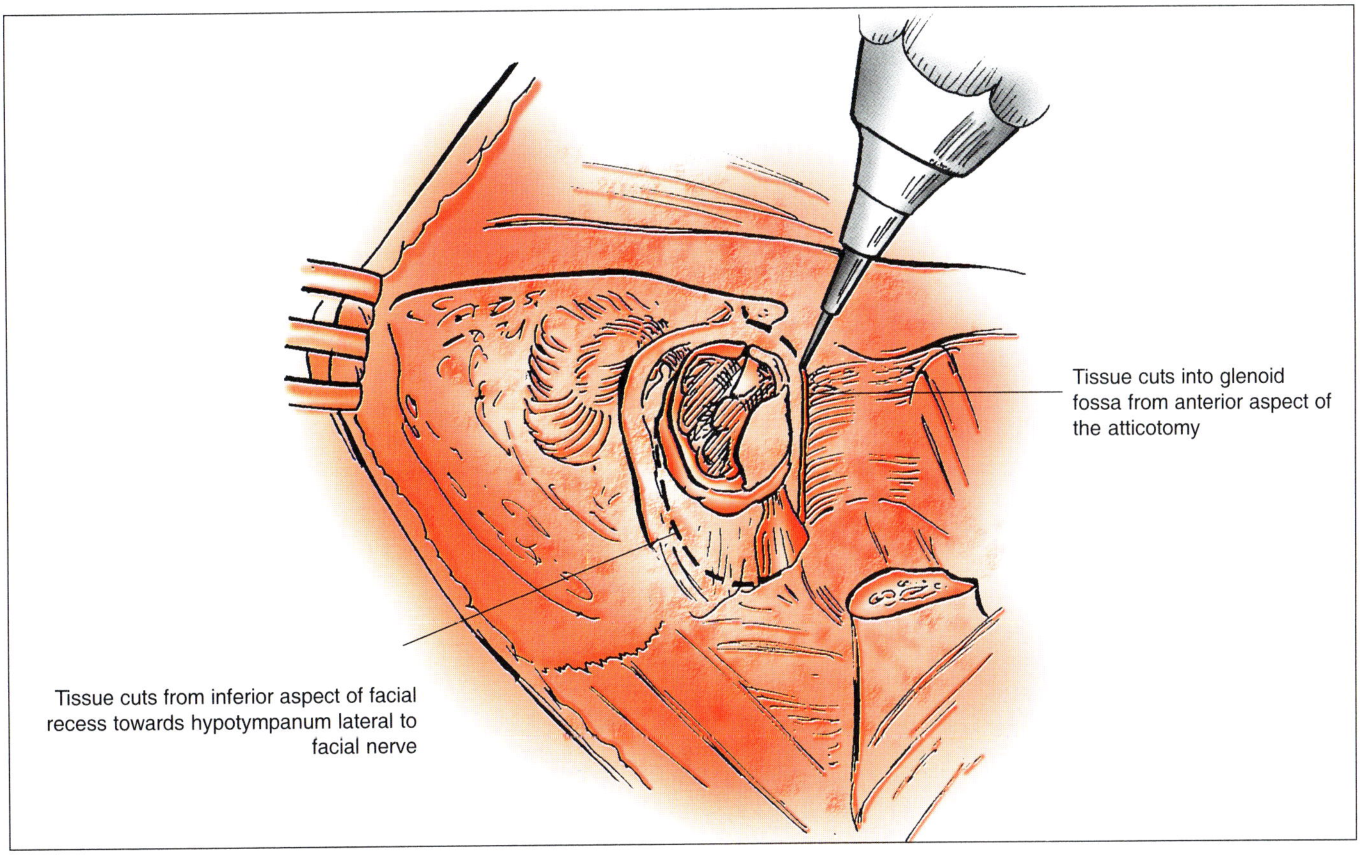

Tissue cuts into glenoid fossa from anterior aspect of the atticotomy
Tissue cuts from inferior aspect of facial recess towards hypotympanum lateral to facial nerve

Fig. 8.38 Showing various bony cuts for lateral temporal bone resection

facial recess toward the hypotympanum, taking care to stay lateral to the facial nerve. In most of the cases, the tympanic membrane requires excision. In those few cases in which the membrane is spared, the fissure cut is made lateral to the tympanic ring. A series of osteotome cuts superiorly, inferiorly, and posteriorly are made.

The final osteotome is placed in the posterior fissure and driven into the glenoid fossa. The specimen fractures away from the main body of the temporal bone and is removed from the last soft tissue attachments at the TMJ. With zygomatic extension, mandibular condylectomy is usually necessary and a more extensive resection is required.

The resection is outlined in. Great care must be taken to stay lateral to the eustachian tube and to come across the mesotympanum close to the tympanic annulus to avoid injury to the internal jugular vein and ICA. Fissures are cut through the glenoid fossa and tympanic bone, connecting the posterior fissure made inferior to the facial recess and the fissure at the zygomatic root. A fascia graft is placed over the stapes in an attempt to reconstruct the tympanic membrane.

Split-thickness skin is applied to the mastoid cavity, and the scalp flap advanced into the defect as well.

Subtotal Temporal Bone Resection

The next most common operation done after the lateral temporal bone resection is the subtotal operation. This procedure is done when tumor invades the middle ear and mastoid.

This operation is based on the principles established by Lewis in the original operation. The importance of his contribution of this procedure-heroic in proportion at the time-cannot be overemphasized. One of the basic modifications to Lewis' original procedure is the use of the highspeed air drill.

A complete mastoidectomy is done despite the fact that the origin of the tumor may have been the auricle or the peri-auricular skin. The first resection block before the mastoidectomy will then be the margin of healthy skin and soft tissue surrounding the tumor and the tumor is amputated at the level of the cartilaginous canal and tumor-breached mastoid cortex. As is mentioned throughout this text, total clearance of tumor by negative frozen-section and eventually negative permanent-section margins ensures total tumor removal and a low incidence of local tumor recurrence. To struggle with a large tumor mass that

interferes with adequate visualization, especially when that necessitates unnecessary sacrifice of normal uninvolved tissue for the sake of the en bloc principle, is unwarranted. A series of "enbloc resections" with tumor only at the deep margin continues until all malignancy is cleared.

Complete encompassment of all disease in the mastoid is effected. Invasion through the tegmen mastoideum and tympani is not uncommon because this route presents a path of least resistance to tumor spread. Tumor may invade the sigmoid sinus or the lateral sinus through the .sigmoid plate. The resection of the lateral sinus must proceed with great care because the vein of Labbe enters the sinus at a variable distance from the top of the sigmoid sinus.

Removal of the vein may result in severe motor deficits or even death, depending upon the integrity of the superior cerebral vein of Trollard.

Below the tentorium, extension of tumor may penetrate the cerebellar dura, and a more extensive removal of the occipital bone will be necessary to provide exposure for resection.

The exposure may require a dissection following the sigmoid sinus to the jugular bulb and even into the neck. Penetration from the jugular fossa into the carotid canal often means the addition of the infratemporal fossa approach for optimal exposure. Exposure of the zygomatic root, mandibular condylectomy, and parotidectomy are done in a similar fashion to the lateral resection. Control of the medial aspect of resection is accomplished by a small, limited middle fossa craniotomy whose size is dictated by the extent of dural invasion.

Temporal craniotomy

The temporal craniotomy is most expeditiously outlined according to the method described by Montgomery. A cutting bur is used to outline a small bony incision in the temporal squama. The incision should extend in a smooth arc from the sinodural angle to a point 4 cm above the EAC, and then arch forward to the cut in the zygomatic arch. Before extending the cut to the dura, the intracranial fluid volume is diminished by extracting CSF through a previously placed lumbar drain, through a lumbar puncture, or by use of an osmotic diuretic such as mannitol. Next, the inner table of skull is carefully cut through and the bone flap carefully dissected from the underlying dura. This is usually fairly easy to do, except in the elderly, in whom the dura is brittle and adherent to the skull. This part of the procedure may be done either by the neurosurgeon or the head and neck surgeon. The author prefers to cut the bone

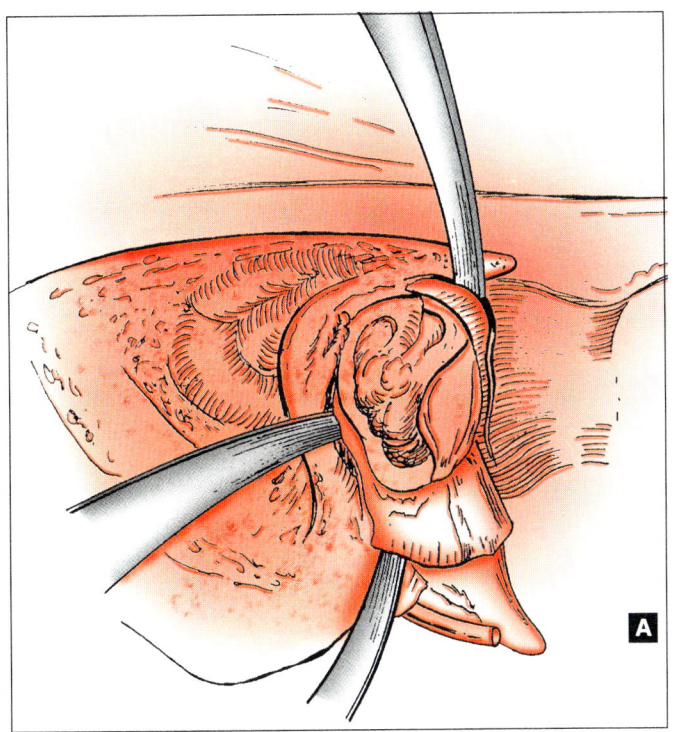

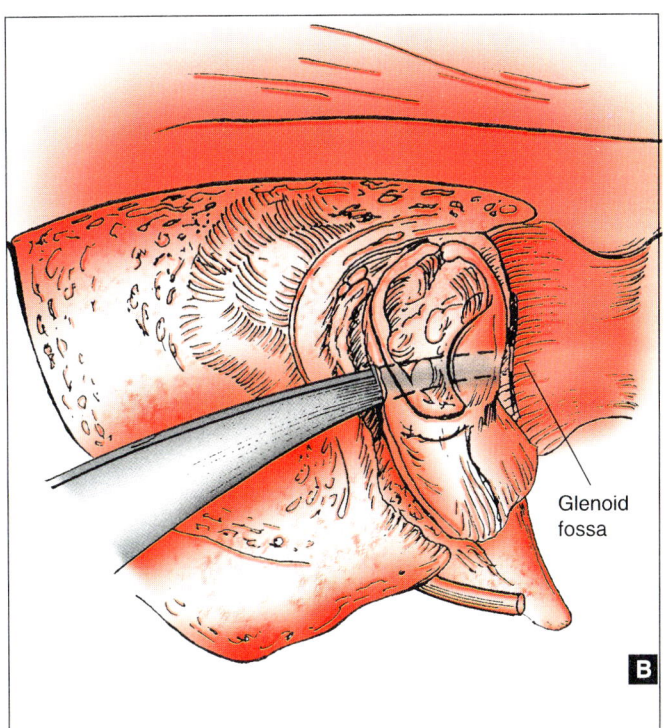

Glenoid
fossa

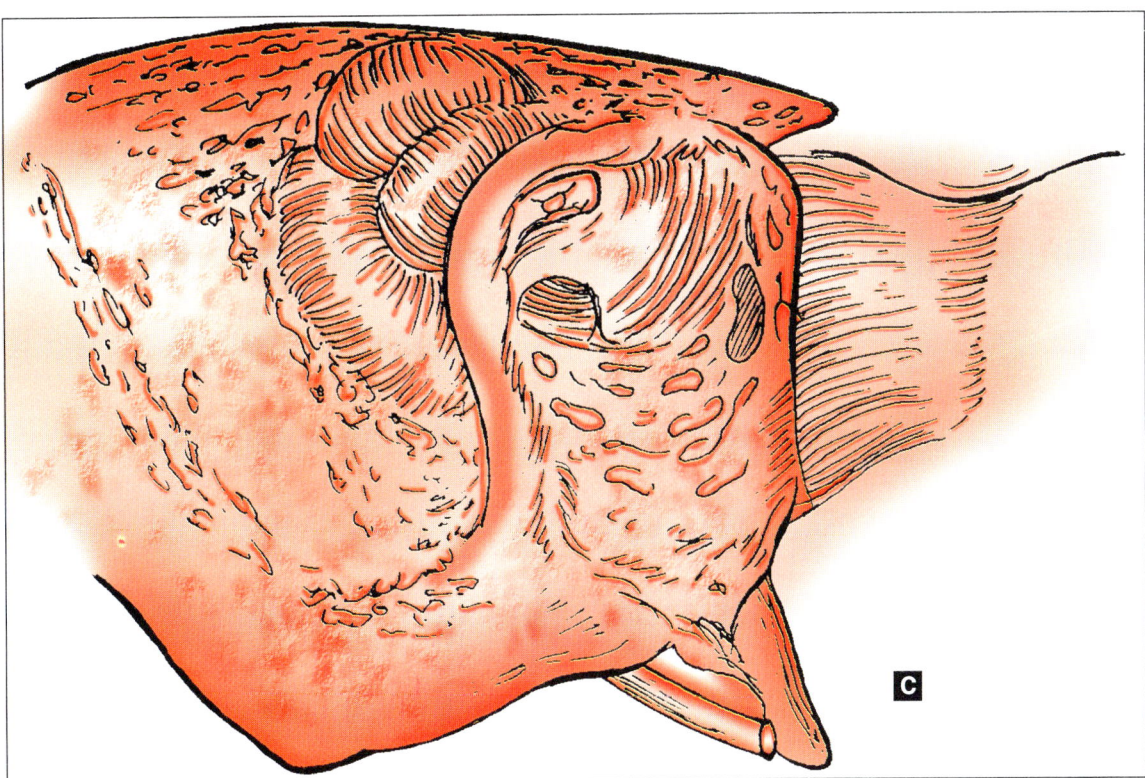

Fig. 8.39 (A, B, C) Lateral temporal bone resection with zygomatic root, condyle and glenoid fossa removed. **A.** Fissure cut and osteotomes placed. Successive cuts being superiorly, inferiorly and finally anteriorly. **B.** An osteotome placed in fissure inferior to the facial recess and driven anteriorly into and through the anterior bony canal into the glenoid fossa. **C.** LTBR resection completed

flap himself and leave the rest to the neurosurgeons, because they seem to think that a bigger craniotomy is desirable. The purpose of this operative step is to control the superior petrosal sinus and the middle meningeal artery, detect and resect any dural invasion or temporal lobe extension if possible, and establish the medial margin of resection. As the temporal lobe dura is elevated from the floor of the middle fossa and retracted with a Teflon-coated retractor,

the superior petrosal sinus is prized from its fissure in the posterosuperior extremity of the temporal bone. This elevation proceeds toward the cavernous sinus and Meckel's cave, judiciously avoiding both. Exposure of the middle fossa floor to the portion of temporal bone medial to the accurate eminence is done with the dural elevator. All aspects of the circumference of the temporal bone are now outlined, and final bony cuts may now be made.

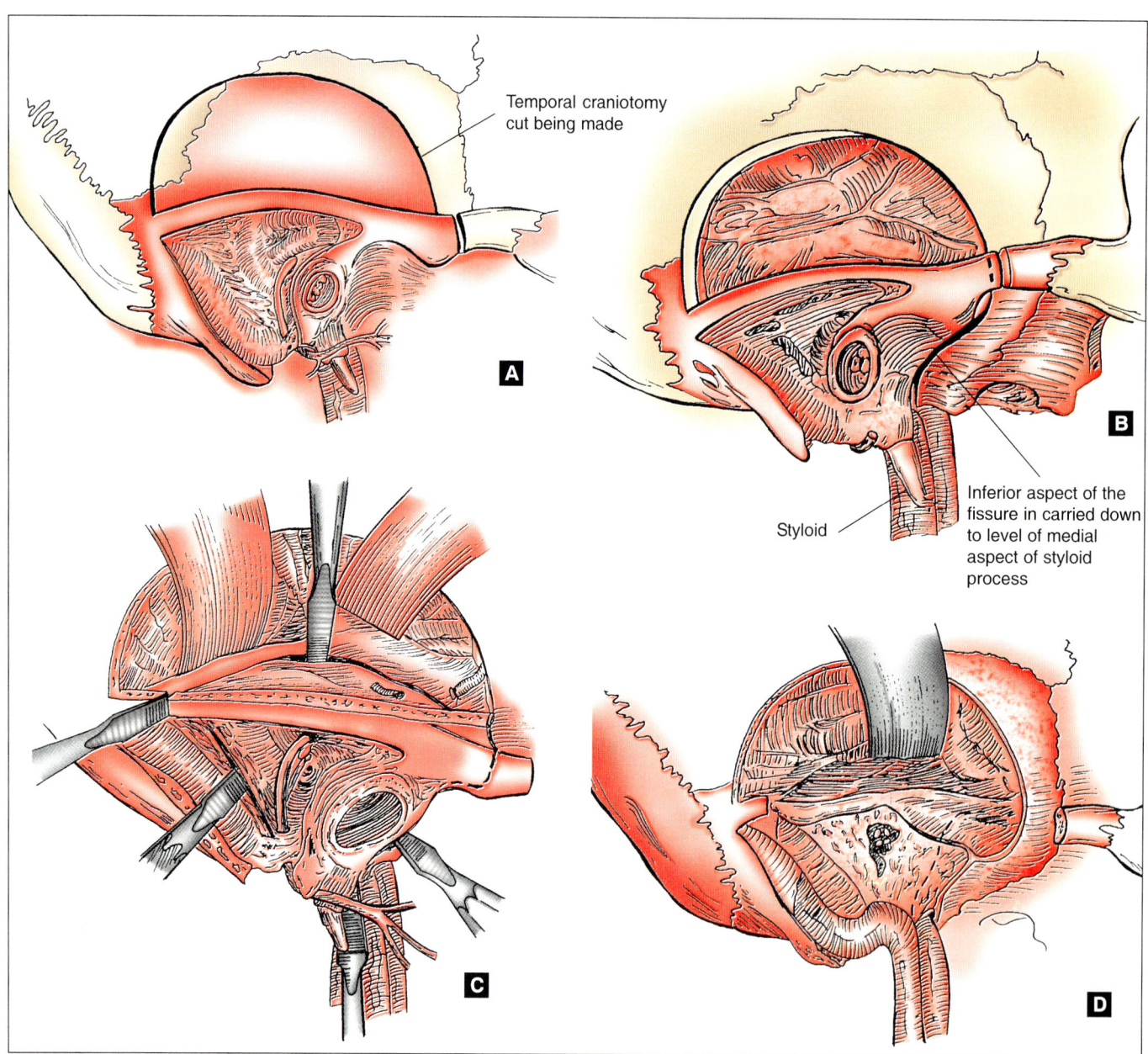

Fig 8.40 (A, B, C, D) Showing steps of total temporal bone resection
A. Temporal craniotomy is outlined with a cutting burr. **B.** Craniotomy flap removed. The glenoid fossa is cut across medially and the incision often transects the Eustachian tube and proceeds into the middle cranial fossa. The inferior aspect of the fissure is carried down to the level of medial aspect of styloid process. **C.** The 5 osteotomes cuts, necessary to excise the bone are outlined. **D.** Defect after excision

Final bony cuts

This critical part of the resection is where most surgical disasters occur. The problem is that the internal cuts that sever the temporal bone from the skull run adjacent to the course of the ICA and the jugular bulb. Injury to the latter structure is no great problem because bleeding can be controlled from below by the umbilical tape and from above through tamponade of the sigmoid or lateral sinuses. However, hemorrhage from a rent in the ICA can be life threatening because bleeding can be only partially controlled in the neck. Moreover, occlusion of the vessel may result in stroke and even death.

Osteotome cuts are initiated at the following sites

- A cut is made posteriorly through the back surface of the bone at its most medial aspect, through the most medial limit of cerebellar plate skeletonization.

- From cut no. 1, a superiorly directed bony incision is made to the sinodural angle. A cut through the tegmen mastoid connects this to the craniotomy and is carried medially.

- A cut is then made inferiorly just lateral to the styloid process and directly lateral to the jugular bulb. This cut is directed superiorly and slightly medially.

- A cut is made anteroinferiorly through the fissure in the glenoid fossa.

- For the "coup de grace," a cut is made superiorly through the floor of the middle fossa, just medial to the arcuate eminence.

These bony incisions are best made with an osteotome. The instrument is guided toward the theoretical center of the temporal bone near the internal acoustic meatus by being angled slightly medially. A gentle tapping with the mallet is followed by a slight twisting of the osteotome. This results in a more controlled type of incision. The cut medial to the arcuate eminence has to penetrate the otic capsule and thus requires a more brisk blow with the hammer.

Anteroinferiorly, the cutting and twisting motion of the osteotome usually results in the bone splitting along the plane of the initial ascending portion of the ICA. The bone is most commonly transected through either the cochlea or the internal auditory canal.

Cavity ablation

If the bone transection is too medial in the internal auditory canal, a CSF leak may result. A fat graft taken from the subcutaneous area of the abdomen and placed at the site of the leak is usually an effective plug. Temporalis muscle flaps may be used to ablate the cavity.

However, the cavity should not be so effaced that possible tumor recurrences might be obscured in their early stages. The most important aspect of closure is the careful replacement of any resected dura with fascia, together with the securing of a watertight closure of any rents.

Hypoglossal-to-facial nerve anastomosis

Full temporal bone resection always necessitates transection of the facial nerve. Although some thought may be given to cable grafting the nerve, this connection must extend from the proximal internal acoustic canal to the transected main trunk near the resected parotid bed. This is a difficult maneuver, and the author elects in most cases to do a hypoglossal-to-facial nerve crossover anastomosis. The hypoglossal nerve is cut as far down in the neck as possible so the anastomosis will be tension free. The approximation is made under microscopic control using 10-0 nylon sutures. Approximately 10 sutures are placed through the epineurium of these nerves (Fig 8.41a & b).

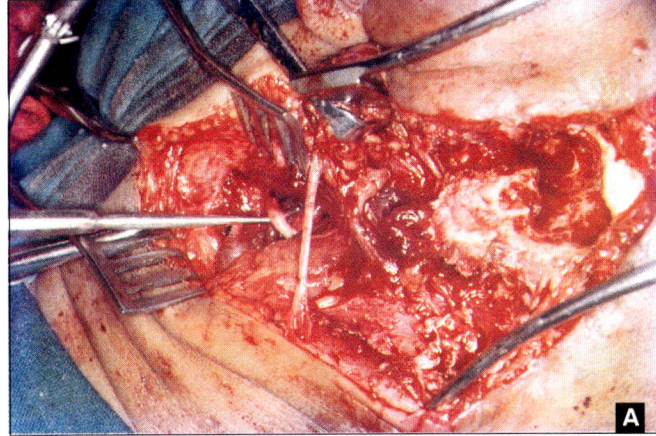

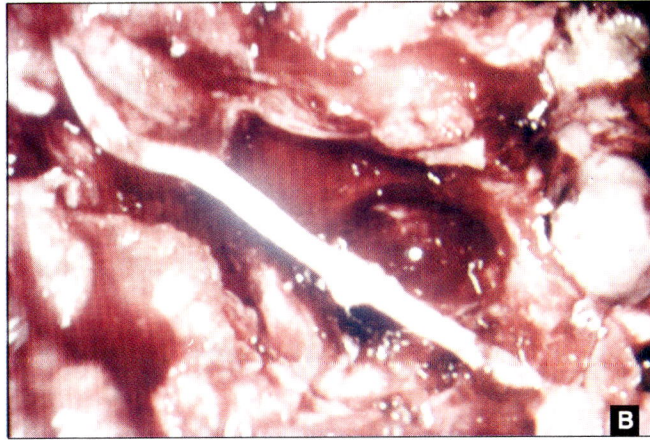

Fig. 8.41a & b Showing the hypoglossal to facial nerve anastomosis

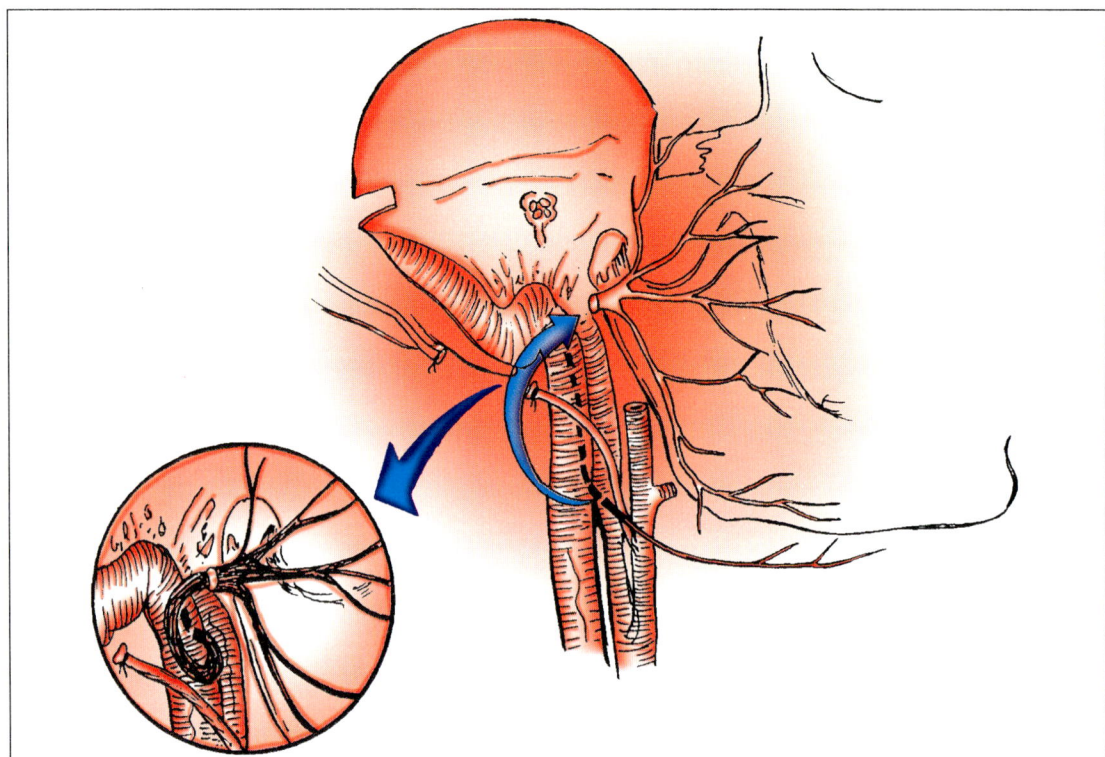

Fig 8.42 Total temporal bone resection with hypoglossal to facial nerve crossover anastomosis

Closure

When a portion of the auricle remains, the flap is returned and the gap created by the conchal and external canal skin excision is bridged with a split-thickness skin graft. The graft is inverted into the cavity and packed with iodoform- or antibiotic- impregnated gauze packing. The graft is sutured to the auricular cut edges, and the remaining wound in the neck and scalp is closed with interrupted sutures. The neck is drained and a large pressure dressing applied, or suction drains are used. Excision of the entire auricle occasionally presents a problem in closure. Because most patients with temporal bone carcinoma are elderly, an elevation of the facial skin similar to that of a face lift enhances flap advancement. When this is not enough, a relaxation incision can be done and a bipedicled scalp flap advanced into the wound. The donor site on the skull is skin grafted, and the wound is closed and drained.

TOTAL TEMPORAL BONE RESECTION

Total petrosectomy + STBR

The most extensive temporal bone cancers are fortunately rarely seen. These tumors involve all or some of the internal acoustic canal, the ICA, the superior or inferior petrosal sinuses, the cavernous sinus, and any of the surrounding dura, the falx, or the temporal lobe of the brain. Controversy continues concerning the advisability of brain, ICA, and cavernous sinus resection. In the authors' experience, the prognosis is adversely affected by involvement of these areas, but resection is still considered warranted even if only as a palliative effort.

The preparation for the resection is similar to that for them subtotal temporal bone resection. Posteriorly, cerebellar plate removal continues to a point just lateral to the porus acusticus. Superiorly, the superior petrosal sinus is elevated to its point of entrance into the cavernous sinus. In the process, Meckel's cave is exposed and the proximity of Dorello's canal is reached. If uninvolved, cranial nerves V and VI are carefully protected. Involvement of the cranial nerve V is not uncommonly seen, and the gasserian ganglion may need to be removed.

Careful elevation of the lateral aspect of the cavernous sinus is necessary so that the final osteotome cut does not lacerate the sinus. The various extensions of the sinus to the foramina of the third and sometimes second divisions of the trigeminal nerve may need to be coagulated with the bipolar cautery and packed off with thrombin-soaked Gelfoam pledgets or hemostatic gauze. Anteriorly, exposure

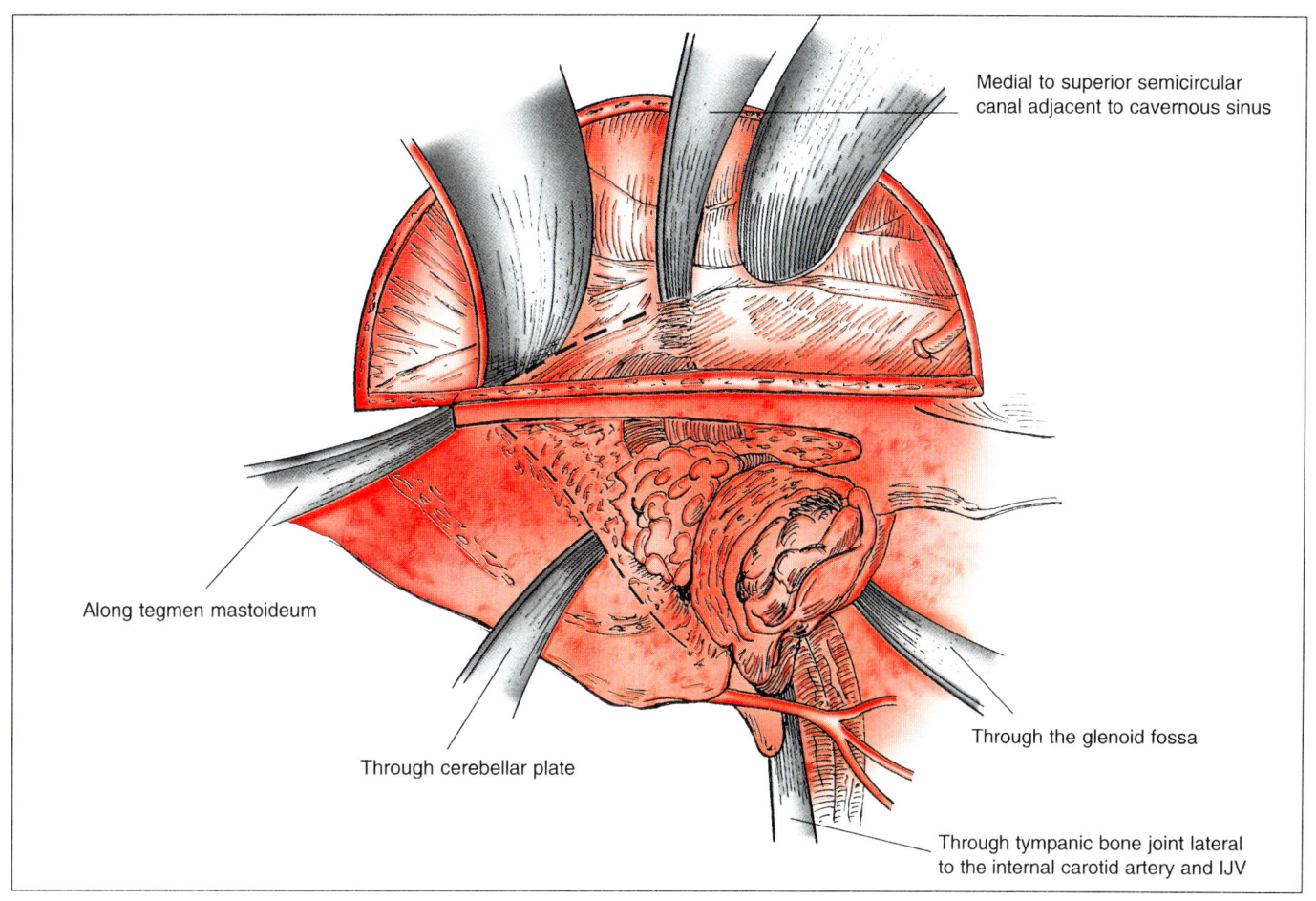

Medial to superior semicircular canal adjacent to cavernous sinus

Along tegmen mastoideum

Through cerebellar plate

Through the glenoid fossa

Through tympanic bone joint lateral to the internal carotid artery and IJV

Fig 8.43 Osteotome cuts for total petrosectomy

of the middle fossa floor provides exposure of the foramen spinosum. The middle meningeal artery can be clipped, tied, or coagulated. Exposure of the foramen ovale requires zygomatic ostectomy to provide infratemporal fossa exposure. Inferiorly, careful attention is given to clear delineation of the ICA and internal jugular vein, and rubber catheters are used to circle these vessels in the neck. If either vessel is invaded at this point, the "modified en bloc" resection principle is invoked, and in the initial phase of total petrosectomy, any tumor involvement of either the vein or artery is left to be addressed at the next phase of resection. Osteotome cuts are made lateral to or just through the most lateral aspect of the internal auditory canal. These are done both posteriorly and superiorly near the petrous apex. The fracture along the carotid canal is even easier in those cases with ICA invasion by tumor. The bone tends to fracture along this line of weakness. With removal of the bone, CSF begins to leak from the internal auditory canal.

With removal of bone, only a rudiment of the petrous apex remains. The remaining bone, and that of its articulation with the sphenoid, is removed with a drill. The carotid canal is drilled away if involved and the carotid removed and grafted. The cavernous sinus is removed by the neurosurgeon. Clival erosion is removed by the drill. Perineural invasion is traced in a central direction until tumor free margins are obtained. Reconstruction involves dural grafting, but a watertight seal between the often incomplete dural closure and the nasopharynx is not uncommon. Complete eustachian tube removal is usually necessary. Closure from the nasopharynx and augmentation of dural closure may occasionally be achieved with fat grafts. Usually a temporalis muscle flap or a rectus abdominis free flap effects closure and seals any CSF leakage. Meticulous postoperative eye care is essential, especially when the facial nerve and trigeminal ganglia have been resected.

Management of the neck

Although metastasis to the neck is uncommon in limited cancers of the temporal bone, neck dissections are routinely performed. With more extensive cancers, dissection of the neck offers staging and provides control of the great vessels and exposure to the skull base. However, the presence of metastasis is associated with a poor prognosis, and neck dissection does not improve survival.

Management of the dura and brain

Although involvement of the dura and brain portend for a poor prognosis, an aggressive approach includes resection of the dura and a small volume of the temporal lobe with a healthy margin.

Reconstruction

Facial nerve grafting is usually not performed in the presence of a malignant lesion. Management of facial nerve paralysis may include CN XII to VII grafting, cross facial grafting, and static procedures. Extensive resections may result in large soft tissue defects. A temporalis muscle flap can be used to fill small to medium defects. The pedicled myocutaneous trapezius flap is an excellent option for reconstruction of the soft tissue and skin defect. The pectoralis flap has limited distant reach to the resected margin. The rectus abdominus free flap and radial forearm flap are particularly suited for the area. Dural defects should be repaired primarily or with graft reconstruction.

Postoperative details: Postoperative care consists of monitoring wound complications, flap viability, intracranial complications, and complications of CN deficits. If the dura was resected and repaired, the wound should be observed for a cerebrospinal fluid leak. Supportive care for dizziness, nausea, and vertigo is needed when the otic capsule is entered during the resection. Eye care should be instituted if postoperative facial paralysis develops or if the facial nerve is resected. Resection of CN X requires swallowing and vocal fold rehabilitation and observation for aspiration or airway complications. If the temporomandibular joint was removed, the mandible should be mobilized early to prevent contralateral dysfunction.

Complications of treatment depend on the extent of resection and the use of adjunctive radiation. Postoperative hearing loss, facial nerve paralysis, vertigo, and other CN deficits (*e.g.*, CN V, VII, VIII, IX, X, XI) may occur. Dural resection may predispose to cerebral spinal fluid leaks, meningitis, or intracranial complications. Significant complications can result from trauma to or resection of the carotid artery. Radiation has known complications of fibrosis of soft tissues, destruction of salivary gland tissue, osteoradionecrosis of the temporal bone, and possibly central nervous system effects if the field of radiation extends to intracranial tissues.

9

Approaches to Posterior Skull Base

Approaches to cerebellopontine angle tumors

Cerebellopontine (CP) angle tumors are an important lesion which can be practiced in our clinical practice. The commonest CP angle tumour being a vestibular schwannoma (acoustic neuroma).

The modern era of surgical removal for CP angle lesions began in 1960's. Prior to this mortality and morbidity rates were quite high using the sub-occipital approach. With the use of the operating microscope, trans labyrinthine and middle fossa approaches have been refined to reduce the morbidity and mortality rates.

The combined trans-labyrinthine and retrosigmoid approach is commonly used now. It is used in cases of large vestibular schwannomas.

The various approaches are

- Translabyrinthine approach
- Retrosigmoid approach
- Combined (translabyrinthine and retrosigmoid) approach
- Transotic approach
- Middle fossa approach

SELECTION OF SURGICAL APPROACH

Following guidelines are used in approach to resection of CP angle tumors.

- *Status of patients hearing:* Hearing conservation approaches are middle fossa and retrosigmoid approaches.

- *The 50:50 rule is followed.* (i.e. hearing pure tone thresholds should be less than 50dB and the speech better than 50% discrimination),

- *Location of tumor:* If lateral one third of the internal auditory canal is involved, middle fossa approach is preferred. If the tumor is more medial in the internal auditory canal and is extending greater than 0.5cm into the CPA, the retrosigmoid approach is used.

- *Tumor size:* Small intracanalicular lesions upto 3.5cm is best accessed by translabyrinthine approach. Large tumors with significant inferior extension is accessed by retrosigmoid approach.

- *Type of CPA tumor:* Tumors other than vestibular schwannomas are accessed best by retrosigmoid approach.

- *Patients age:* Translabyrinthine is the preferred approach for elderly patients.

TRANSLABYRINTHINE APPROACH

Indications

- Small intracanalicular tumors like acoustic neuromas and medium-sized lesions upto 3.5 cm in diameter in the CPA.

- Other lesions of the internal acoustic meatus and cerebellopontine angle such as congenital cholesteatoma, meningioma, angioma or neuromas arising from V, VII, IX, X or XI may also be removed provided VIII nerve function is permanently lost.

- Useful in patients who have persistent symptoms from idiopathic endolymphatic hydrops and who have irreversible loss of auditory function on the affected side.

- This procedure is sometimes required, after stapedectomy failure or following sudden spontaneous hearing loss, provided there is no useful function and when distracting tinnitus cannot be relieved by antidepressants.

- This approach can also be used to drain pus in very rare instances of chronic suppurative petrositis and labyrinthitis with recurrent meningitis and posterior fossa arachnoiditis.

Preoperative procedure

- MRI scan with gadolinium enhancement.

- Antibiotics started preoperatively.

- Hair is shaved 3 cm above and 6 cm posteriorly to the pinna along with left lower quadrant of abdomen.

- Inj. Dexamethasone 0.1 mg/kg body weight is given.

- Inj. Mannitol 1 g/kg body weight is given.

- Patient is intubated, positioned in supine position with head turned to opposite side by 45 degrees and neck is slightly extended.

- 2 ml of 1% xylocaine with adrenaline is infilterated in the postauricular region and 4 quadrants of EAC.

Procedure

- A curved postauricular incision is made from the mastoid tip upto a point 1cm above the auricle. Posteriorly, the incision is placed 3 cm posterior to the postauricular crease (Fig. 9.1). The incision is carried down through the skin and the subcutaneous tissue. The postauricular skin flap is elevated forward upto the skin of the external auditory canal. An incision is made through the periosteum 2 cm posteriorly along the inferior temporal line. A second incision 1.5 cm inferior to the inferior temporal line is created parallel to this initial incision. The two parallel incisions are connected posteriorly with a perpendicular incision, creating an anteriorly pedicled periosteal flap attached to the EAC (Fig. 9.2).

- The periosteum posterior to the ear canal is elevated upto the ear canal.

- The skin of the bony external auditory canal is elevated down to the level of the annulus and the tympanic membrane is elevated.

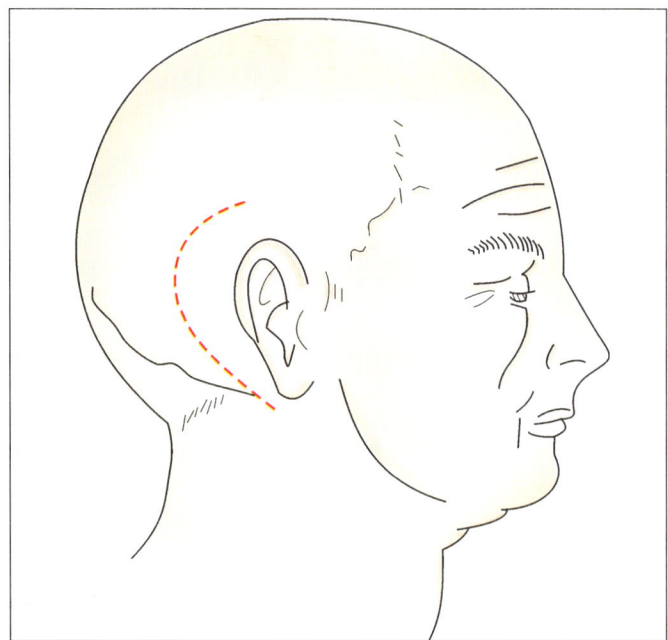

Fig 9.1 Curved postauricular incision

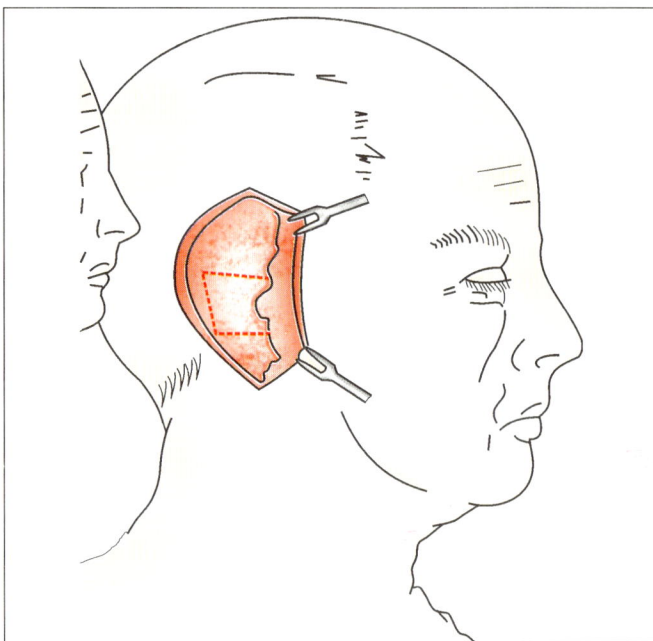

Fig 9.2 Two parallel incison connected posteriorely with a parpendicular incision

- A complete mastoidectomy is performed, skeletonizing the tegmen superiorly and the sigmoid sinus posteriorly (Fig. 9.3).

- The entire sigmoid sinus is skeletonized, leaving a thin sheet of bone covering the sinus laterally known as the "BILL'S ISLAND". Dura is exposed anterior and 2cm posterior to the sigmoid sinus (Fig. 9.4).

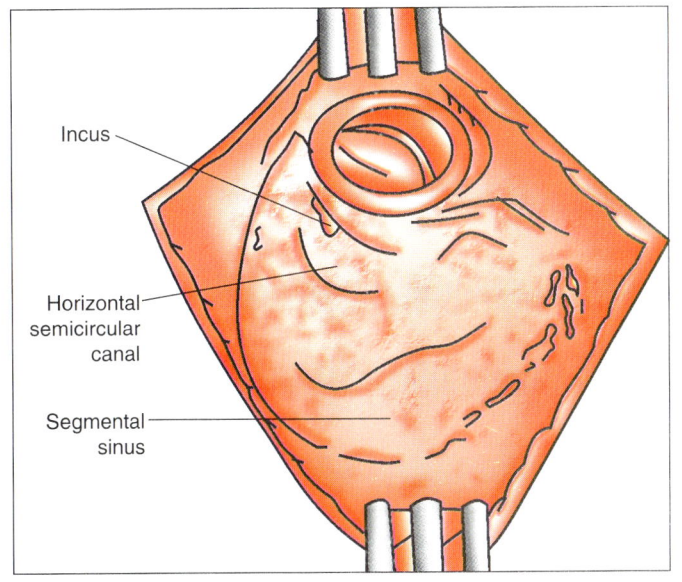

Fig 9.3 Complete mastoidectomy

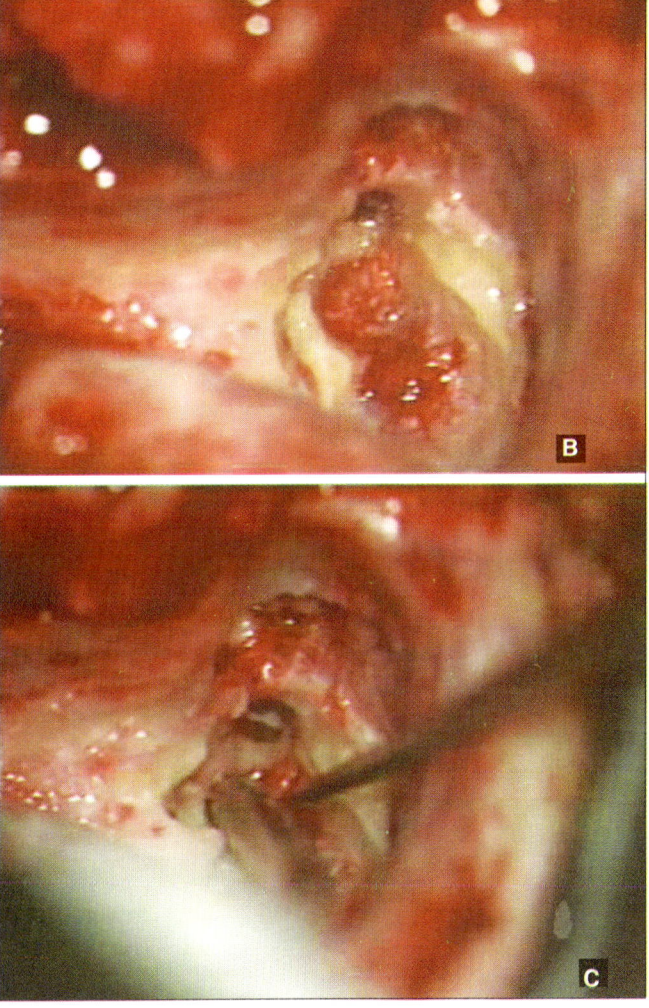

Fig 9.4 Dura is reposed and sigmoid sinuses skeletonized

- A labyrinthectomy is performed beginning with the horizontal followed by the posterior and then finally the superior semicircular canals. The vestibule is opened (Fig. 9.5a, b & c).

- The internal auditory canal is skeletonized 210 degrees along the superior, posterior and inferior circumference. Inferiorly, the dissection proceeds between the jugular bulb and the inferior aspect of the internal auditory canal. All the remaining bone covering the posterior 210 degrees of the internal auditory canal is elevated off the dura and removed (Fig. 9.6a & b).

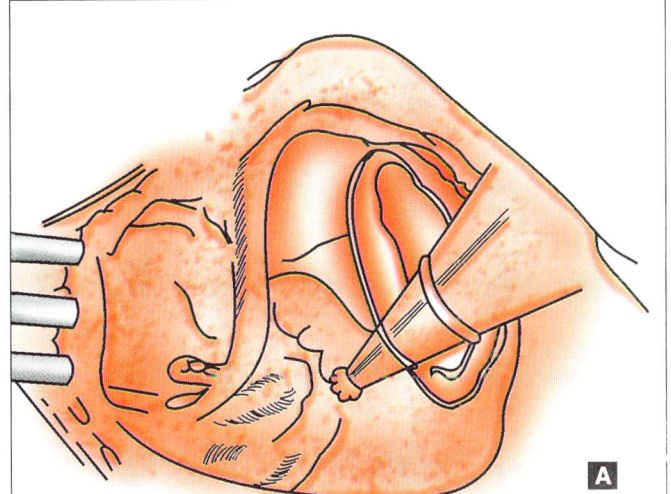

Fig 9.5 a, b, c Labyrinthectomy being performed

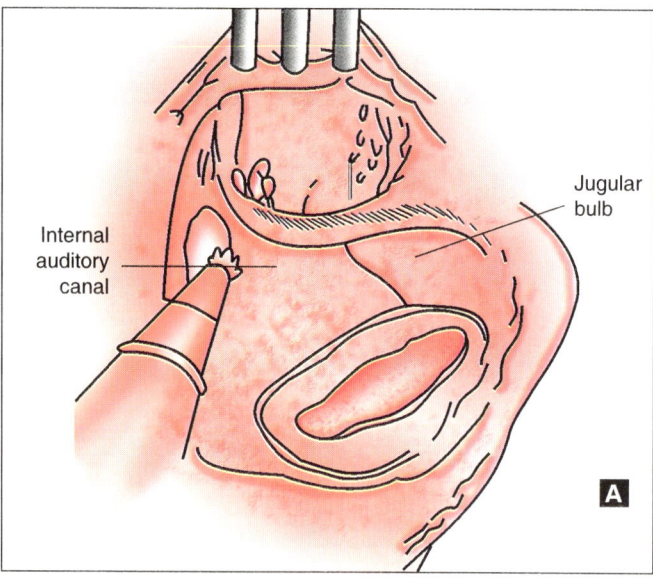

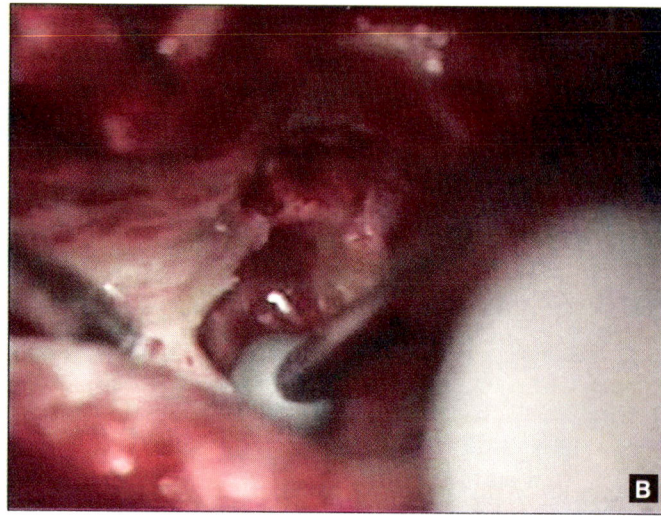

Fig 9.6 a & b Dissection proceeds between the jugular bulb and inferior aspect of internal auditory canal

- An incision is made in the dura extending from the sigmoid sinus to the porus austicus (Fig. 9.7).

- The facial nerve is easily identified in it's intralabyrinthine segment. Verification of the position of the facial nerve is aided by the stimulation using a nerve probe set. Once the facial nerve is identified, the superior vestibular nerve is separated from it. The vestibular schwannoma along with the distal free end of the vestibular nerve are dissected out of the internal auditory canal. Vestibulocochlear nerve is cauterized as it exits the tumor (Fig. 9.8a, b & c).

- In cases of large tumors, additional exposure can be achieved by gentle retraction of the cerebellum 1 to 2 cm posteriorly.

- After the dissection, facial nerve can be visualized extending from the brainstem into the intralabyrinthine portion of the fallopian canal. The lower cranial nerves entering the jugular foramen can also be visualized (Fig. 9.9a & b).

- The mucosa of the middle ear and protympanum is removed. The mucosa, lining the eustachian tube, is inverted. A small piece of temporalis fascia is harvested and inserted into the Eustachian tube, filling the entire lumen. A small piece of temporalis fascia is then placed over the Eustachian tube. The flaps of posterior fossa dura are reapproximated and a large piece of temporalis fascia is placed over the dura and draped over the facial nerve. The abdominal fat graft is trimmed to fill the entire mastoid cavity and middle ear cleft.

- The mastoid periosteum is sutured with 3-0 vicryl, skin is sutured with 4-0 silk. Pressure dressing is applied.

- The abdominal fat graft site is closed.

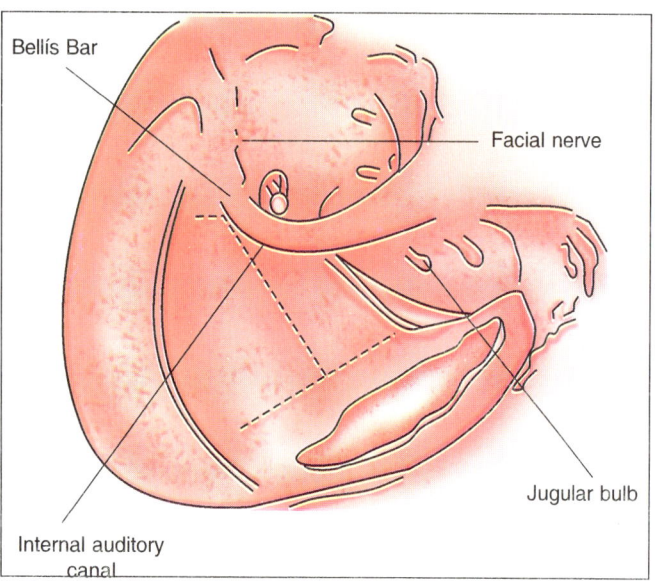

Fig 9.7 Incision over dura is made

Advantages

- Excellent access to CPA without retraction of the cerebellum.

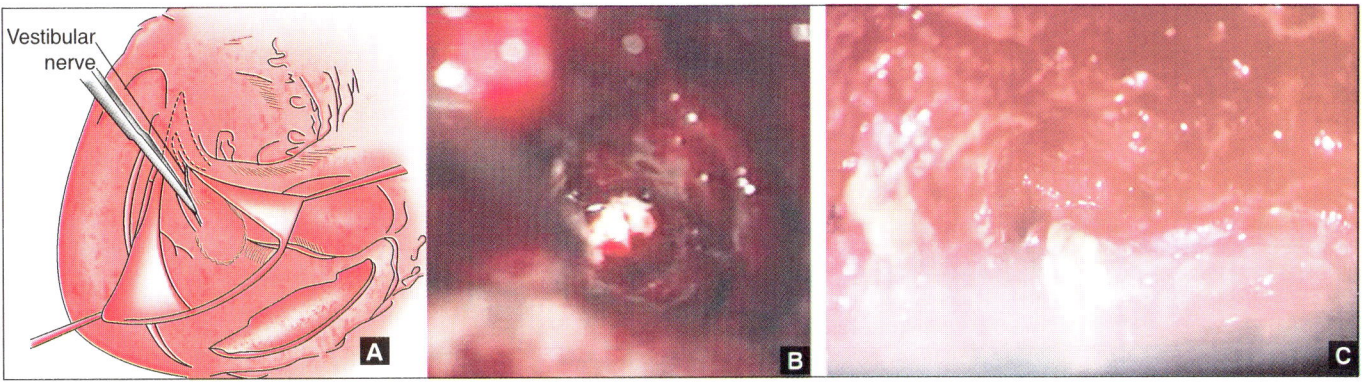

Fig 9.8 a, b, c The vestibular schwannoma identified

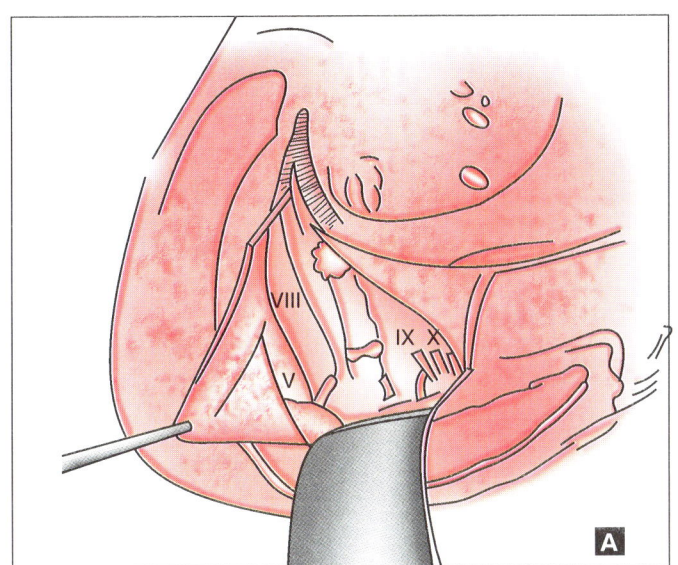

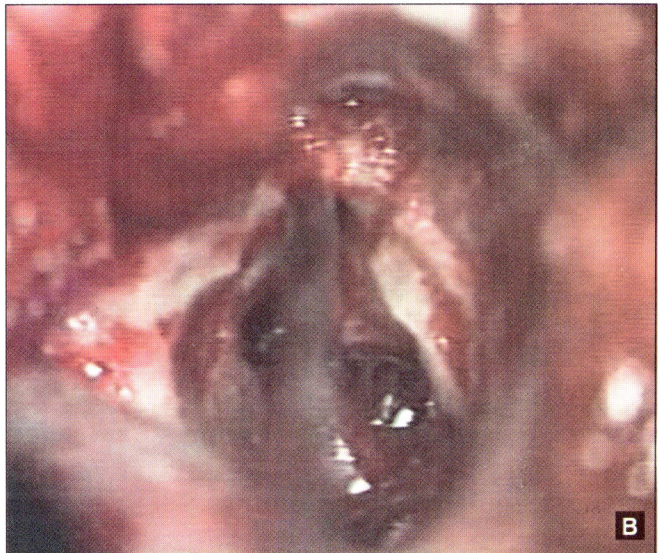

Fig 9.9 a, b Lower cranial nerves entering the jugular foramen visualized

- Easy identification of facial nerve which is in a constant location before tumor dissection with the help of bony landmarks like Bill's Bar.

- Minimizes the risk of recurrence of tumor.

- Risk of CSF fistula is less due to current techniques of Eustachian tube obliteration.

- Reduction of post-operative headache.

Disadvantages

- Reduced exposure in patients with high jugular bulb or significantly contracted mastoid air cell system.

- Hearing is sacrificed

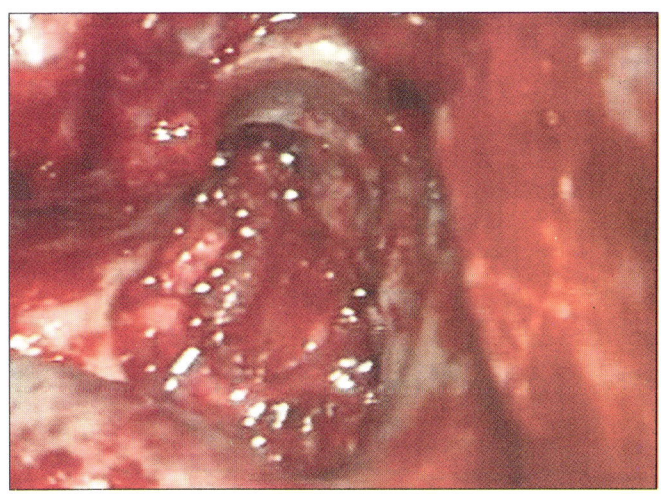

Fig 9.10 The graft is placed to fill entire mastoid cavity

Retrosigmoid Approach

The retrosigmoid approach to the posterior cranial fossa is the latest of numerous modifications of the classic suboccipital approach.

Indications

- Patients who have near-normal hearing

- When the tumor involves the medial two-third of the internal auditory canal and also if there is extension into the CPA (>5mm).

- Patients with contracted mastoid cavities or high jugular bulbs.

- Patients with CPA tumors other than vestibular schwannoma.

Procedure

Position

- A "LAZY-S" incision is created four fingerbreadths behind the postauricular crease (Fig. 9.11).

- The skin and subcutaneous flaps are elevated and retracted (Fig. 9.12).

- The periosteum is elevated off the lateral mastoid and occiput along with the muscular attachments.

- A 4x4cm craniotomy is created with the sigmoid sinus as the anterior border and the transverse sinus as the superior border (Fig. 9.13).

- The transverse sinus and sigmoid sinus are skeletonized (Fig. 9.14).

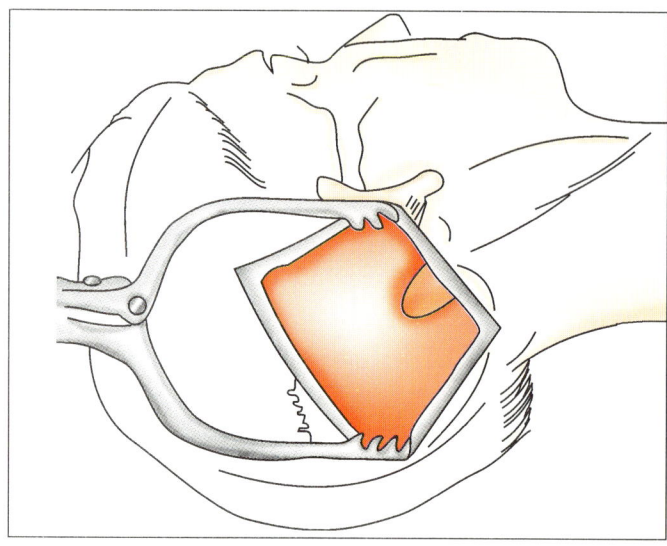

Fig 9.12 Skin and subcutaneous flaps are elevated

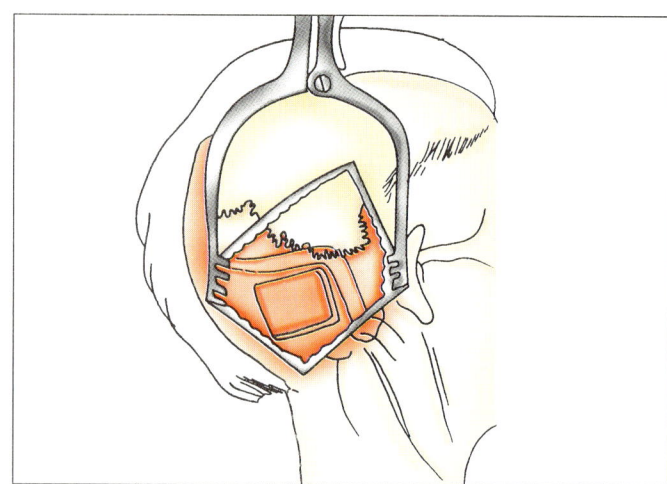

Fig 9.13 4x4 craniotomy created with the sigmoid sinus anteriorly and the transverse sinus superiorly

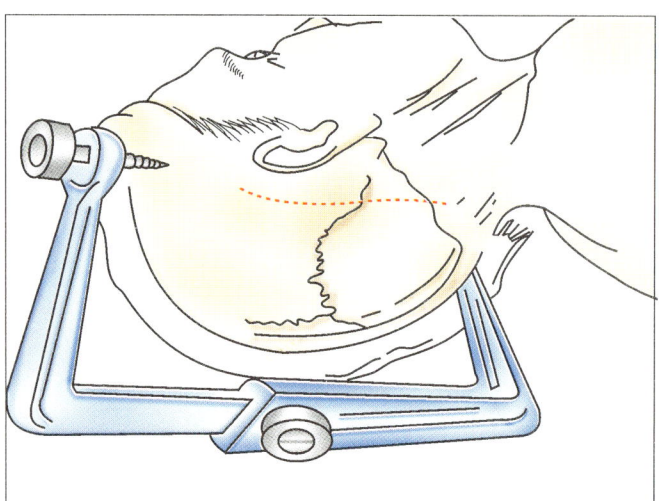

Fig 9.11 "LAZY-S" incision

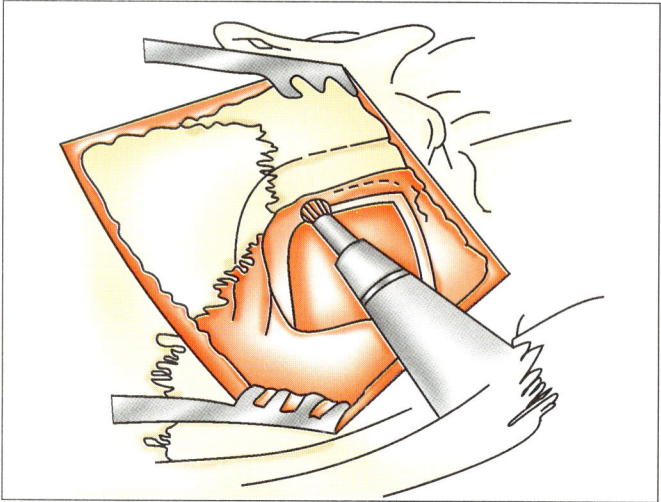

Fig 9.14 Transverse and sigmoid sinuses are skeletonized

- Mastoid cells anterior or lateral to the sigmoid sinus are removed.

- Dural incisions form an anteriorly pedicled dural flap that is secured with silk suture (Fig. 9.15).

- The cerebellum is gently retracted and the arachnoid tissue is incised. Adhesions between the cerebellum and dura are lysed and the tumor in the cerebellopontine angle is visualized.

- Cranial nerves VII and VIII are seen passing from the brainstem into the internal auditory canal (Fig. 9.16).

- Incisions are created in the dura over the petrous bone, creating superiorly and inferiorly based flaps (Fig.9.17a,b).

- The intracapsular tumor in the cerebellopontine angle is debulked (Fig.9.18).

- The internal auditory canal is skeletonized using operculum (a bony projection along the posterior face of the petrous bone at which point the endolymphatic duct enters the bone) and endolymphatic duct as the landmarks. Dissection of the bone is performed medial and anterior to the endolymphatic duct to avoid inadvertent entry into the vestibule and posterior semicircular canal. In general, up to 7 mm of bone can be removed safely from the medial aspect of the internal auditory canal (Fig.9.19).

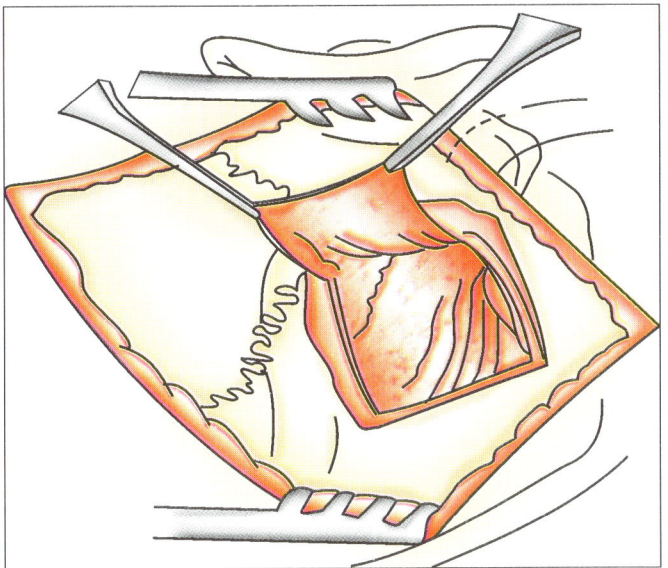

Fig 9.15 Dural incisions form an anteriorly pedicled dural flaps

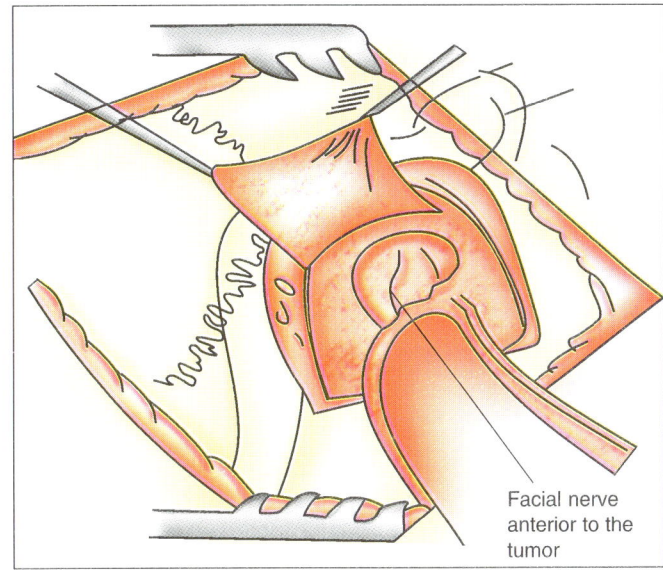

Facial nerve anterior to the tumor

Fig 9.16 Facial nerve seen passing from brain stem

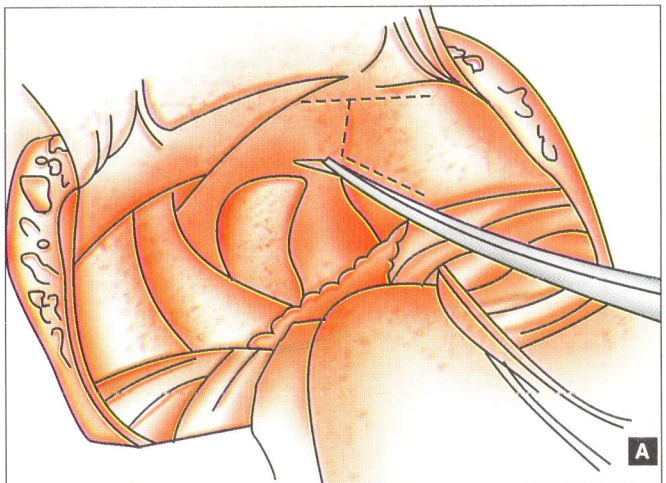

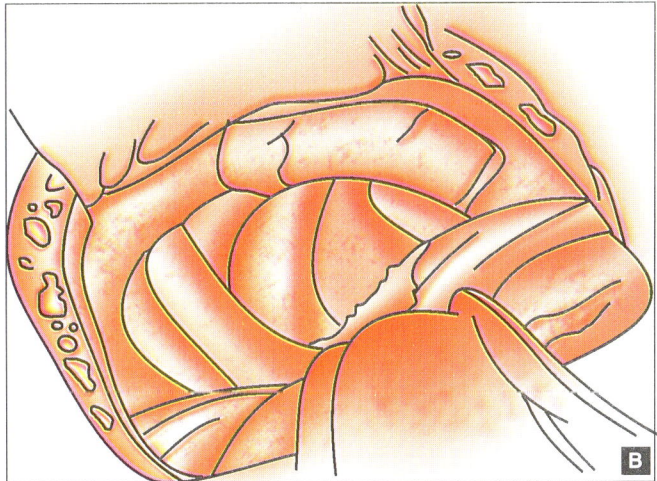

Fig 9.17 a, b Incisions are created in the dura over the petrous bone

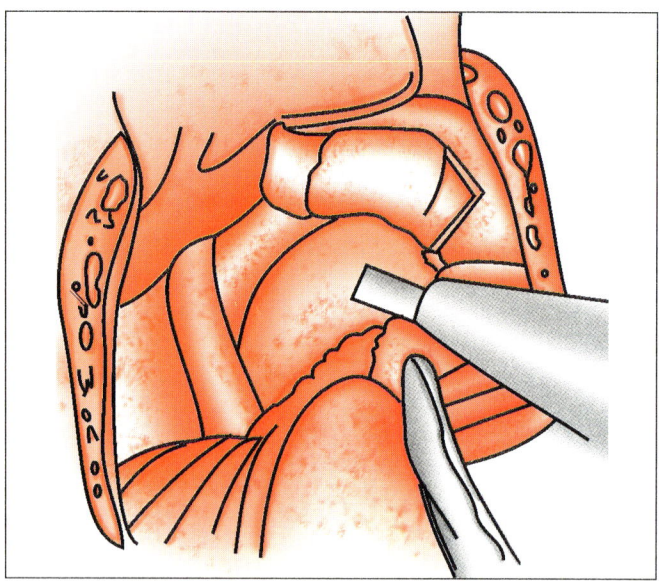

Fig 9.18 Intracapsular tumor in the CPA is debulked

- The dura of the internal auditory canal is incised along the edges of the canal. The superior vestibular nerve is removed from its attachments to the labyrinth, and retracted medially. Dissection of the tumor and the vestibular nerve proceeds in a lateral to medial direction along the length of the canal.

- After removal of the intracanalicular portion of the tumor, the cerebellopontine component of the tumor is debulked. As the contents of the tumor are excised, the capsule is rolled inward and dissected off the underlying facial and cochlear nerves. As the

debulking progresses, the brainstem origin of cranial nerves VII and VIII of the brain stem is identified and the tumor is dissected off the brainstem (Fig. 9.20).

- Hemostasis is secured.

- Bone wax is placed into all air cells around the internal auditory canal and the mastoid air cells at the edge of the craniotomy to prevent CSF leak through the mastoid and the middle ear (Fig. 9.21a,b).

- The dura that had originally been on the face of petrous apex, overlying the internal auditory canal, is reflected into the surgical defect.

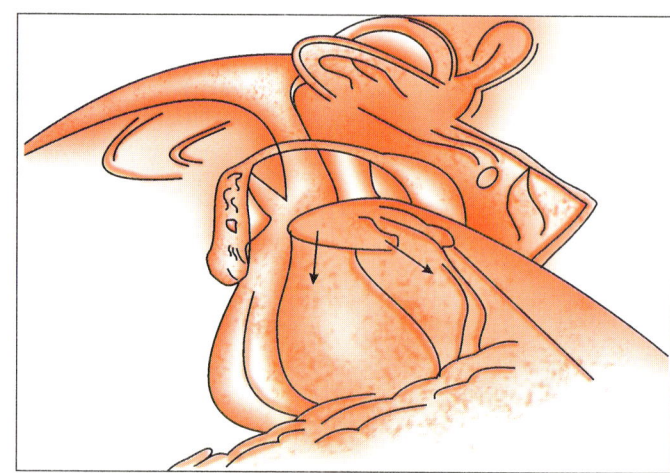

Fig 9.20 Tumor capsule is rolled inward and dissected off the underlying facial and cochlear nerves

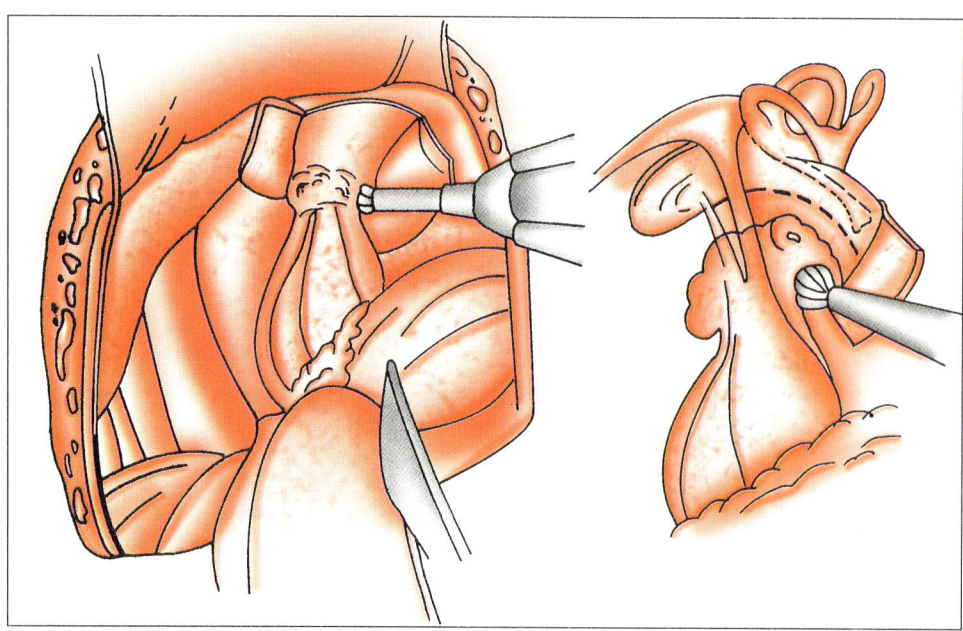

Fig 9.19 Internal auditory canal skeletonized

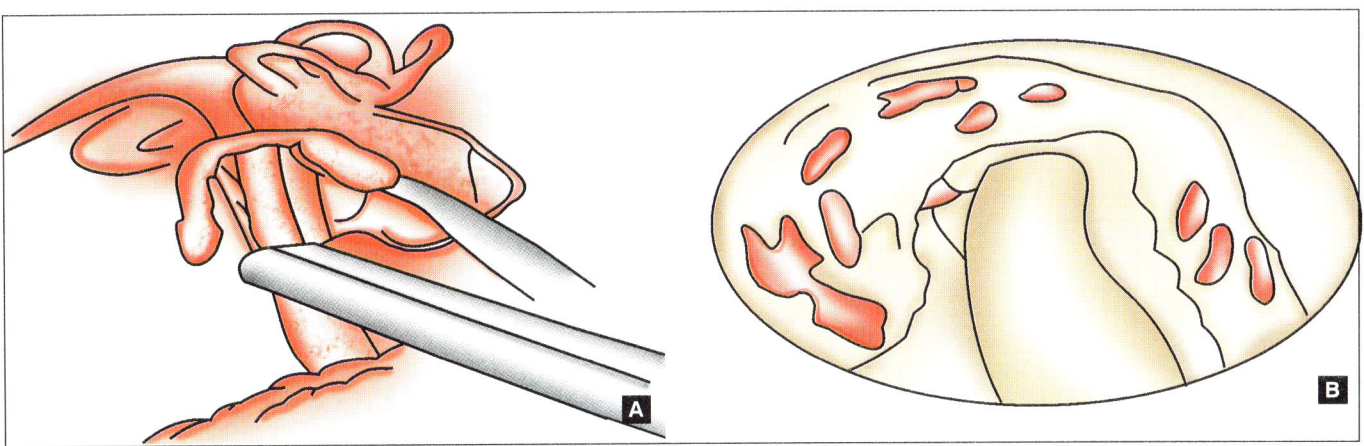

Fig 9.21 a, b Bone wax is placed into the air cells

- A piece of temporalis fascia is then placed over the internal auditory canal. The large anteriorly based dural flap is closed with 4-0 silk.

- The craniotomy bone flap and bone chips are replaced into the craniotomy defect before wound closure (Fig. 9.22).

- The attachments of the neck musculature are reattached to the skull by suspension sutures, which pass through holes at the edge of the craniotomy.

- The skin is sutured in three layers; galea, subcutaneous and skin.

- A pressure dressing is applied.

Advantages

- Hearing is preserved.

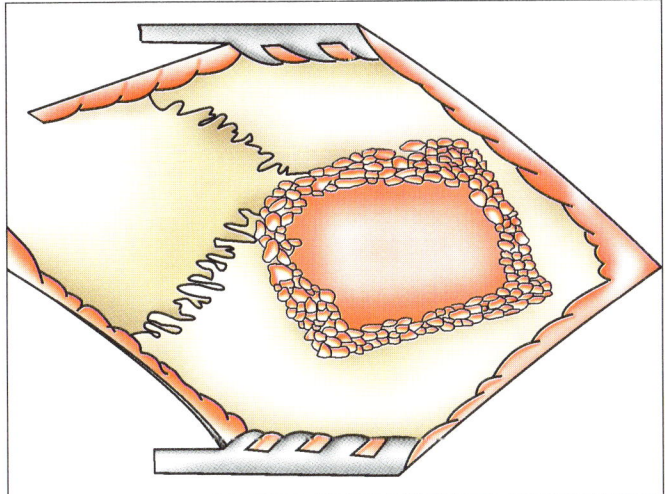

Fig 9.22 Craniotomy bone flap and bone cheps are replaced into the craniotomy defect

- This approach can be used in patients with contracted mastoid cavities and high jugular bulbs.

- All CPA tumors can be accessed.

Disadvantages

- Lack of constant bony landmarks to identify the facial nerve.

- Difficult to excise complete tumor if it extends into the lateral portion of internal auditory canal.

Transotic Approach

Transotic approach is an extension beyond the translabyrinthine technique.

Preoperative procedure is the same as in Translabyrinthine approach.

Indications

- Tumors upto 2.5 cm in size that are not adherent to the brainstem.

- Facial nerve grafting or hypoglossal-facial anastomosis may be incorporated into the procedure at the time of tumor resection.

Procedure

- The step upto elevation of the periosteum posterior to the ear canal is done as in translabyrinthine approach. Paul. J. Donald et al have achieved the blind sac procedure by the following technique. The ear canal is severed at the bony cartilaginous junction. The lateral canal skin is elevated and reflected out of the external auditory canal. The skin is sutured laterally

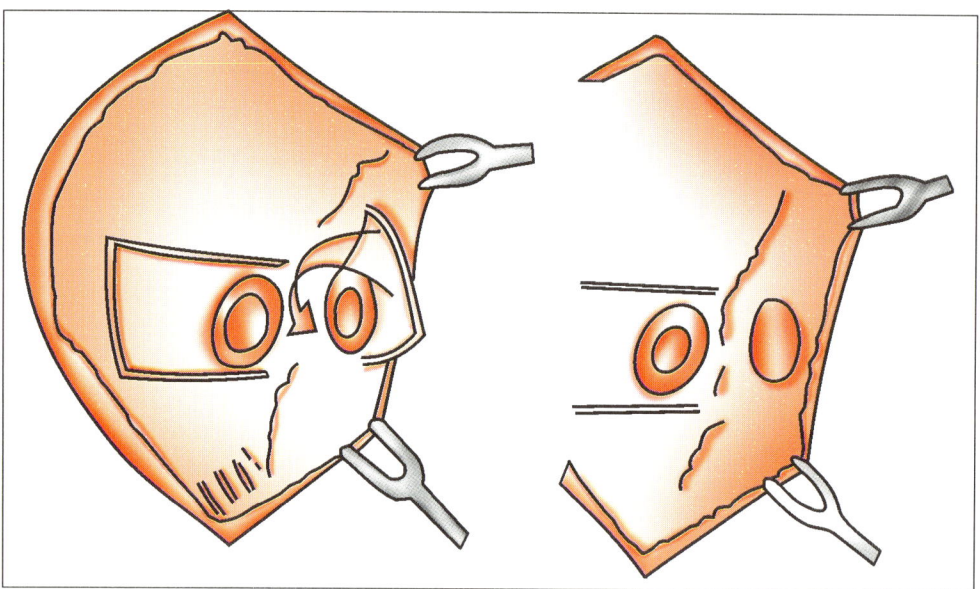

Fig 9.23 Ear canal is sutured at bony cartilage junction and lateral canal is elevated

and the periosteal flap is reflected over the medial aspect of the canal and sutured anterior to the anterior lip of the canal, creating a two layered closure (Fig.9.23).

- The skin of the bony external auditory canal is elevated down to the level of the annulus and the tympanic membrane is elevated. The incudo stapedial joint is separated and the incus, malleus and tympanic membrane are resected (Fig. 9.24).

- The cochlea is removed, skeletonizing the internal carotid artery anteriorly, the jugular bulb inferiorly and the internal auditory canal posteriorly and superiorly. The internal auditory canal is skeletonized 300 degrees around its circumference (Fig. 9.25).

- An incision in the dura is created to extend from anterior to the sigmoid sinus through the posterior ring of fibrous tissue of the porus acousticus which is severed anteriorly and then the dura is cut anteroinferiorly to the internal auditory canal. The dural edges are reflected and sutured.

- Dissection anterior to the facial nerve reveals the facial nerve as it is splayed anteriorly before entering the porus acousticus.

- Tumor dissection is performed.

- A large piece of temporalis fascia is placed over the exposed area of dura and dural defect. A second smaller piece of fascia is placed anterior to the facial nerve over the dural defect.

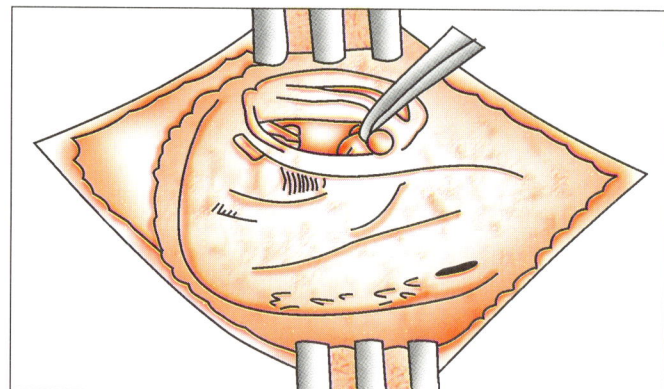

Fig 9.24 Incudo stapedial joint is separated, incus, malleus and tympanic memebrane are resected

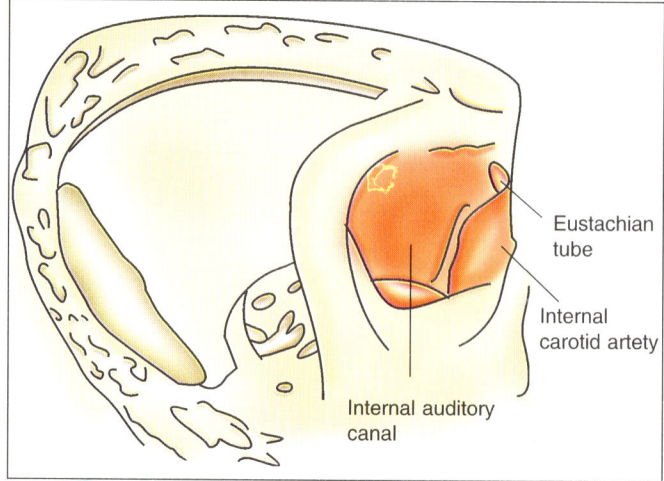

Fig 9.25 Anterior auditory canal skeletonized and cochleas removed

- After inversion of the eustachian tube mucosa into the eustachian tube, muscle is inserted into the orifice. The muscle is wedged in place with the modified incus.

- A third piece of temporalis fascia is then placed over the protympannum, covering the Eustachian tube orifice.

- An abdominal graft is divided into two pieces; one is wedged firmly under the bony canal of the facial nerve and is used to obliterate the medial portion of the mastoid cavity; the second one is placed lateral to the first graft and hence the remainder cavity is obliterated.

- The skin is closed in two layers and a pressure dressing is applied.

Advantages

- Wider surgical access with a circumferential exposure of the internal auditory canal and the porus acousticus.

- Direct visualization and access to the anterior CPA where the facial nerve is usually tenuous and most vulnerable.

- Permanent closure of ear canal and Eustachian tube with complete obliteration of the surgical cavity, minimizing the CSF leak.

Disadvantage

- Hearing is sacrificed.

Middle fossa approach
Indications

- Used in patients with near- normal hearing in the involved ear.

- If tumor is located in the lateral one third of the internal auditory canal and does not protrude greater than 5mm into the CPA.

Pre-operative procedure

- MRI Scan with gadolinium enhancement

- Antibiotics to be started

- Dexamethasone and mannitol is administered intravenously similar to translabirintine approach.

- The scalp has to be shaved from the ipsilateral mid-pupillary line, to the vertex, and extending to the occipital condyle.

- The surgeon is positioned at the vertex of the patient's head. The patient is positioned supine with the head turned so the affected ear is upward.

Procedure

- A "LAZY-S" (FRAZIER) skin incision extends from the preauricular crease toward the vertex. The incision is carried down to the temporalis fascia, which is elevated and reflected inferiorly. The temporalis muscle is split vertically, anterior to the plane of the external auditory canal (Fig.9.26)

- A 4x4cm window is created in the squamosal portion of the temporal bone. Two-thirds of the window is anterior to the vertical plane of the external auditory canal, and one third is posterior to the canal (Fig.9.27).

- Dura tethered to the under surface of the edges of the craniotomy is dissected free around the perimeter of the window (Fig. 9.28).

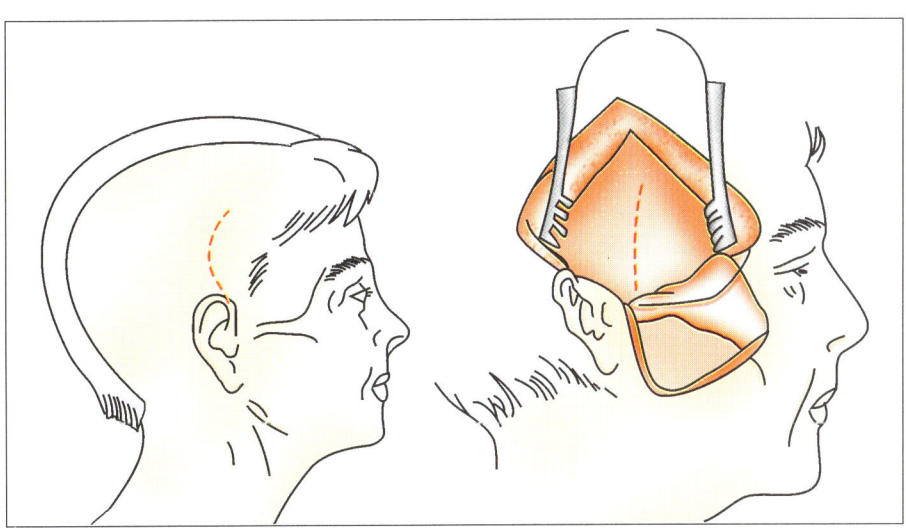

Fig 9.26 Frazier incision

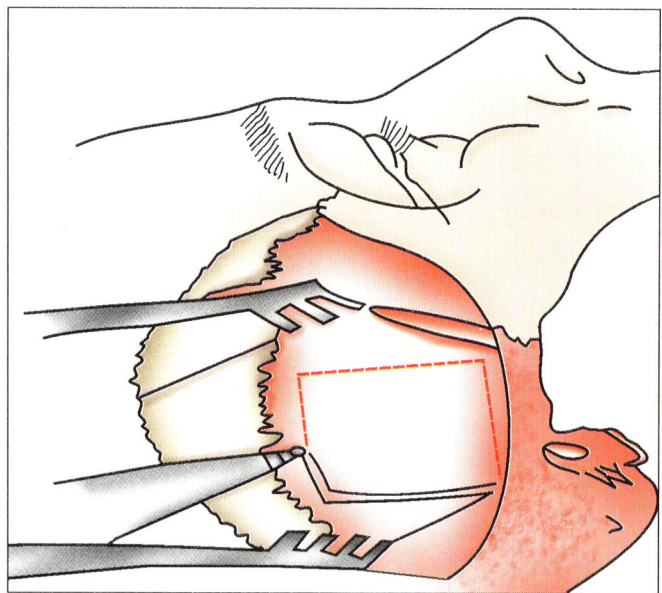

Fig 9.27 4x4 cm window created in the squamosal portion of temporal bone

- Bone rongeur is used to remove the remaining portion of the squamosal bone down to the level of the tegmen. Removal of this lip of bone provides an optimal surgical line of site with minimal temporal bone retraction (Fig. 9.29).

- Dura of the middle cranial fossa is elevated off the petrous bone. The landmarks in the middle fossa are the middle meningeal artery at the foramen spinosum, the greater superficial petrosal nerve at the facial hiatus and the arcuate eminence (Fig. 9.30).

- The geniculate ganglion may be exposed without a bony covering on the floor of the middle fossa, so care should be exercised during dural elevation.

- The landmark for superior semicircular canal is the arcuate eminenece. The tegmen tympani is removed which exposes the malleus and body of the incus. These additional landmarks can be helpful when the arcuate eminence is not appreciated and the superior semicircular canal has not been located (Fig. 9.31).

- Once the "blue-line" of the semicircular canal has been identified, dissection proceeds over the meatal plane superior to the internal auditory canal. The internal auditory canal lies within a 60 degree angle from the blue-lined semicircular canal (Fig. 9.32).

- The internal auditory canal is skeletonized around the superior 180 degrees of its circumference. In the lateral aspect of the internal auditory canal, "Bill's Bar"

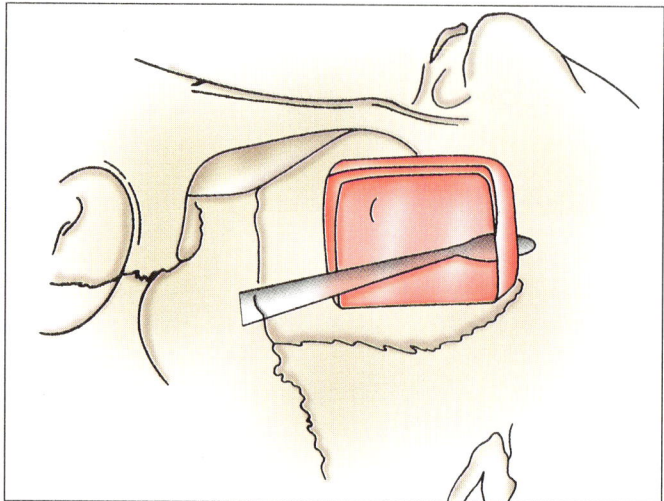

Fig 9.28 Edges of craniotomy dissected free

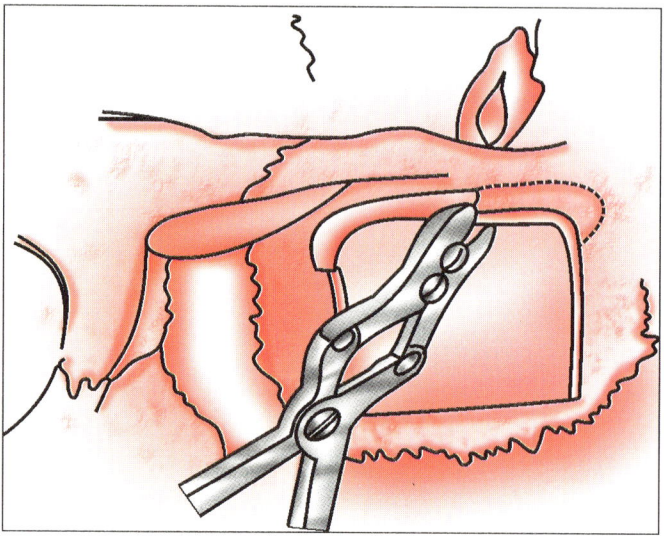

Fig 9.29 The remaining portion of the squamous bone removed

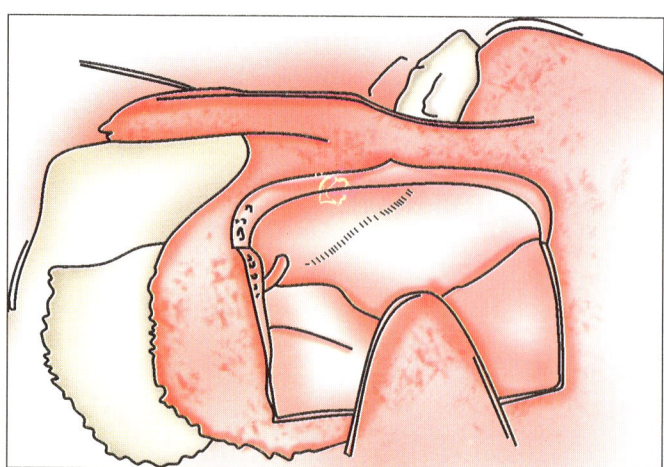

Fig 9.30 Middle meninged artery identified at foramen spinosum

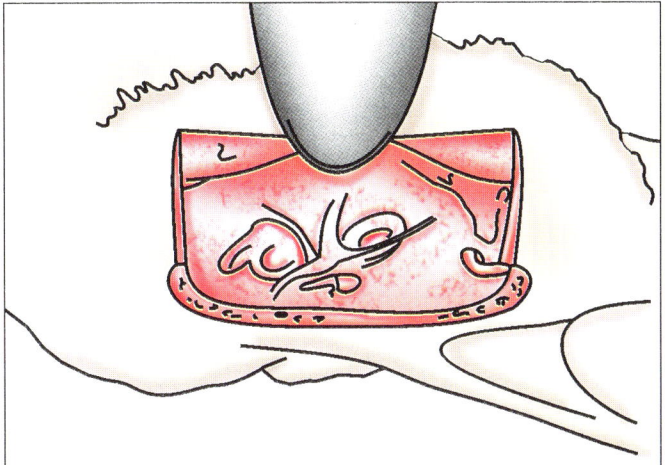

Fig 9.31 Blue line of semi auricular canal has been identified

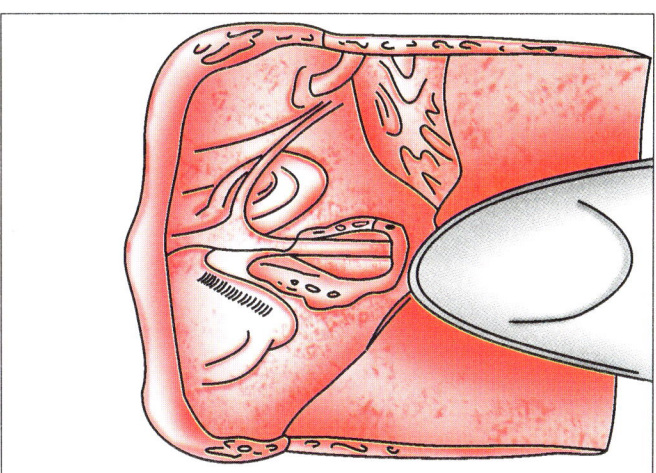

Fig 9.33 The internal auditory canal is skeletonized

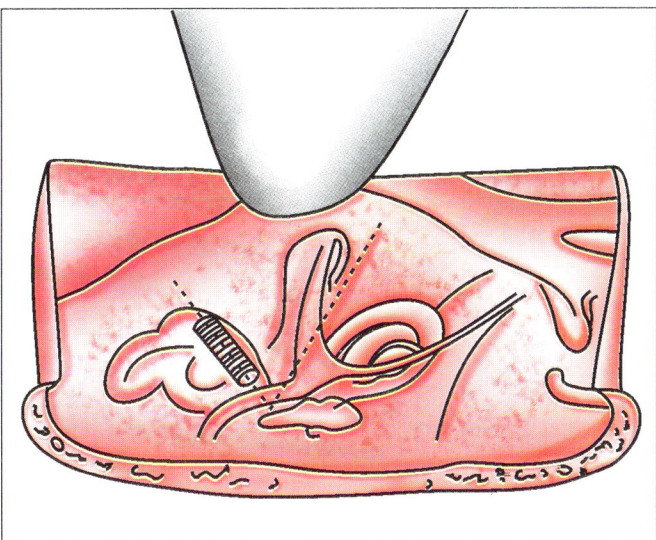

Fig 9.32 Tegment tympanic removed

separates facial nerve anteriorly from the vestibular nerve posteriorly (Fig. 9.33)

- The dura of the internal auditory canal is incised in a longitudinal fashion, along the posterior edge, away from the facial nerve. Dura is reflected. Tumor and the facial nerve will be visualized at this point. Facial nerve is usually expected to be anterior or superior to the body of the tumor.

- The superior vestibular nerve is then removed from its lateral attachment to the labyrinth and is retracted medially. The tumor and the vestibular nerve is

dissected from the facial and the cochlear nerves, in a lateral to medial direction.

- Hemostasis is secured.

- Bone wax is used to fill the exposed air cells. A piece of temporalis muscle is placed in the bony defect and the pedicled temporalis fascia flap is reflected over the floor of the middle cranial fossa. The temporal lobe compressing the fascia over the bony defect is released. The bone flap is secured to the edges of the craniotomy with sutures.

- The temporalis muscle is closed superiorly, leaving a gap inferiorly where the temporalis fascia is passing.

- The skin is closed in two layers pressure dressing is applied.

Advantages

- Full visualization of the entire internal auditory canal.

- Hearing can be preserved.

Disadvantages

- Temporal lobe stroke ; injury to middle meningeal artery and petrosal sinus.

- Elderly are poor candidates due to the tenuous nature of their dura. Even a little retraction of the temporal lobe can cause seizures.

- Tumor from inferior vestibular nerve cannot be resected as facial nerve comes in between and hence it will have to be sacrificed.

10

Common Complications of Skull Base Surgery

INTRAOPERATIVE

- Injury to cranial nerves. Commonest is facial nerve followed by lower cranial nerves, then comes the trigeminal and abducent nerves.

- Bleeding due to injury to sigmoid sinus and other arterial bleeders.

- Brain edema, commonly seen with retrosigmoid approach due to cerebellum retraction.

- Venous air embolism can occur when air is sucked into a venous sinus or an emissary vein. It can further cause death if the embolus reaches the right heart due to corpulmonale. Air embolism is diagnosed by fluctuant blood pressure and a characteristic churning heart murmur.

- Cardiac arrythmias can be caused due to tumor dissection from the brainstem patient may develop tachycardia and hypertension.

- Giant vestibular schwannomas may cause hydrocephalus (owing to compression of the fourth ventricle), leading to intraoperative herniation.

POSTOPERATIVE

- Hemorrhage can be epidural, subdural or intraparenchymal (due to overzealous retraction of cerebellum).

- Brain edema with increased intracranial pressure, confusion and altered mental status.

- Infarction may be secondary to arterial or venous occlusion. Commonly see is the infarction of pons (lateral pontomedullary syndrome). LPS consists of unilateral labyrinthine infarction, cerebellar infarction, ipsilateral facial and contralateral body sensory loss, contralateral hemiparesis

- Cerebrospinal fluid leak occurs usually secondary to translabyrinthine and retrosigmoid approaches. Patients with well pneumatized temporal bones are at an increased risk. Incidence of CSF leak is around 10% -15% after vestibular schwannoma removal.

- Meningitis usually occurs secondary to CSF leak or due to retained bone dust and other irritants. Patient presents with fever, headache, neck and back stiffness, photophobia and mental status changes.

- Tension pneumocephalus due to air trapping within the cranial cavity and may present with symptoms of increased intracranial pressure and mental status changes.

- Other complications like DVT and postoperative pneumonia can develop.

POST OPERATIVE CARE

When to extubate?

Once these variables are assessed and judged to be satisfactory, the patient is extubated.

- The patients who have sufficiently recovered from anesthesia to follow commands are usually extubated.

- Recovery from anesthesia is expedited by the use of short-acting, low solubility inhalational agents and infusions of potent narcotic agents.

- Respiratory parameters have to be adequate and the patient should be able to maintain blood O_2 saturation while intubated and spontaneously breathing.

- As mentioned previously, excessive blood loss leading to large fluid and blood replacement could produce excessive airway edema, especially when the patient is prone. This would negate attempts at extubation.

- Cranial nerve deficits including injury to the vagus nerve producing vocal cord paralysis may occur after skull base surgery. Even though this would produce unilateral vocal cord paralysis, the patient should be awake and able to handle secretions so as to avoid the risk of aspiration.

In view of the potential for complications in cranial base surgery, patients should be monitored postoperatively.

- All the patients are initially admitted to an intensive care unit staffed by nurses experienced in neurosurgical and head-neck surgical care.

- Consultants in critical care medicine, internal medicine and other specialties actively precipitate when required.

- Patients should be under continuous monitoring of ECG, oxygenation via pulse oximeter and systemic blood pressure.

- Central venous lines are used to assess cardiovascular status and fluid balance.

- Close monitoring of hematologic and biochemical parameters is essential.

- Appropriate replacement of blood to maintain oxygen delivery and to prevent coagulopathy.

- It is advisable to keep the patient relatively flat in bed for the first 4 postoperative days.

- Advice not to blow nose for few days in post operative period.

- Watch for any signs of CSF rhinorrhea.

- Antibiotics.

- Antacids to prevent stress ulcer.

- Anticonvulsants to prevent seizures

- *Role of Analgesics therapy:* The incidence, magnitude, and duration of acute pain experienced after skull base resection is not well known or characterized. Patient-controlled analgesia is extremely valuable after skull base surgical procedures. Patient-controlled analgesia has been found to be subjectively better for patients. Morphine in a dosing regimen of 1.5 mg morphine/dose with an 8-minute lockout period. The total dose of morphine in 4 hours should not exceed 40 mg.

- *Role of antiemetic therapy:* Common associated discomfort and a reason for dissatisfaction with patient-controlled analgesia is the development of postoperative nausea and vomiting Nausea and vomiting has been a frequent and important postoperative morbidity, which is of particular concern to the skull base surgical patient. Beyond the extreme discomfort, postoperative nausea and vomiting can lead to increased intracranial pressure, systemic hypertension, increased bleeding, worsening cerebrospinal fluid leaks, and an increased risk of aspiration, especially with postsurgical vocal cord dysfunction. Ondansetron (4-8 mg intravenously) given 30 to 60 minutes before awakening from anesthesia has been of some benefit.

- Postoperative day 1 CT scan if cranial vault has been opened.

- Prophylaxix against deep vein thrombosis and pulmonary embolism.

- A tracheostomy (for tracheal toilette) and a Gastrostomy tube (for nutrition and hydration) are often necessary during the peri and postoperative period.

COMPLICATIONS OF SKULL BASE SURGERY

Complications of surgery can generally be classified into

- Neurologic
- Wound-related
- Cosmetic
- Perioperative

Neurologic

- Neurologic complications include cranial nerve injuries and other morbidities affecting the CNS. Cranial nerve injuries can occur to any cranial nerve in proximity to the surgical field. Stretch or traction injury, thermal injury from electrocautery, or sharp transection of nerves can occur. Cranial nerves displaced by or under tension from tumor growth are prone to injury. Therefore, the location of the tumor determines which cranial nerve is at risk.

- Concurrent injury to multiple cranial nerves can be devastating. Injuries to cranial nerves V and VII may cause the eye to be insensate and may make the patient unable to close the eye, which puts the eye at risk for corneal ulceration and infection and, ultimately, loss of the eye. Tumors in the cerebellopontine angle, such as acoustic neuromas, can involve both of these nerves when the tumors are very large. Injury to the lower cranial nerves can lead to swallowing difficulties and can put the patient at risk for aspiration and pneumonia. Foramen magnum meningiomas and chordomas of the lower clivus can grow in close proximity to these nerves.

- Intraoperative cranial nerve monitoring alerts the surgeon to times that the nerves are at risk of damage and may lead to an improved outcome. The facial nerve is monitored frequently with electroneuronography and the auditory nerve can be monitored with brainstem-evoked auditory responses. Cranial nerves II-XII can be monitored intraoperatively.

Other morbidities affecting the CNS include the following

- Pneumocephalus
- Intracranial hemorrhage
- Cerebral contusion
- Meningitis
- CSF leakage
- Cerebral edema
- Stroke
- Epidural abscess
- Seizures
- Diabetes insipidus
- Altered mental status
- Anosmia

CSF leaks occur if the dura is violated either intentionally or because of tumor invasion. Many areas of the skull base dura are thin and difficult to repair. Dura overlying the cribriform plate can be troublesome because the olfactory nerves travel through it to the nasal cavity. The use of pericranial flaps to repair holes in the dura decreases the incidence of CSF leaks. Other vascularized flaps (*e.g.*, temporalis muscle flaps, trapezius muscle

flaps, free radial forearm flaps, free rectus abdominus muscle flaps) must be considered in select situations. The problems associated with CSF leakage include poor wound healing and the risk of meningitis.

Wound-related

Wound complications include the following:

- Cellulitis
- Infected cranial bone flap or osteomyelitis
- Coronasal fistula
- Necrosis of a pericranial flap
- Encephalocele
- Crusting of nasal cavity

Because the nasal cavity may be included in the wound, chronic sinusitis from infection, loss of sinus mucociliary transport, and stenosis of the sinus ostia can occur. In addition, nasal airway stenosis may occur.

Cosmetic

Cosmetic complications include enophthalmos, facial scar, burr hole, and ocular dystopia. Cosmetic deformity is a risk that is especially associated with anterior surgical approaches. After surgery, maintaining the position of the eye and the contour of the facial structures is important. Various reconstructive techniques, including free flaps and bony reconstruction with miniplate fixation, have been developed to address these issues.

Perioperative

Blood loss at surgery is an issue because of the extensive dissections necessary for these approaches and the vascularity of the scalp, skull and dura. Blood loss should be monitored closely, and packed red blood cells, clotting factors, and platelets should be replaced aggressively.

Cranial neuropathies

Deficits of the trigeminal nerve are the most common morbidity of surgery of the ITF. The loss of corneal sensation, especially in someone with facial nerve dysfunction, greatly increases the risk of a corneal abrasion or exposure keratitis. Facial anesthesia may predispose the patient to self-inflicted injuries, including neurotrophic ulcers. The loss of motor function of the mandibular nerve causes asymmetry of jaw opening and decreased force of mastication on the operated side, which may be further impaired by resection of the TMJ or mandibular ramus. Fisch reports recovery of fifth nerve function after iatrogenic transection in a significant proportion of his cases.

Temporary or permanent facial nerve dysfunction is common after transposition for ITF dissection and tumor removal. The facial nerve can suffer an ischemic injury due to devascularization of its infratemporal segment or because of traction to the extratemporal segments. Expect a temporary paresis of the facial nerve with mobilization of the mastoid segment of the facial nerve. Frontal branches of the facial nerve are at risk of injury during elevation of the temporal scalp flap. Injury is usually the result of a dissection in a plane that is superficial to the superficial layer of the deep temporal fascia or the result of compression during retraction of the flap.

Trismus

Postoperative trismus is a common occurrence due to postoperative pain and scarring of the pterygoid musculature and TMJ. Trismus improves dramatically if patients regularly perform stretching exercises for the jaw using devices such as the Therabite appliance. In severe cases, a dental appliance may be fabricated that gradually opens with a screw.

Infections

Infectious complications are rare. Predisposing factors include communication with the nasopharynx, seroma or hematoma, and CSF leaks. In general, obliterate the dead space to prevent fluid collection, which subsequently can be infected. Separate the cranial cavity from the sinonasal tract. The use of vascularized tissue flaps is preferred, especially when dissection of the ICA or resection of the dura mater has been performed.

Wound necrosis of the scalp flap

This situation is rare. Poorly designed incisions and prolonged use of hemostatic clamps may result in areas of ischemia, particularly around the auricle, that can make the tissue susceptible to secondary infection.

Neurovascular complication

Postoperative cerebral ischemia may result from surgical occlusion of the ICA, temporary vasospasm, and thromboembolic phenomenon. Surgical dissection of the ICA can injure the vessel walls, resulting in immediate or delayed rupture and hemorrhage. In the event that a repair of the ICA is not possible, permanently occlude it by ligation or by the placement of a detachable balloon or vascular coil. Perform the occlusion as distal as possible (near the origin of the ophthalmic artery). The potential for thrombus formation decreases with a short column of stagnant blood above the level of occlusion.

Cerebrospinal fluid leak

A watertight dural closure may be difficult to achieve around nerves and vessels. Most CSF leaks can be managed nonsurgically by placement of a pressure dressing and a spinal drain to diminish the CSF pressure. Surgical exploration and repair of the dural defect may be necessary if the CSF leak does not resolve within a week.

The authors have encountered patients who develop profuse unilateral rhinorrhea in the postoperative period, which was misinterpreted as a CSF leak. These cases were all associated with surgical dissection of the petrous ICA and probably are due to loss of the sympathetic fibers that travel along the ICA en route to the nasal mucosa. This situation produces vasomotor rhinitis that may be treated with the use of anticholinergic nasal sprays or botulinum toxin injections. However, testing of the fluid for beta-2 transferrin is mandatory to rule out a CSF leak.

11

Instruments

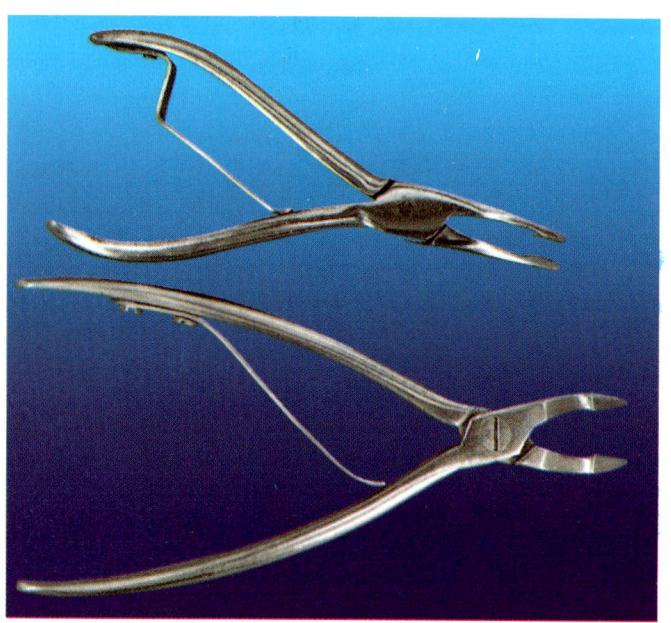

Fig 11.1 Bone roungers

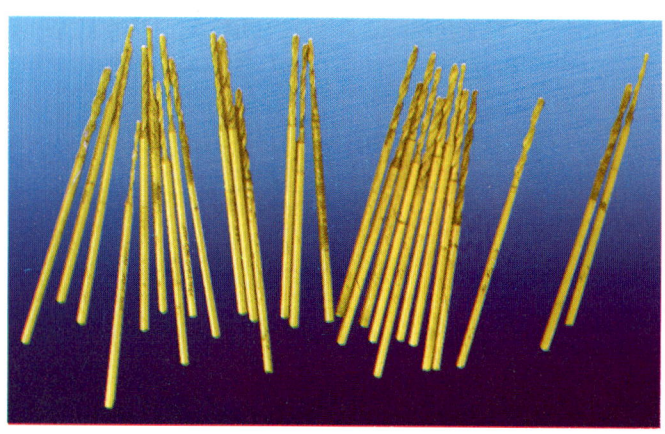

Fig 11.2 Drill bits

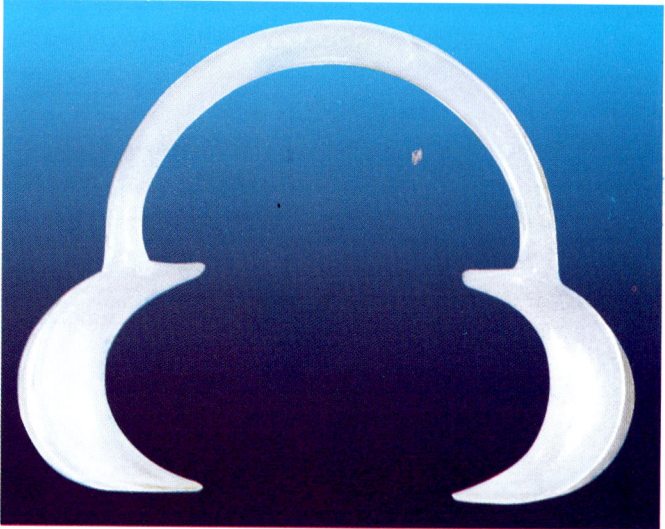

Fig 11.3 Cheek retractor

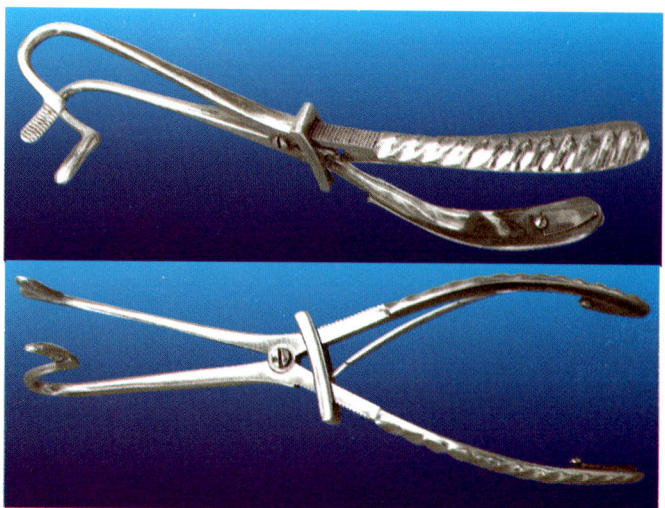

Fig 11.4 Ferguson mouth gag

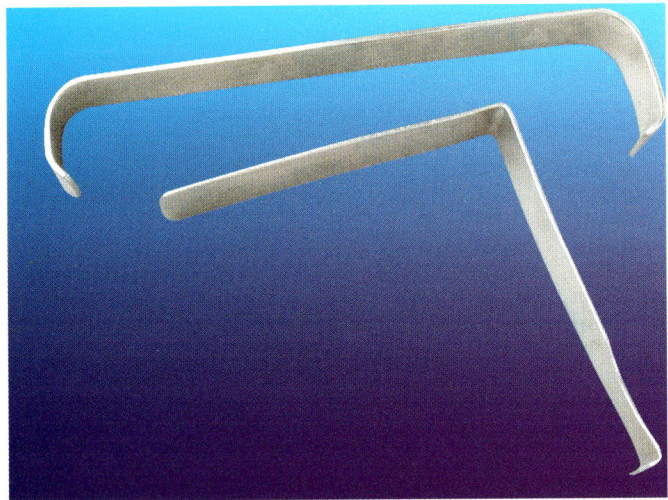

Fig 11.5 Retractors

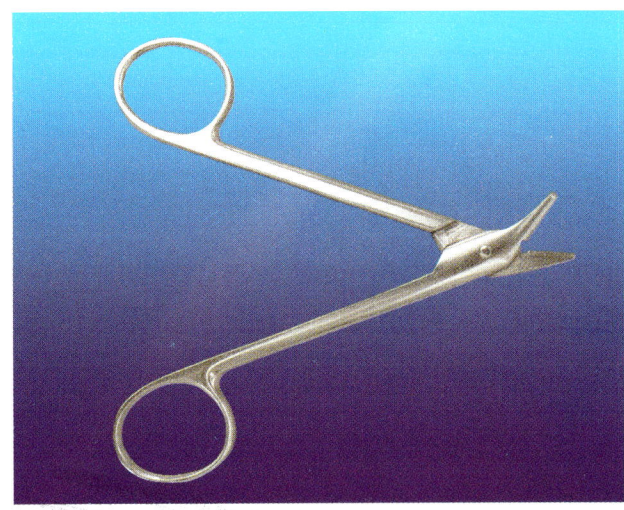

Fig 11.8 Wire cutter

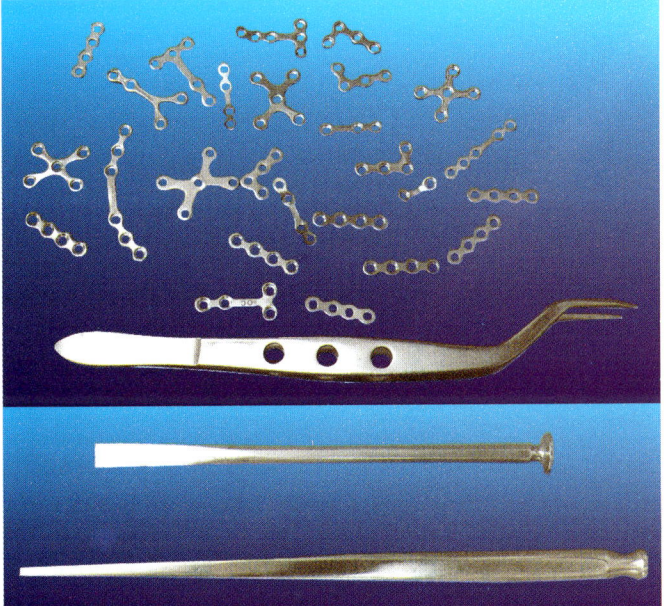

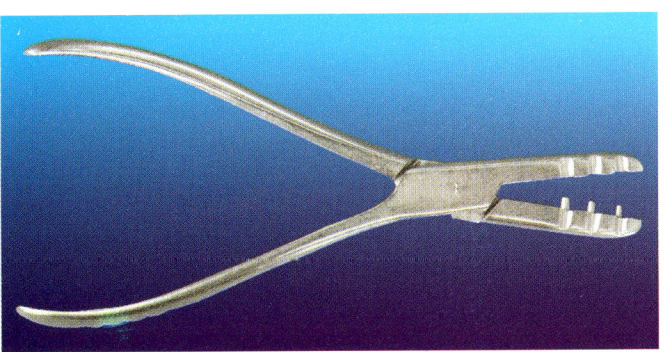

Fig 11.6 Plate holder and mini plates

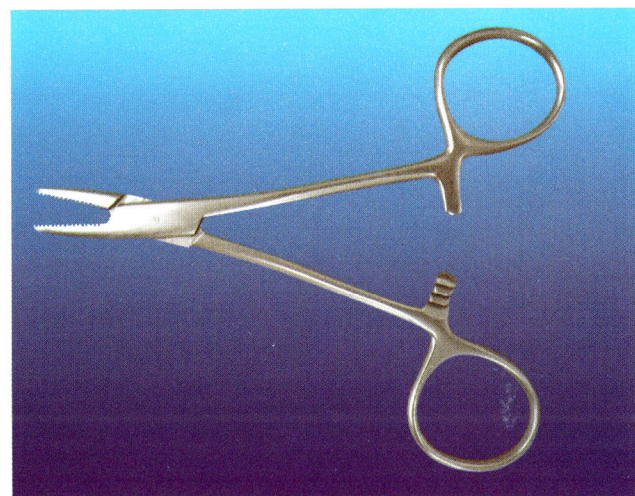

Fig 11.9 Wire twister

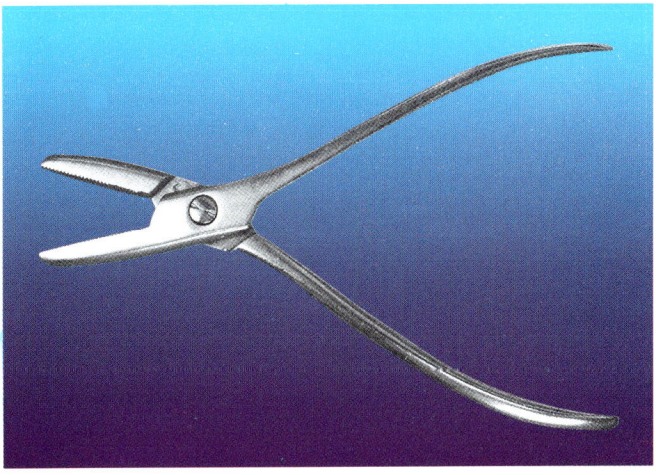

Fig 11.7 Plate bender

Fig 11.10 Plate bender

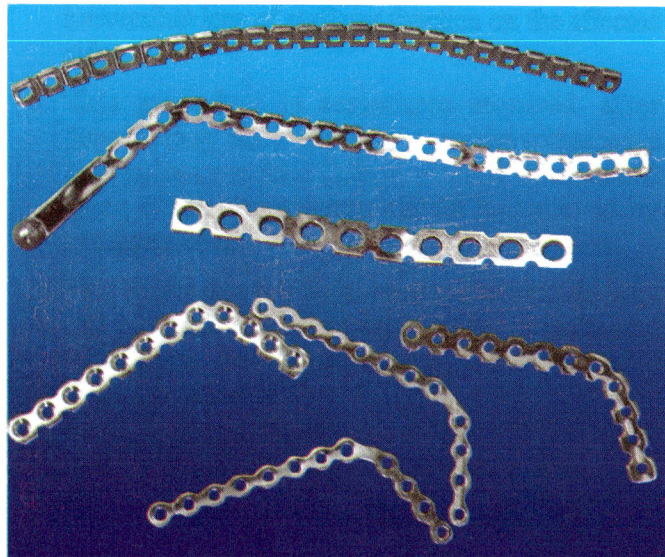

Fig 11.11 Reconstruction plate

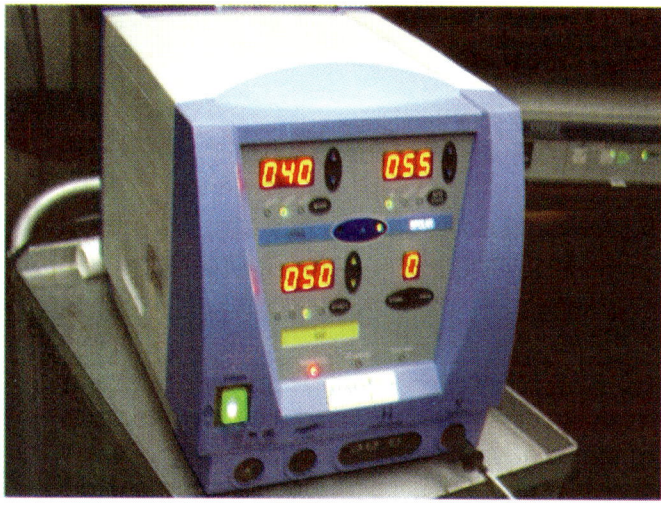

Fig 11.12 Diathermy (monopolar / bipolar)

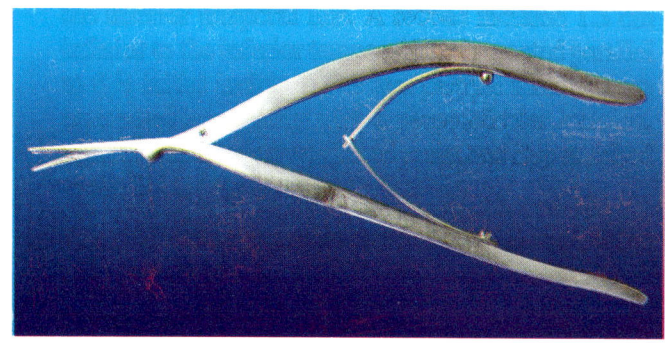

Fig 11.13 Roweris clamp

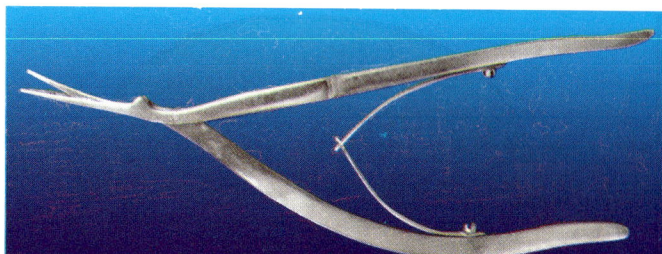

Fig 11.14 Roweris clamp

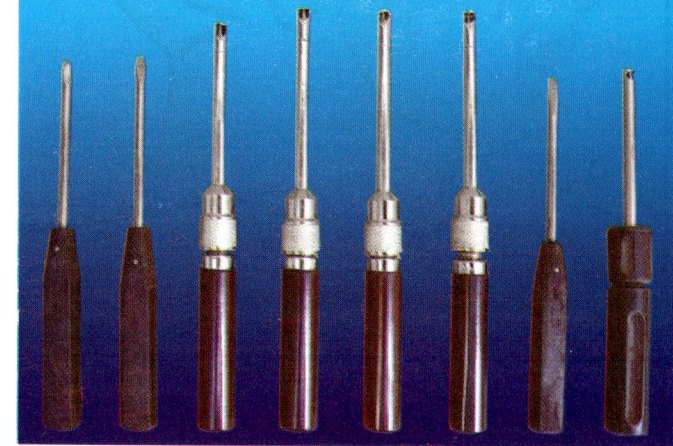

Fig 11.15 Screw holder

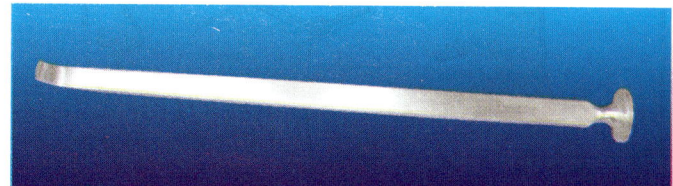

Fig 11.16 Pterygoid chisel

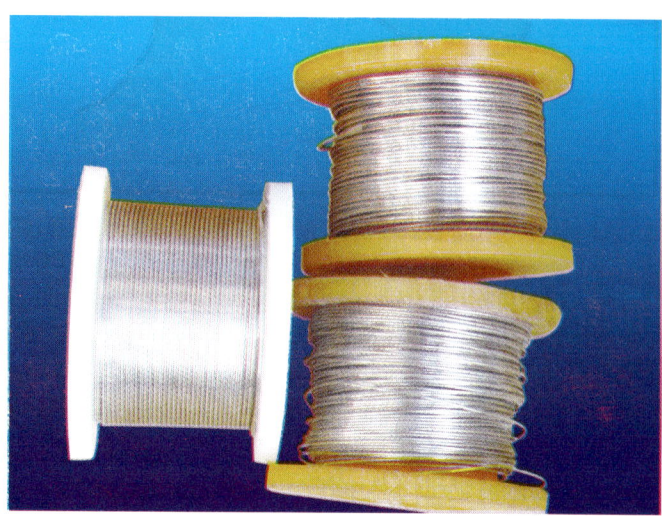

Fig 11.17 Wires - 24, 26, 28

Bibliography

1. Primary Malignant Fibrous Histiocytoma of Ethmoid Sinus - Indian Journal of Cancer, 22: 76-84, 1985. Produl Hazarika, R.G. Nayak & V. Balasundaram.

2. Carotid Body Tumour - Indian J. of Otolaryngology, 37, No.3, 111-112,1985. Hazarika, P.S. Murty & M. Chandran.

3. Schwannoma of Jugular Foramen - Infra Temporal Fossa approach - Indian Journal of Otolaryngology and Head and Neck, Vol. 1, No. 3, 133-135, 1992. Hazarika & A. Kumar.

4. Myxomas of Paranasal Sinuses - Indian Journal of Otolaryngology and Head and Neck, Vol. 1, No.2, 76-78, 1992.P.S. Murty, P. Hazarika, Kevin Periera & Ravikala Rao.

5. Surgical Treatment of Lateral Skull Base Tumours - Our Experience - Indian Journal of Otolaryngology and Head and Neck Surgery, Vol. 2, No.1, 19-22, 1993. P. Hazarika, Jaspal Singh Sahota, Sajeev George & A.Raja.

6. Parapharyngeal Space tumours in Children - Proceedings C.M.E. Association of Paediatric Otolaryngologists of India, Sponsored by Medical Council of India, New Delhi, 75-76, 1995. Deepak Murthy K., Hazarika P & Dipak Ranjan Nayak.

7. Anterior Skull Base Surgery - Our experience Indian Journal of Otolaryngology & Head & Neck Surgery, 40(4), 353-359, 1997.P. Hazarika, Dipak Ranjan Nayak, Deepak Murty, Miklu Senapathi, Ashwamed Singh & Raja.

8. Malignant tumours of the skull base and CFR - Proceedings of Asia-Pacific Congress, International Federation of Head and Neck Oncologic Societies, sponsored by Indian Society of Head and Neck Oncology, Mumbai, P.34, December 1997. Nayak R., Hazarika P., Balakrishnan R. & Raja A.

9. Olfactory Neuroblastoma - our experience - Proceedings of Asia-pacific congress, International Federation of Head and Neck Oncologic Societies, sponsored by Indian Society of Head and Neck Oncology, Mumbai, P.50, December 1997. Balakrishnan R., Hazarika P., Nayak D.R. & Raja A.

10. The Indications and complications of Pectoralis Major Myocutaneous Flap reconstruction Head & Neck Surgery - Our experience - Indian Journal of Otolaryngology and Head & Neck Surgery, Vol. 50, No.4 (October - December 1998), P. 362-367. Shalabh Sharma, P.S.N. Murty, Produl Hazarika, Dipak R. Nayak & Surabhi Sharma.

11. Anterior Skull Base Surgery - our experience - The Indian Journal of Otolaryngology and Head & Neck Surgery, Vol. 50, No.4 (October - December 1998), P.338-344. Produl Hazarika, Dipak Ranjan Nayak, K. Deepak Murty, Miklu Senapati, Ashwamedsing Dinassing & A. Raja.

12. Olfactory Neuroblastoma - Our experience - The Indian Journal of Otolaryngology and Head & Neck Surgery, Vol. 51, No.1, Jan-March 1999, P. 68 - 73. Shalabh Sharma, Jaspal Singh Sahota, Produl Hazarika, Surabhi Sharma & A. Raja.

13. Synovial Sarcoma of the Head and Neck - A report of 3 cases - Indian Journal of Otolaryngology and Head & Neck Surgery, Vol. 51, No. 4, P. 36-41, Sept.-Doc. 1999. Produl Hazarika, Parul Shah, Kailesh Pujary & Balakrishnan R.

14. Carcinoma of External Auditory Canal - Indian Journal of Otolaryngology & Head Neck Surgery, Vol. 53, No.3, PP. 229-230, July-Sept. 2001. Aditya Shenoy, Shubha Jyothy, K. Koteshwer Rao & Hazarika P.

15. Schwannoma of the Nose and Paranasal Sinuses - Indian Journal of Otolaryngology and Head and Neck Surgery, Vol. 55, No.1, PP. 34-38, Jan.-March 2003.

16. P. Hazarika, D.R. Nayak, K. Pujary & L. Rao. Solitary Malignant Schwanoma of Para Pharyngeal Space - Indian Journal of Otolaryngology and Head and Neck Surgery, Vol. 55, No.4, PP. 277- 280, October -December 2003. P. Hazarika.

17. Nasopharyngeal Haemangiopericytoma in a child - International J. of Paediatric Otolaryngology (USA), 4: 267-271, 1982. P. Hazarika & Dr. P.L.N.G. Rao.

18. Extra-Nasopharyngeal Extension of Juvenile Angiofibroma - The Journal of Laryngology and Otology (UK), 99: 813-817, 1985. P. Hazarika, R.G. Nayak & M. Chandran.

19. Our Experience with the Management of malignant tumour of the Maxilla - Ear, Nose & Throat Journal (USA), 65: 575, 1986. P. Hazarika, P. Satyanarayana Murty, Rajamma Rajan & V. Balasundaram.

20. Neurogenic tumours of the Parapharyngeal Space in the Paediatric Age Group - International Journal of Paediatric Otorhinolaryngology (USA), 22 (1991) 195-200. Kumar, P. Hazarika & R.P. Kapadia.

21. Congenital Internal Carotid Artery Aneurysm - International Journal of Paediatric Otorhinolaryngology (USA), 28, 63-68, 1993. P. Hazarika, J.S. Sahota, D.R. Nayak & S. George.

22. Osteogenic Sarcoma of Sphenoid Bone - An extended lateral skull base approach - The Journal of Laryngology & Otology, Vol. 109, 1101-1104, 1995. P. Hazarika, D.R.Nayak, J.Sahota, D.Rao & R.D.Kapadia.

23. Osteolipoma of the Skull Base a case report - The Journal of Laryngology & Otology, U.K.Vol. 115, PP.136-139, Feb. 2001 P. Hazarika, Kailesh Pujary, Harish G. Kundaje & P. Lakshmi Rao.

24. Surgical Access to Parapharyngeal space tumours - The Manipal Experience. P. Hazarika, R.N. Dipak, P. Parul & P. Kailesh Med. J Malaysia Vol. 59, No. 3, PP. 323 - 329, August 2004.

25. Surgery of the skull base : Paul J.Donald ; Lippincott - Raven.

26. Lore' & Medina An Atlas Of Head & Neck Surgery (Fourth Edition)

27. Kumar A, Valvassori G, Jafar J, Mafee M. Skull base lesions: a classification and surgical approaches. Laryngoscope. 1986 Mar; 96(3):252-63.

28. Dandy WE: Orbital Tumors: Results Following The Transcranial Operative Attack. New York: O Piest, 1941

29. Frazier CH: An approach to the hypophysis through the anterior cranial fossa. Ann Surg 57:145-150, 1913

30. Ray BS, McLean JM: Combined intracranial and orbital operation for retinoblastoma. Arch Ophthalmol 30:437-445, 1943

31. Smith RR, Klopp CT, Williams JM: Surgical treatment of cancer of the frontal sinus and adjacent areas. Cancer 7:991-994, 1954

32. Ketcham AS, Hoye RC, Van Buren JM, et al: Complications of intracranial facial resection for tumors of the paranasal sinuses. Am J Surg 112:591-596, 1966

33. Van Buren JM, Ommaya AK, Ketcham AS: Ten years' experience with radical combined craniofacial resection of malignant tumors of the paranasal sinuses. J Neurosurg 28:341-350, 1968

34. Simpson D: The recurrence of intracranial meningiomas after K. R. Bulsara, T. Fukushima, and A. H. Friedman 10 Neurosurg. Focus / Volume 13 / October, 2002 surgical treatment. J Neurol Neurosurg Psychiatry 20:22-39, 1957

35. Johns ME, Winn HR, McLean WC, et al: Pericranial flap for the closure of defects of craniofacial resection. Laryngoscope 91: 952-959, 1981

36. Evine PA, McLean WC, Cantrell RW: Esthesioneuroblastoma: the University of Virginia experience 1960-1985. Laryngoscope 96:742-746, 1986

37. Essier P, Guiot G, Derome P: Orbital hypertelorism. II. Definite treatment of orbital hypertelorism (OR.H.) by craniofacial or by extracranial osteotomies. Scand J Plast Reconstr Surg 7: 39-58, 1973

38. Derome P: [Spheno-ethmoidal tumors. Possibilities for exeresis and surgical repair.] Neurochirurgie 18 (Suppl 1):1-164, 1972

39. Derome PJ, Tessier P: Craniofacial reconstruction in patients with craniofacial malformations: the neurosurgical approach. Clin Neurosurg 24:642-652, 1977

40. Colli B, Al-Mefty O: Chordomas of the craniocervical junction: follow-up review and prognostic factors. J Neurosurg 95: 933-943, 2001

41. (Management of Malignant Tumors of the Anterior Skull Base: Experience With 76 Patients from Neurosurgical Focus Posted 11/19/2002 Ketan R. Bulsara, M.D., Takanori Fukushima, M.D., D.M.Sc., Allan H. Friedman, M.D.)

42. Blacklock JB, Weber RS, Lee YY, et al: Transcranial resection of tumors of the paranasal sinuses and nasal cavity. J Neurosurg 71:10-15, 1989

43. Janecka IP, Nuss DW, Sen CN: Midfacial split for access to the central base. Acta Neurochir Suppl 53:199-203, 1991

44. Skinner DW, Van Hasselt CA, Tsao SY: Nasopharyngeal carcinoma: modes of presentation. Ann Otol Rhinol Laryngol 100:544-551, 1991Skinner DW, Van Hasselt CA, Tsao SY: Nasopharyngeal carcinoma: modes of presentation. Ann Otol Rhinol Laryngol 100:544-551, 1991

45. Mehta S, Verma A, Mann SB, et al: Rhabdomyosarcoma of head and neck -- an analysis of 24 cases. Indian J Cancer 33: 37-42, 1996

46. Aulino AC, Simon JH, Zhen W, et al: Long-term effects in children treated with radiotherapy for head and neck rahbdomyosacroma. Int J Radiat Oncol Biol Phys 48:1489-1495, 2000

47. Lang J: Anterior cranial base anatomy, in Sekhar LN, Schramm VL Jr (eds): Tumors of the Cranial Base: Diagnosis and Treatment. Mt. Kisco, NY: Futura, 1987, pp 247-264

48. Stern SJ, Hanna E. Cancer of the nasal cavity and paranasal sinuses. In: Myers EN, Suen JY, eds. Cancer of the Head and Neck. 3rd ed. Philadelphia, Pa: WB Saunders Co; 1996:205-233.

49. Danks RA, Kaye AH. Carcinoma of the paranasal sinuses. In: Kaye A, Laws ER Jr, eds. Brain Tumours: An Encyclopedic Approach. New York, NY: Churchill Livingstone; 1995:809-824.

50. Management of Malignant Tumors of the Anterior and Anterolateral Skull Base from Neurosurgical Focus Thomas C. Origitano, M.D., Ph.D., Guy J. Petruzzelli, M.D., Ph.D., Darl Vandevender, M.D., Bahman Emami, M.D.

51. J Oral Maxillofac Surg. 1998 May;56(5):578-84 A surgical approach to extensive tumors in the pterygopalatine fossa extending into the maxillary sinus. Jian XC, Chen XQ, Wang CX. Rhinology. 1991 Jun;29(2):105-10.

52. Technique and indications of extended sublabial rhinotomy ("midfacial degloving") Berghaus A, Jovanovic S.

53. The role of midfacial degloving in modern rhinological practice David J Howard, Valerie J Lund. The Journal of Laryngology and Otology. London: Oct 1999.Vol.113, Iss. 10; pg. 885, 3 pgs

54. Hussain A, Hulmi OJ, Murray DP. Lateral rhinotomy through nasal aesthetic subunits. Improved cosmetic outcome. J Laryngol Otol. 2002 Sep;116(9):703-6

55. The safety and effectiveness of the Le Fort I approach to removing central skull base lesions Michael P Colreavy, Tim Baker, Matthew Campbell, Michael Murphy, Bernard Lyons. Ear, Nose & Throat Journal. New York: May 2001.Vol.80, Iss. 5; pg. 315, 4 pgs

56. Le Fort 2 osteotomy and skull base tumors: A pediatric experience Tyler M Lewark, Gregory C Allen, Khalid Chowdhury, Kenny H Chan. Archives of Otolaryngology - Head & Neck Surgery. Chicago: Aug 2000.Vol.126, Iss. 8; pg. 1004, 5 pgs

57. Hendryk S; Czecior E; Misio?ek M; Namys?owski G; Mrówka R. Surgical strategies in the removal of malignant tumors and benign lesions of the anterior skull base. Neurosurg Rev. 2004; 27(3):205-13 (ISSN: 0344-5607)

58. Surgical approaches to the skull and near skull base neoplasms from Lin Chuang Er Bi Yan Hou Ke Za Zhi - Dec 2002 - Wanjun Chen, Tianduo Wang, Ying Chen, et. al.

59. Jackson et al: Malignant neoplasm of nasal cavity and paranasal sinuses. Laeynfoscope 1976 June, 86: 726-736.

60. Har EL et al: Pathology of nasal cavity and paranasal sinuses. Ed, Otolaryngol, Vol 2: New York, 1984. Harpent Raw Publishers Inc.

61. Bush et al: Carcinoma of the paranasal sinus. Cancer 1982; 50: 154-158.

62. Miyaguchi et al: Symptoms in patients with maxillary sinus. Cancer JLO 1980 July; 104: 557-559.

63. Sakai et al: Multidisciplinary treatment maxillary sinus carcino. a Cancer 52: 1360, 1983.; 89: 1077-1091.

64. Richtsmeir WJ et al: Complications and early outcome of anterior craniofacial resection. Otolaryngol Head and Neck Surg 1992; 118: 913-917.

65. Alfred S Ketcham, John M Van Buren: Tumors of the paranasal sinuses: A therapeutic challenge. The American Journal of Surgery 1985 Oct; 150: 406-413.

66. Schramm et al: Anterior skull base surgery for benign and malignant disease. Laryngoscope 197

67. Sisson GA. et al: Carcinoma of the paranasal sinuses and cranial-facial resection. J Laryngol Otol 1976; 90: 59-68.

68. Cousins VC, Lund VJ, Cheesman AD: Craniofacial resection of extensive benign lesions of hte anterior skull base, Aust N Z J Surg 57 (8): 515-520.

69. Barrs DM: Temporal bone carcinoma. Otolaryngol Clin North Am 34:1197-1218, 2001

70. Boyle JO, Shah KC, Shah JP: Craniofacial resection for malignant neoplasms of the skull base: an overview. J Surg Oncol 69:275-284, 1998

71. Cantu G, Solero CL, Mariani L, et al: Anterior craniofacial resection for malignant ethmoid tumors -- a series of 91 patients. Head Neck 21:185-191, 1999

72. Cushing H: Meningiomas: Their Classification, Regional Behaviour, Life History, and Surgical End Results. Springfield, IL: Thomas, 1938

73. Dandy WE: Orbital Tumors; Results Following the Transcranial Operative Attack. New York: O Piest, 1941

74. Gal TJ, Futran ND, Bartels LJ, et al: Auricular carcinoma with temporal bone invasion: outcome analysis. Otolaryngol Head Neck Surg 121:62-65, 1999

75. Harrison LB, Pfister DG, Kraus D, et al: Management of unresectable malignant tumors at the skull base using concomitant chemotherapy and radiotherapy with accelerated fractionation. Skull Base Surg 4:127-131, 1994

76. Irish JC, Gullane PJ, Gentili F, et al: Tumors of the skull base: outcome and survival analysis of 77 cases. Head Neck 16: 3-10, 1994

77. Ketcham AS, Wilkins RH, Van Buren JM, et al: A combined intracranial facial approach to the paranasal sinuses. Am J Surg 106:698-703, 1963

78. Malecki J: New trends in frontal sinus surgery. Arch Otolaryngol 50:137-140, 1959 (Reference unverified)

79. Pensak ML, Gleich LL, Gluckman JL, et al: Temporal bone carcinoma: contemporary perspectives in the skull base surgical era. Laryngoscope 106:1234-1237, 1996

80. Rae BS, McLean JM: Combined intracranial and orbital operation for retinoblastoma. Arch Ophthalmol 30:437-445, 1943 (Reference unverified)

81. Raveh J, Laedrach K, Speiser M, et al: The subcranial approach for fronto-orbital and anteroposterior skull-base tumors. Arch Otolaryngol Head Neck Surg 119:385-393, 1993

82. Shah JP: Anterior and middle cranial fossa surgery: U.S. experience, in Bloom HJG, Hanham IWF (eds): Head and Neck Oncology. New York: Raven Press, 1986, pp 159-165 15. Shah JP: Head and Neck Surgery; ed 2. London: Mosby- Wolfe, 1996, pp 85-141

83. Shah JP: Head and Neck Surgery; ed 2. London: Mosby-Wolfe,1996, pp 85-141

84. Shah JP, Galicich JH: Craniofacial resection for malignant tumors of ethmoid and anterior skull base. Arch Otolaryngol 103:514-517, 1977

85. Shah JP, Galicich JH: Surgical approach to carcinoma of the nasal cavity and paransal sinuses with extension to the base of the skull. Cancer Bull 8:61-66, 1978

86. Shah JP, Kraus DH, Bilsky MH, et al: Craniofacial resection for malignant tumors involving the anterior skull base. Arch Otolaryngol Head Neck Surg 123:1312-1317, 1997

87. Shah JP, Sundaresan N, Galicich J, et al: Craniofacial resections for tumors involving the base of the skull. Am J Surg 154: 352-358, 1987

88. Smith RR, Klopp CT, Williams JM: Surgical treatment of cancer of the frontal sinus and adjacent areas. Cancer 7:991-994, 1954 (Reference unverified)

89. Al-Mefty O, Anand VK: Zygomatic approach to skull-base lesions. J Neurosurg 73:668-673, 1990

90. Al-Mefty O, Borba LA: Skull base chordomas: a management challenge. J Neurosurg 86:182-189, 1997

91. Alshail E, Rutka JT, Drake JM, et al: Utility of frameless stereotaxy in the resection of skull base and basal cerebral lesions in children. Skull Base Surg 8:29-38, 1998

92. Amirjamshidi A, Mehrazin M, Abbassioun K: Meningiomas of the central nervous system occurring below the age of 17: report of 24 cases not associated with neurofibromatosis and review of literature. Childs Nerv Syst 16:406-416, 2000

93. Ariel IM, Verdu C: Chordoma: an analysis of twenty cases treated over a twenty-year span. J Surg Oncol 7:27-44, 1975

94. Azzarelli A, Quagliuolo V, Cerasoli S, et al: Chordoma: natural history and treatment results in 33 cases. J Surg Oncol 37:185-191, 1988

95. Barnes L, Kapadia SB: The biology and pathology of selected skull base tumors. J Neurooncol 20:213-240, 1994

96. Baskin DS, Wilson CB: Surgical management of craniopharyngiomas. A review of 74 cases. J Neurosurg 65:22-27, 1986

97. Beham A, Beham-Schmid C, Regauer S, et al: Nasopharyngeal angiofibroma: true neoplasm or vascular malformation? Adv Anat Pathol 7:36-46, 2000

98. Bejjani GK, Sekhar LN, Riedel CJ: Occipitocervical fusion following the extreme lateral transcondylar approach. Surg Neurol 54:109-116, 2000

99. Belmont JR: The Le Fort I osteotomy approach for nasopharyngeal and nasal fossa tumors. Arch Otolaryngol Head Neck Surg 114:751-754, 1988

100. Bluestone CD, Klein JO: Intratemporal complications and sequelae of otitis media, in Bluestone CD, Stool SE, Kenna MA (eds): Pediatric Otolaryngology, ed 3. Philadelphia: WB Saunders, 1996, Vol 1, pp 604-635

101. Borba LA, Al-Mefty O, Mrak RE, et al: Cranial chordomas in children and adolescents. J Neurosurg 84:584-591, 1996

102. Bremer AM, Nguyen TQ, Balsys R: Therapeutic benefits of combination chemotherapy with vincristine, BCNU, and procarbazine on recurrent cystic craniopharyngioma. A case report. J Neurooncol 2:47-51, 1984

103. Browne JD, Jacob SL: Temporal approach for resection of juvenile nasopharyngeal angiofibromas. Laryngoscope 110: 1287-1293, 2000

104. Camilleri AE: Craniofacial fibrous dysplasia. J Laryngol Otol 105:662-666, 1991

105. Carlotti CG Jr, Drake JM, Hladky JP, et al: Primary Ewing's sarcoma of the skull in children. Utility of molecular diagnostics, surgery and adjuvant therapies. Pediatr Neurosurg 31: 307-315, 1999

106. Cass SP, Hirsch BE, Stechison MT: Evolution and advances of the lateral surgical approaches to cranial base neoplasms. J Neurooncol 20:337-361, 1994

107. Cass SP, Sekhar LN, Pomeranz S, et al: Excision of petroclival tumors by a total petrosectomy approach. Am J Otol 15: 474-484, 1994

108. Catton C, O'Sullivan B, Bell R, et al: Chordoma: long-term follow-up after radical photon irradiation. Radiother Oncol 41:67-72, 1996

109. Chao KS, Kaplan C, Simpson JR, et al: Esthesioneuroblastoma: the impact of treatment modality. Head Neck 23: 749-757, 2001

110. Coffin CM, Swanson PE, Wick MR, et al: Chordoma in childhood and adolescence. A clinicopathologic analysis of 12 cases. Arch Pathol Lab Med 117:927-933, 1993

111. Crockard A, Macaulay E, Plowman PN: Stereotactic radiosurgery. VI. Posterior displacement of the brainstem facilitates safer high dose radiosurgery for clival chordoma. Br J Neurosurg 13:65-70, 1999

112. Cummings BJ, Blend R, Keane T, et al: Primary radiation therapy for juvenile nasopharyngeal angiofibroma. Laryngoscope 94:1599-1605, 1984

113. Cummings BJ, Esses S, Harwood AR: The treatment of chordomas. Cancer Treat Rev 9:299-311, 1982

114. de Divitiis E, Cappabianca P, Gangemi M, et al: The role of the endoscopic transsphenoidal approach in pediatric neurosurgery. Childs Nerv Syst 16:692-696, 2000

115. Di Rocco C, Marchese E, Velardi F: Fibrous dysplasia of the skull in children. Pediatric Neurosurgery 18:117-126, 1992

116. Economou TS, Abemayor E, Ward PH: Juvenile nasopharyngeal angiofibroma: an update of the UCLA experience, 1960-1985. Laryngoscope 98:170-175, 1988

117. Elkon D, Hightower SI, Lim ML, et al: Esthesioneuroblastoma. Cancer 44:1087-1094, 1979

118. Fagan JJ, Snyderman CH, Carrau RL, et al: Nasopharyngeal angiofibromas: selecting a surgical approach. Head Neck 19: 391-399, 1997

119. Ferry AP, Haddad HM, Goldman JL: Orbital invasion by an intracranial chordoma. Am J Ophthalmol 92:7-12, 1981

120. Fisch U, Pillsbury HC: Infratemporal fossa approach to lesions in the temporal bone and base of the skull. Arch Otolaryngol 105:99-107, 1979

121. Fischer EG, Welch K, Shillito J Jr, et al: Craniopharyngiomas in children. Long-term effects of conservative surgical procedures combined with radiation therapy. J Neurosurg 73: 534-540, 1990

122. Forsen JW: Chronic disorders of the middle ear and mastoid, in Wetmore RF, Muntz HR, McGill TJ (eds): Pediatric Otolaryngology: Principles and Practice Pathways. New York: Thieme, 2000, pp 293-303

123. Fournier H, Mercier P: A limited anterior petrosectomy with preoperative embolization of the inferior petrosal sinus for ventral brainstem tumor removal. Surg Neurol 54:10-18, 2000

124. Fucci MJ: Skull base, petrous apex, tumors. eMedicine J 2(7):2001

125. Fuller DB, Bloom JG: Radiotherapy for chordoma. Int J Radiat Oncol Biol Phys 15:331-339, 1988

126. Gadwal SR, Fanburg-Smith JC, Gannon FH, et al: Primary chondrosarcoma of the head and neck in pediatric patients: a clinicopathologic study of 14 cases with a review of the literature. Cancer 88:2181-2188, 2000

127. Garap JP, Dubey SP: Canal-down mastoidectomy: experience in 81 cases. Otol Neurotol 22:451-456, 2001

128. Gates GA, Rice DH, Koopmann CF Jr, et al: Flutamide-induced regression of angiofibroma. Laryngoscope 102: 641-644, 1992

129. Glasscock ME III, Woods CI III, Poe DS, et al: Petrous apex cholesteatoma. Otolaryngol Clin North Am 22:981-1002, 1989

130. Goepfert H, Cangir A, Lee YY: Chemotherapy for aggressive juvenile nasopharyngeal angiofibroma. Arch Otolaryngol 111:285-289, 1985

131. Gonzales-Pardo L, Brackett CE, Lansky LL: Facial nerve schwannoma in a 16-year-old girl. Childs Brain 7:220-224, 1980

132. Gonzales-Portillo G, Tomita T: The syndrome of inappropriate secretion of antidiuretic hormone: an unusual presentation for childhood craniopharyngioma: report of three cases. Neurosurgery 42:917-922, 1998

133. Gsponer J, De Tribolet N, Deruaz JP, et al: Diagnosis, treatment, and outcome of pituitary tumors and other abnormal intrasellar masses. Retrospective analysis of 353 patients. Medicine 78:236-269, 1999

134. Gullane PJ, Davidson J, O'Dwyer T, et al: Juvenile angiofibroma: a review of the literature and a case series report. Laryngoscope 102:928-933, 1992

135. Haines SJ, Duvall AJ III: Transzygomatic and transpalatal excision of juvenile nasopharyngeal angiofibroma with intracranial extension: the surgical procedure, in Sekhar LN, Janecka IP (eds): Surgery of Cranial Base Tumors. New York: Raven Press, 1993, pp 477-484

136. Haisa T, Ueki K, Yoshida S: Toxic effects of bleomycin on the hypothalamus following its administration into a cystic craniopharyngioma. Br J Neurosurg 8:747-750, 1994

137. Hamilton HB, Voorhies RM: Tumors of the skull, in Wilkins RH, Rengachary SS (eds): Neurosurgery, ed 2. New York: McGraw-Hill, 1996, Vol 2, pp 1503-1528

138. Harada K, Nishizaki T, Adachi N, et al: Pediatric acoustic schwannoma showing rapid regrowth with high proliferative activity. Childs Nerv Syst 16:134-137, 2000

139. Harwick RD, Miller AS: Craniocervical chordomas. Am J Surg 138:512-516, 1979

140. Hoffman HJ, De Silva M, Humphreys RP, et al: Aggressive surgical management of craniopharyngiomas in children. J Neurosurg 76:47-52, 1992

141. Hoffman HJ, Hendrick EB, Humphreys RP, et al: Management of craniopharyngioma in children. J Neurosurg 47: 218-227, 1977

142. Honegger J, Buchfelder M, Fahlbusch R, et al: Transsphenoidal microsurgery for craniopharyngioma. Surg Neurol 37: 189-196, 1992

143. Howard DJ, Lund VJ: The role of midfacial degloving in modern rhinological practice. J Laryngol Otol 113:885-887, 1999

144. Jacob HE: Chemotherapy for cranial base tumors. J Neurooncol 20:327-335, 1994

145. Jafek BW, Krekorian EA, Kirsch WM, et al: Juvenile nasopharyngeal angiofibroma: management of intracranial extension. Head Neck Surg 2:119-128, 1979

146. Jennett B, Bond M: Assessment of outcome after severe brain damage. Lancet 1:480-484, 1975

147. Jones NF, Schramm VL, Sekhar LN: Reconstruction of the cranial base following tumor resection. Br J Plast Surg 40: 155-162, 1987

148. Kaatsch P, Rickert CH, Kuhl J, et al: Population-based epidemiologic data on brain tumors in German children. Cancer 92:3155-3164, 2001

149. Kadish S, Goodman M, Wang CC: Olfactory neuroblastoma. A clinical analysis of 17 cases. Cancer 37:1571-1576, 1976

150. Karakousis CP, Park JJ, Fleminger R, et al: Chordomas: diagnosis and management. Am Surg 47:497-501, 1981

151. Kawahara N, Sasaki T, Nibu K, et al: Dumbbell type jugular foramen meningioma extending both into the posterior cranial fossa and into the parapharyngeal space: report of 2 cases with vascular reconstruction. Acta Neurochir 140:323-331, 1998

152. Kennedy JD, Haines SJ: Review of skull base surgery approaches: with special reference to pediatric patients. J Neurooncol 20:291-312, 1994

153. Kirazli T, Oner K, Ovul L, et al: Petrosal presigmoid approach to the petroclival and anterior cerebellopontine region (extended retrolabyrinthine, transtentorial approach). Rev Laryngol Otol Rhinol 122:187-190, 2001

154. Kristensen IB, Sunde LM, Jensen OM: Chondrosarcoma. Increasing grade of malignancy in local recurrence. Acta Pathol Microbiol Immunol Scand [A] 94:73-77, 1986

155. Landolt AM, Zachmann M: Results of transsphenoidal extirpation of craniopharyngiomas and Rathke's cysts. Neurosurgery 28:410-415, 1991

156. Lang DA, Neil-Dwyer G, Evans BT, et al: Craniofacial access in children. Acta Neurochir 140:33-40, 1998

157. Laws ER Jr: Transsphenoidal microsurgery in the management of craniopharyngioma. J Neurosurg 52:661-666, 1980

158. Laws ER Jr: Transsphenoidal removal of craniopharyngioma. Pediatr Neurosurg 21 (Suppl 1):57-63, 1994

159. Lee JP, Tsai MS, Chen YR: Orbitozygomatic infratemporal approach to lateral skull base tumors. Acta Neurol Scand 87: 403-409, 1993

160. Lewark TM, Allen GC, Chowdhury K, et al: Le Fort I osteotomy and skull base tumors: a pediatric experience. Arch Otolaryngol Head Neck Surg 126:1004-1008, 2000

161. Lippman CR, Jallo GI, Feghali JG, et al: Aneurysmal bone cyst of the temporal bone. Pediatr Neurosurg 31:219-223, 1999

162. Liu JM, Garonzik IM, Eberhart CG, et al: Ectopic recurrence of craniopharyngioma after an interhemispheric transcallosal approach: case report. Neurosurgery 50:639-645, 2002

163. Locatelli D, Castelnuovo P, Santi L, et al: Endoscopic approaches to the cranial base: perspectives and realities. Childs Nerv Syst 16:686-691, 2000

164. Long DM: Surgical approaches to tumors of the skull base: an overview, in Wilkins RH, Rengachary SS (eds): Neurosurgery, ed 2. New York: McGraw-Hill, 1996, Vol 2, pp 1573-1584

165. Low Y, Foo CL, Seow WT: Childhood temporal bone osteoblastoma: a case report. J Pediatr Surg 35:1127-1129, 2000

166. Macfarlane R, Rutka JT, Armstrong D, et al: Encephaloceles of the anterior cranial fossa. Pediatr Neurosurg 23:148-158, 1995

167. Mandai K, Tamaki N, Kurata H, et al: [The clinical analysis of pediatric meningioma: 5 cases.] No Shinkei Geka 25: 131-136, 1997 (Jpn)

168. Mazzoni A, Calabrese V, Danesi G: A modified retrosigmoid approach for direct exposure of the fundus of the internal auditory canal for hearing preservation in acoustic neuroma surgery. Am J Otol 21:98-109, 2000

169. McDermott MW, Durity FA, Rootman J, et al: Combined frontotemporal-orbitozygomatic approach for tumors of the sphenoid wing and orbit. Neurosurgery 26:107-116, 1990

170. McLendon RE: Epidermoid and dermoid tumors: pathology, in Wilkins RH, Rengachary SS (eds): Neurosurgery, ed 2. New York: McGraw-Hill, 1996, Vol 1, pp 959-964

171. Megerian CA, Chiocca EA, McKenna MJ, et al: The subtemporal-transpetrous approach for excision of petroclival tumors. Am J Otol 17:773-779, 1996

172. Mendel RC, Brumback RA, Leech RW, et al: Pediatric eighth cranial nerve schwannoma without evidence of neurofibromatosis. J Child Neurol 14:67-69, 1999

173. Moore KD, Couldwell WT: Craniopharyngioma, in Bernstein M, Berger MS (eds): Neuro-Oncology: The Essentials. New York: Thieme Medical Publishers, 2000, pp 409-418

174. Morita A, Ebersold MJ, Olsen KD, et al: Esthesioneuroblastoma: prognosis and management. Neurosurgery 32: 706-715, 1993

175. Morita A, Piepgras DG: Tumors of the skull base, in Vecht CJ (ed): Handbook of Clinical Neurology. Amsterdam: Elsevier Science, 1997, pp 465-496

176. Morita A, Sekhar LN: Skull base tumors, in Bernstein M, Berger MS (eds): Neuro-Oncology: The Essentials. New York: Thieme Medical Publishers, 2000, pp 419-433

177. Mortensen A, Bojsen-Moller M, Rasmussen P: Fibrous dysplasia of the skull with acromegaly and sarcomatous transformation. Two cases with a review of the literature. J Neurooncol 7:25-29, 1989

178. Mortini P, Mandelli C, Franzin A, et al: Surgical excision of clival tumors via the enlarged transcochlear approach. Indications and results. J Neurosurg Sci 45:127-140, 2001

179. Moulin G, Chagnaud C, Gras R, et al: Juvenile nasopharyngeal angiofibroma: comparison of blood loss during removal in embolized group versus nonembolized group. Cardiovasc Intervent Radiol 18:158-161, 1995

180. Nelson GA, Bastian FO, Schlitt M, et al: Malignant transformation in craniopharyngioma. Neurosurgery 22:427-429, 1988

181. O'Conor GT Jr, Drake CR, Johns ME, et al: Treatment of advanced esthesioneuroblastoma with high-dose chemotherapy and autologous bone marrow transplantation. A case report. Cancer 55:347-349, 1985

182. Polonowski JM, Brasnu D, Roux FX, et al: Esthesioneuroblastoma. Complete tumor response after induction chemotherapy. Ear Nose Throat J 69:743-746, 1990

183. Posnick JC, Goldstein JA, Armstrong D, et al: Reconstruction of skull defects in children and adolescents by the use of fixed cranial bone grafts: long-term results. Neurosurgery 32: 785-791, 1993

184. Pownell PH, Wright CG, Robinson KS, et al: The effect of cyclophosphamide on development of experimental cholesteatoma. Arch Otolaryngol Head Neck Surg 120:1114-1116, 1994

185. Prescott CA: Cholesteatoma in children -- the experience at The Red Cross War Memorial Children's Hospital in South Africa 1988-1996. Int J Pediatr Otorhinolaryngol 49: 15-19, 1999

186. Razis DV, Tsatsaronis A, Kyriazides I, et al: Chordoma of the cervical spine treated with vincristine sulfate. J Med 5: 274-277, 1974

187. Reddy KA, Mendenhall WM, Amdur RJ, et al: Long-term results of radiation therapy for juvenile nasopharyngeal angiofibroma. Am J Otolaryngol 22:172-175, 2001

188. Regine WF, Kramer S: Pediatric craniopharyngiomas: long term results of combined treatment with surgery and radiation. Int J Radiat Oncol Biol Phys 24:611-617, 1992 Chang CY, O'Rourke DK, Cass SP: Update on skull base surgery. Otolaryngol Clin North Am 1996 Jun; 29(3): 467-501.

189. Jackson IT: Craniofacial osteotomies to facilitate the resection of tumors of the skull base. Neurosurgery 1996; II: 1585-602.

190. Kokkino AJ, Abdel Aziz KM, Tew JM Jr: Honored guest presentation: contemporary treatment of skull base meningiomas. Clin Neurosurg 2000; 46: 554-74..

191. Levine PA, McLean WC, Cantrell RW: Esthesioneuroblastoma: the University of Virginia experience 1960-1985. Laryngoscope 1986 Jul; 96(7): 742-6.

192. Levine PA, Scher RL, Jane JA, et al: The craniofacial resection--eleven-year experience at the University of Virginia: problems and solutions. Otolaryngol Head Neck Surg 1989 Dec; 101(6): 665-9.

193. Long DM: Surgical approaches to the skull base: an overview. Neurosurgery 1996; II: 1573-84.

194. Sampson JH, Wilkins RH: Paragangliomas of the carotid body and temporal bone. Neurosurgery 1996; II: 1559-72.

195. Scher RL, Richtsmeier WJ: Craniofacial resection of anterior skull base tumors. Neurosurgery 1996; II: 1603-10.

196. Sekhar LN, Swamy NK, Jaiswal V, et al: Surgical excision of meningiomas involving the clivus: preoperative and intraoperative features as predictors of postoperative functional deterioration. J Neurosurg 1994 Dec; 81(6): 860-8.

197. Sekhar LN, Gay E, Wright DC: Chordomas and chondrosarcomas of the cranial base. Neurosurgery 1996; II: 1529-44.

198. Van Tuyl R, Gussack GS: Prognostic factors in craniofacial surgery. Laryngoscope 1991 Mar; 101(3): 240-4.

Index